Baseball Injuries

Case Studies, by Type, in the Major Leagues

W. Laurence Coker, M.D.

McFarland & Company, Inc., Publishers
Jefferson, North Carolina, and London

LIBRARY OF CONGRESS CATALOGUING-IN-PUBLICATION DATA

Coker, W. Laurence, 1953–
    Baseball injuries : case studies, by type, in the major leagues /
W. Laurence Coker, M.D.
        p.   cm.
    Includes bibliographical references and index.

    ISBN 978-0-7864-6868-3
    softcover : acid free paper ∞

    1. Baseball injuries — Case studies.   2. Baseball injuries.
3. Sports medicine.   I. Title.
RC1220.B3C65 2013
617.1'0276357 — dc23
                                                    2013004733

BRITISH LIBRARY CATALOGUING DATA ARE AVAILABLE

Cover illustration © 2012 Frederick R. Matzen

Manufactured in the United States of America

McFarland & Company, Inc., Publishers
    Box 611, Jefferson, North Carolina 28640
    www.mcfarlandpub.com

Baseball Injuries

In memory of my dad,
Dr. Grady N. Coker, Jr.,
who got me interested in the sport of baseball
both as a participant and a fan

Table of Contents

Preface

There is considerable interest in the subject of sports in the United States. Injuries are a major factor in sports, often determining who will win and who will lose on any given day. Through my discussions with acquaintances of mine whom I know are interested in sports, I saw that there might be some interest in a book about sports injuries.

But my book would not be a general book about sports injuries. It would have a unique viewpoint. Most sports injury books look just at injuries and their treatment. There are many medical books for healthcare professionals and lay people that present this slant on the subject of injuries. A classic example of this is a book I read while I was an active runner: *Dr. George Sheehan's Medical Advice for Runners*.[1] This book is a discussion of running injuries, what are the possible causes, and what to do about them. Within the book there are questions that individuals submitted to Sheehan during the time he was an acting editor for *Runner's World* magazine. The contents: the book presents information in a systematic fashion from head to toe. The people submitting questions are for the most part listed anonymously, except the author, who discusses his own injuries.

Another example of a book that discusses sports injuries, and more in line with the content of this present book, is *Injuries in Baseball* by Andrews, Zarins, and Wilk. *Injuries in Baseball* looks at almost all possible aspects of baseball injuries, including surgical techniques and rehabilitation.[2] But once again there are no specific players' names mentioned.

I wanted to look at specific individuals with specific injuries. I wanted to tie a name to an injury as an example of the injury. The emphasis would be more on the individual. There are numerous articles on the Internet and in newspapers covering the material presented in this book, but I am unaware of any books *solely devoted* to looking at types of injuries through examination

1

of specific cases. There are biographies that discuss individuals' injuries, but in context of the person's total life. There are books about specific teams and events, but once again the injuries are often just small parts of the total picture.

In this book I have combined the interest in sports injuries with the general interest in sports figures. Our society regards many of our sports figures as celebrities and heroes. There is much interest in these individuals' lives. Why not look at these people and the injuries they have suffered while participating in their sports? Why not look at injuries that affected their lives?

Another point: a baseball player's career ultimately ends. There are three main ways this can happen. First, as the player ages he gets more injuries, some of which are career altering. Second, as the player ages his performance in the field declines by decreased quickness (i.e., the pitcher can't throw the ball as fast, the hitter can't swing the bat as fast, or the fielder can't get to the ball as fast as before, etc.). Along with decreased quickness, power and strength decline with age. Last, a player may simply lose motivation and desire to continue his career. Certainly injuries or decreased performance can factor into decreased motivation, but off-field issues, such as family concerns, can also factor into the equation.

A good example of this is Don Mattingly (discussed in more detail later), who developed back problems starting in 1987. Because of the back injury and subsequent pain he endured, he was forced to alter his usual swing to a less effective swing. His work ethic was affected by back pain issues, as he was just not able to practice as much in the batting cage as he did before the back issues arose.[3] Decreased performance and daily back pain, as well as all the exercises and physical therapy directed at coping with his back pain, sapped Mattingly's desire to continue playing baseball. Finally, family matters and other commitments influenced Mattingly's decision not to continue with his career.[4]

Why write a book on sports injuries? Well, I have several reasons. First, I have had a life-long interest in sports both as a participant and a fan. Second, as a participant, especially as a runner, I have had my share of personal sports injuries. Third, even though my professional training is as a Family Practice doctor, I have had, and still do have, a special interest in sports medicine problems. It is not unusual for a family doctor, involved in all aspects of medical care, to have a special interest in one specific aspect of medical practice without actually specializing in that particular area. To add credence to this special interest, the Family Practice Board actually offers *extra* board certification in Sports Medicine.

From my interest in sports as a physician, participant, and sports fan came my inspiration for writing a book initially called *Famous Sports Injuries*. The idea was to cover many different sports, though mainly baseball, football, and basketball. The book would be about specific injuries in specific sports and the famous and sometimes not-so-famous players having those particular injuries.

While gathering material to write the section of the book concerning baseball injuries, I realized that there was more than enough material on that topic alone to constitute a book-length study, leading to the present work.

When I talk about injuries I limit my discussion to significant injuries. These are usually ones where the player goes on the DL (disabled list), unable to play. There are many injuries a player can play through, not missing practice or games, but the majority of injuries I want to discuss involve a trip to the DL. This trip may include the need for surgery to correct the injury. Some baseball injuries can be severe in nature: loss of consciousness, immediate consequences that lead to hospitalization, or even death. Fortunately death is a very rare event. Some of the injuries may have long-term consequences leading to decreased performance on the baseball field or even leading to early retirement (e.g., Tony Conigliaro's early retirement secondary to an impact injury to the eye from a beaning).

I make no attempt to discuss every famous injury and many injuries I present are not so famous. These latter injuries are mainly presented for two reasons. First, they are classic examples of the types of injuries associated with the game of baseball as opposed to other sports. Second, many of the not-so-famous injuries I cite occurred in the last several years, making information about them more accessible through newspaper and Internet searches. Also, good diagnostic tests to confirm the diagnosis of an injury have been presented.

On the flip side of the equation, players from the distant past are discussed less in this book. Information is less accessible or diagnoses are often given in vague terms. It's impossible to discuss an injury with any precision if one doesn't know what, exactly, the problem was. Often only the symptoms are mentioned (e.g., the pitcher had arm pain), and injury diagnoses are referred to in generic terms (e.g., the pitcher had a "bad arm").

A case in point is *The Old Ball Game: How John McGraw, Christy Mathewson, and the New York Giants Created Modern Baseball,* by Frank Deford. This book was published more recently, 2005, but most certainly relied on older references as the basis of its text (Hall of Fame player Mathewson pitched from 1900 to 1916 with career record of 373 wins against 188 losses).[5] The book spends very little text discussing Mathewson's injuries at the end of his career. I surmise one reason for this is because so little information about the nature of Mathewson's injuries was available. Ray Robinson's book on Christy Mathewson, *Matty: An American Hero, Christy Mathewson of the New York Giants,* is similar in its lack of discussion about Christy Mathewson's injuries.[6]

Even in a more scholarly work such as Jack Smiles' *Big Ed Walsh: The Life and Times of a Spitballing Hall of Famer* (career from 1904 to 1917 with a record of 195 wins against 126 losses), where more text is devoted to the discussion of injuries, injuries from references are discussed in generic terms. Words used are "sore arm," "bad wing," or "ligament displaced in the shoulder and in my arm where it is attached to the bone at the elbow."[7] Any delving into a clearer diagnosis with Walsh, such as possible "rotator cuff tear," is based purely on speculation by a consulting orthopedic surgeon who researched available records on Walsh.[8]

The vast majority of injuries I note are at the major league level. I cite a few minor league injuries, two of which resulted in deaths — a coach and a player. I confess I have more examples of injuries of St. Louis Cardinals players as compared to other teams. This skewed result is directly related to my familiarity with the Cardinals, having followed them closely as a fan since their World Series championship season of 1967. Even though I check multiple Internet and newspaper sites on a daily basis looking for injuries, I regularly check familiar Cardinals team sites before I check any other references.

In many cases there have been so many players experiencing a particular injury or mechanism of injury it is only possible to scratch the surface in discussing cases. I make no attempt to give examples in numbers that would reflect the frequency of the injury. Example: In the case of hamstring injury, there are just too many possible cases, as this is one of the most common baseball injuries. But the hamstring injury is not unique to baseball. Hamstring injuries occur in many other sports. More time here is spent discussing injuries that are more specific to baseball. For example, I devote considerable discussion to impact injuries caused by being hit by the baseball or to ulnar collateral ligament injuries of the elbow leading to Tommy John surgery.

There is some grouping here of the discussion by the manner in which injuries occurred (e.g., sliding injuries). Sliding injuries can lead to a large variety of problems, some depending on whether the slide is head-first or feet-first. Sliding injuries sometimes involve attempts by the runner to bowl over the fielder, deliberately trying to knock the ball out of the fielder's hand. The sliding collision causes the injuries, though different types of injuries can occur, most of them traumatic in nature. In my discussion I group some of the diverse injuries under a common mechanism of the injury.

With the injury examples are intermittent discussions of innovations in the game of baseball. These innovations such as batting helmets or padded outfield walls, more often than not occurred as a result of injuries (e.g., beanings and outfield wall collisions).

Finally, there is some discussion of innovations in medicine, both in diagnosis and treatment, that have prolonged players' careers. Regrettably, there have been a few innovations that may have shortened careers (e. g., excessive use of cortisone shots to treat medical conditions).

A cortisone shot, an anti-inflammatory treatment, helps to decrease pain and to clear inflammation of a joint and soft tissue (tendons and ligaments). The bad part: if used excessively (too frequently), cortisone can lead over time to weakening of tissues and in the long run actually increase tendon, ligament, and joint damage. The excessive use of cortisone was especially a problem between 1947 and 1979.[9] Sandy Koufax, for example, received way too many cortisone shots in his elbow to relieve pain, especially in 1966, as will be discussed in further detail.

Who knows how many careers, though possibly made better in performance over the short run by anabolic steroids and growth hormones, were ultimately cut short by injuries or health issues related to the use of these medications? The exact incidence and prevalence of injuries caused by anabolic steroids or HGH is difficult to estimate. One reason is that few players who have taken these medications ever admit to having used them. Also, with steroid use, most information on short-term and long-term consequences of drug use has been obtained *anecdotally.*[10] The ideal evaluation of injuries caused by steroid use by *controlled scientific studies* will in all likelihood never be done. These scientific studies, if done, would more accurately pinpoint the true incidence and prevalence of steroid-induced injuries.

Introduction

Injuries in baseball players mainly fall into two categories: overuse and traumatic injuries. Overuse injuries in baseball are common as baseball involves many repetitive activities. Pitchers and fielders throw and catch the baseball over and over, both during the game and in practice to prepare for games. Batters swing the bat during the game and then spend hours in the batting cage refining their technique. Running is a major part of baseball. There are no marathons here as most running in baseball involves short busts of speed on the basepaths and in the field, often after a period of relative inactivity. The legs need to be in good condition to help the overall performance of the player. All these activities lead to acute and chronic stress and damage to the joints, bones, and soft tissues (tendons, muscles, and ligaments) and can even lead to damage to nerves and blood vessels. All these are part of overuse injuries. When you look at spring training and add the 162 games in the major league season, it is easy to see why overuse injuries are common in baseball at the major league level.

One can break down acute *non-traumatic* soft tissue injuries into tendon, ligament, and muscle tears. Quite often with acute ligament or tendon tears, where no trauma is involved, the tears are preceded by some weakening of anatomic structures due to overuse. After the tendon or ligament is torn it is difficult to determine if overuse had anything to do with it, unless a biopsy of the damaged tendon or ligament is done at the time of repair.

There have been scientific studies done where biopsies have been taken at the time of surgery performed to repair a torn tendon. Freddie H. Fu, MD, in his excellent book *Sports Injuries: Mechanisms-Prevention-Treatment*, cites two studies that looked at the issue of overuse changes in acute tears.[1] One of these studies in the *Journal of Bone and Joint Surgery* (December 1991) showed degenerative changes present in 97 percent of biopsies of the 891 acute tendon ruptures examined.[2]

A classic example of a tendon tear of this nature would be Joel Zumaya's 2007 flexor finger tendon tear (discussed later). The tear occurred spontaneously on a thrown ball. There is a good chance that weakening of the tendon occurred prior to the acute tear in this pitcher who regularly throws his fastball in the 100mph range.[3]

Then there is the pop or snap that often happens as the medial collateral ligament in the elbow tears completely. Yes, the injury can be acute, but here more often than not there is overuse-induced weakening of the ligament before the acute elbow ligament tear. As with many tendon tears, unless the injury is traumatic, some weakening of the ligament occurs before the acute tear.

Muscle strains involve some tearing of the muscle fibers. With many muscle strains no weakening of the muscle precedes the strain. The injury is acute.

Exceptions are repeat injuries. If a muscle strain has not healed completely, then the muscle is more susceptible to tearing in exactly the same place. This is the reason the team has the player go on the DL until management is absolutely sure the player's muscle tear has healed. Even after pain symptoms (at rest and with activity) resolve, it is prudent to delay taking the player off the DL.

With the initial muscle injury, quite often an MRI is obtained. MRIs are very good for looking at soft-tissue injuries (muscle, tendons and ligaments). Often a follow-up MRI is done to assess healing of the original injury before the player is permitted to return to play, as an extra precaution. That an MRI is expensive isn't much concern when one considers major league players are paid millions of dollars. A team's success during the season often hinges greatly on a correct decision to return the player to the field. An aggravation of a previous injury, one not completely healed, could be even worse than the initial injury.

Another consideration is that with muscle tears, if the tear is significantly severe, it may never completely heal. With severe tears sometimes new muscle never completely fills in the gap where the original muscle tear was. Scar tissue may form. In this case the muscle is more susceptible to tearing in exactly the same location where the scar tissue formed. Though infrequent, severe muscle tears can result in surgery to remove the scar tissue.

Surgery may also be necessary when the muscle tears at its tendon attachment and the tendon is involved, whether scar tissue formed or not.

For purposes of this book, some muscle injuries, especially ones not involving the shoulder or elbow, are discussed at the same time as tendon injuries. That might seem odd, since as previously stated quite often tendon injuries have overuse changes prior to tearing and many muscle injuries do not. However, the muscle/tendon structure functions as a unit. When a muscle tears, most often it tears exactly where it joins the tendon. There may be some involvement of the tendon. Also, when the tendon tears off the bone it is the muscle/tendon structure pulling the tendon off the bone. When the tendon splits or tears in half, it is the muscle contracting against a force that leads to the tear.[4]

Traumatic injuries are not as common as overuse injuries in baseball. In other sports, especially football, traumatic injuries make up a much larger percentage of overall injuries. Still, baseball has its fair share of trauma. Unique to baseball are injuries caused by players being hit by the baseball, either by a thrown ball or a hit ball. Collisions, though not as common as in football, do occur. Players run into the fixed bases on the basepaths, walls around the field, equipment next to the field or in the dugout, and even into each other. There are collisions with the ground that occur as players dive to catch a ball. A player can dig his spikes into the ground sliding for a base. There are infrequent occasions where players are hit by the bat or a piece of the bat. Players can even be hit by debris thrown from the stands, though fortunately this doesn't occur very often. Then there is that occasional bench-clearing brawl resulting in injury.

A significant portion of the research for this book was done in the years 2006 to 2010. From this research it is very evident there are a tremendous number of injuries in baseball, and these injuries significantly affect a team's performance in any given year. Any attempt to discuss the various injuries only touches the surface of the problem, but in doing so there is hope to give some good examples of these injuries in well-known and not-so-well-known players. Discussion of overuse injuries is first, followed later by the discussion of traumatic injuries.

PART I. OVERUSE INJURIES

Chapter 1

Shoulder

Shoulder injuries are primarily throwing injuries; pitchers practice to get their mechanics correct, increase muscle strength, improve flexibility, and improve throwing speed. Pitchers throw more than anyone else on the field and generally, when they do throw, throw harder than other positions on the baseball field. Thus, it is not surprising that they have the highest incidence of repetitive throwing injuries to the elbow and shoulder. The other positions that require the most throwing in frequency, effort, and distance, and therefore have more injuries are shortstop and third base. The second baseman does not throw as hard or as far as the shortstop, even if he throws just as often. It is not unusual to move a shortstop to second base later in his career when arm strength begins to decrease. The shortstop has great demands put on him in the throwing department, and often the best athlete (non-pitcher) with the strongest and most accurate arm is positioned at shortstop. It should not be surprising, therefore, that some players who are shortstops early in their career end up as pitchers (Woody Williams, former Cardinal, comes to mind). If a player with a strong arm can't make it as a shortstop, turn him into a pitcher. The reverse is rarely true.

Outfielders do throw farther than infielders, and often with greater effort, but they definitely don't have to throw nearly as often. The outfielder who has to throw the farthest the most often is the right fielder. His throw from the right field corner to third base is a common occurrence. Thus the right fielder usually has the strongest and most accurate arm of the three outfield positions.

Upper extremity (shoulder and elbow) injuries are common in the throwing athletes of several sports (baseball, football quarterback, volleyball, water polo, and javelin). Of all sports, baseball has a highest frequency of throwing injuries. With nine positions on the field for defense, all participate in throwing activities, though the pitcher by far throws the most often and the hardest.

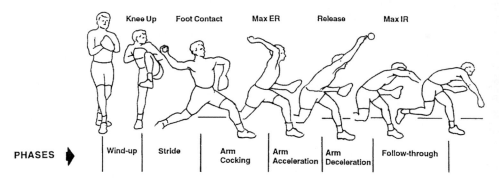

PHASES ▶ Wind-up | Stride | Arm Cocking | Arm Acceleration | Arm Deceleration | Follow-through

The six phases of the pitching motion are indicated. (This is a modification of an image appearing in Fleisig, et al., "Biomechanics of Overhand Throwing with Implications for Injuries," *Sports Medicine* 21, 6 [1996]: 421–437, Fig. 1, reproduced by the permission of the publisher, Wolters Kluwer, and the author.)

Many agree that throwing is not an activity that the arm was structurally meant to do. It creates violent torque (stress) on the shoulder and elbow.

There are six phases in throwing. There is a windup (I), stride (II), arm cocking (III), acceleration (IV), deceleration (V), and follow-through (VI).

At the professional level the entire motion usually takes less than two seconds. Proper mechanics are necessary to prevent injury, and this should be emphasized from the Little League level up. An example of good mechanics: a pitcher's front foot lands first with the foot properly pointing toward the target. Any other position for foot landing, such as a heel landing or landing with the front foot not pointing towards the target, increases the stress on the shoulder (and elbow) by not allowing for a more fluid motion. With excessive stress come excessive injuries.

Shoulder injuries, and other overuse injuries, occur with high frequency in baseball, especially with pitchers. Quite often, all pitchers on a team's staff have had shoulder problems at some point in their career. The shoulder allows for considerable more range of motion compared to the anatomically similar structure of the lower extremity, the hip. The shoulder has a very shallow bone and cartilage socket as compared to the hip joint.

The shoulder is held in place

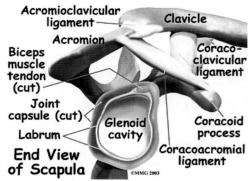

Here is a cross-section (end on) view of the shoulder with humerus bone removed, showing key anatomical structures (used by permission of Medical Multimedia Group LLC).

mainly by cartilage (labrum), muscles, ligaments, and tendons. Shoulder movement is restricted superiorly (upward) by the scapula (shoulder blade) and clavicle (collar bone).

When you raise your hand, the scapula does rotate upward with the shoulder to decrease this restriction somewhat; otherwise it would be very difficult to throw a ball overhand. The rotation upward of the structures of the shoulder when throwing overhand is not 100 percent, thus there is a greater chance of getting some rubbing (called impingement) on the tendons and ligaments between the acromium (part of scapula) that forms the top part of the shoulder, causing damage with repeated use. Fortunately within the shoulder there is a lubricating fluid (synovial fluid) within the joint itself and a fluid filled sac containing the same fluid called a bursa sac under the acromium. If the bursa sac gets excessive use or gets injured, you can have what is called bursitis.

The whole shoulder is enclosed in a sac called a capsule. There is no connection to outside the capsule except via blood vessels. This is good as it helps to prevent infections from moving to the joint from outside the shoulder capsule. A joint infection is a very serious problem that requires very aggressive treatment. It is a clear indication for hospitalization. An infection in a joint can lead to dire consequences. It can destroy the synovial fluid cells, leading to decreased lubrication and premature arthritis. The capsule itself is very flexible and allows for considerable movement of the joint. Four ligaments are part of the capsule, running from humerus to labrum. The ligaments, cartilage rim, and muscles with tendons provide the most support for the shoulder, with some support by the acromium, the part of the scapula that sits on top of the shoulder joint. If there was just the capsule with ligaments and labrum rim, the shoulder would easily come out of its socket, a condition called a shoulder dislocation.

Anything that disrupts any of the support structures of the shoulder (cartilage rim, muscles, tendons, or capsule and ligaments) can result in subluxation (sliding out and then back in of the humerus, the upper arm bone) or shoulder dislocation (humerus comes completely out of its socket).

In baseball recently there has been an example of shoulder subluxation due to damage to the shoulder cartilage rim (labrum) that supports the humerus bone head (top): third baseman Scott Rolen (discussed more fully later on with references cited). He injured the cartilage of the socket rim after running into Dodgers first baseman Hee-Seop Choi in 2005. It was his non-throwing shoulder and didn't cause problems throwing, but it did cause problems batting. Physical therapy to strengthen the muscles to support the shoulder helped some, but ultimately he had to have surgery on the shoulder to repair the labrum. This was a traumatic injury (see later discussion).

Another example of shoulder subluxation, but not due to trauma, is the pitching shoulder of Orel Hershiser. After three straight years of 250-plus innings, his anterior shoulder gave out in 1990 because of damage to the anterior capsule and ligaments that attached to the labrum in front of the shoulder. He, like Scott Rolen, needed surgical repair to correct an unstable shoulder (see later discussion).

The rotator cuff surrounds the shoulder and consists of tendons and muscles attached to those tendons. The tendons attach to the bones around the shoulder and have some attachment to the labrum and capsule surrounding the shoulder. A rotator cuff injury can include a labrum injury. As opposed to the knee's cruciate ligaments within the knee's capsule, there are no ligaments inside the shoulder capsule. There are four outer ligaments that help to reenforce the capsule.

Rotator Cuff Tendonitis (or Tendonosis) or Bursitis

Rotator cuff tendonitis is much more common than rotator cuff tears. Tendonosis is a more correct term. Pathological specimens reveal very little inflammation ("-itis"). Instead there is damage to the fibers of the tendon ranging from microscopic injury all the way up to observable tears, the most severe going completely through the tendon (e.g., biceps tendon tear). Most tendonosis is treated with rest first, then ice, followed by physical therapy. A cortisone shot to relieve pain is sometimes helpful, though cortisone itself does little to aid in the tendon healing process. The shot mainly helps relieve pain so therapy and rehabilitation can proceed.

Any of the four tendons of the rotator cuff can have tendonosis. These are the supraspinatis, infraspinatis, subscapularis, or biceps tendon. The supraspinatis is especially prone to injury as the blood circulation to that particular tendon is the poorest of the four. Thus, injury to that tendon is slowest to heal.[1]

Rotator Cuff Tears

Before talking about rotator cuff tears, it should be noted that it is very common to have some damage to the labrum at the same time as a rotator cuff tear (the labrum being the cartilage surface of the scapula the humerus bone articulates with). This should not be surprising as there are fibrous connections between the rotator cuff as it attaches to the scapula bone and to the labrum.

Rotator cuff tears can be **traumatic** in the case of a player falling and landing on his shoulder when diving to catch a ball, or in a collision, such as often occurs at home plate where a runner tries to score and meets the only slightly movable catcher blocking home plate, but usually rotator cuff tears occur due to **chronic overuse** in throwing motions. Naturally, pitchers have more rotator cuff tears than other position players. These tears can be partway through the rotator cuff, or completely through. Partial tears in the rotator cuff can often be career-threatening injuries. A complete tear, or almost complete tear, in the rotator cuff is a career-ending injury (especially if there is also damage to the labrum).

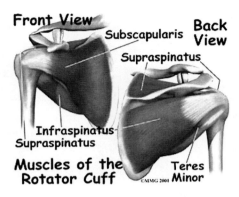

Listed are rotator cuff muscles. Most often with rotator cuffs tears, the supraspinatus muscle tendon is torn near its attachment to the humerus bone (used by permission of Medical Multimedia Group LLC).

ROBB NEN

The classic example of a severe tear in the rotator cuff with a concomitant labral tear is Robb Nen of the Giants. In 2002 he helped San Francisco get to the playoffs and World Series. He recorded 43 saves that year with a 2.20 ERA. He pitched with pain at the end of the season and during the playoffs and World Series. He probably had a partial rotator cuff tear near the end of the season, but continued to pitch through the pain, probably extending a partial tear to a severe tear (the exact percentage of Nen's tear is debated — one article said Nen had a 70 percent tear, another article said 75 percent, and still another article said it was only 40 percent, still a very significant rotator cuff tear for a pitcher). After three years of trying to make a comeback and three surgeries to try and fix the problem, he decided to hang up the glove and retire. His situation in 2002 illustrates that it is not always a good idea to continue to pitch in pain.[2]

Nen had three surgeries but never had the tear completely closed (something rarely ever done for a pitcher if he wants to continue to pitch). The first surgery, in November 2002, by Dr. Lewis Yocum, was mainly to clean up loose particles and debris in the shoulder. He had a second surgery, a diagnostic procedure done by Dr. Yocum in April 2003, which revealed a torn labrum as well as damage to Nen's capsule near his rotator cuff. The labrum tear was repaired by Dr. Craig Morgan of Delaware in May of 2003. Whether the labrum tear was there after the initial injury is controversial, as apparently this labral tear was in an area difficult to see. Dr. Morgan also cut into the posterior (back of the) joint capsule to allow more space for Nen's arm movement, something successfully done to Curt Schilling in 1999. Nen had developed shoulder movement restriction, possibly from scar tissue. Restricted movement in a pitcher's shoulder is a very bad thing.[3]

The rest is history. Nen never came back from his injury. A fourth surgery was never seriously considered.

MARK MULDER

Mark Mulder's case is another example of a rotator cuff tear significant enough to require some repair of his tear. Many pitchers with partial tears of the rotator cuff just need trimming of frayed, damaged tissue. That is the best case scenario. Unfortunately this was not the case with Mulder (see articles cited later).

Mulder started off the 2006 season in April well, but struggled considerably in May and June. His ERA by the June 22 was 6.09, and he was 1–4 with an ERA of 11.39 in his last six starts. He was put the DL on June 22, 2006, for the first time in his career, with the diagnosis of left shoulder strain. An MRI on June 25 showed rotator cuff irritation, shoulder impingement, inflammation and slight fraying of the labrum.[4]

Non-surgical methods of rehabilitation were tried first to get him back in playing condition. After a period of rest where there was no throwing at all and anti-inflammatory medications were administered, Mulder began rotator muscle strengthening exercises. The next step was to start throwing; Dave Duncan, the Cardinals' pitching coach, probably helped Mulder work on his mechanics (normal throwing motion and proper release point). After a period of time he was to throw simulated pitching situations with a batter in the box, using a pitcher's mound and rubber to push off. When all that went well, he was sent the weekend after August 2, 2006, to pitch in minor league games. You can see there was a gradual return to normal pitching after rest, muscle strengthening, and working on proper throwing mechanics.

Mulder pitched in the minor leagues with fair results and returned to the big leagues, coming off the DL on August 23. He pitched two games, first giving up nine runs in three innings against the Mets on August 23 and then five runs in one and two-thirds innings against Florida on August 29, before being put on the DL again August 31. It was apparent that conservative (non-surgical) treatment was a failure in Mulder's case.

Arthroscopy

What is an arthroscope? The word has two parts. "Arthro" is from the Greek word "arthron," meaning "joint." "Scope" is from the Greek word "skopein" which means to examine. Thus we have "arthroscopy," to look at or examine a joint. Today the arthroscopy is a procedure in which a rigid fiber optic scope (not much bigger than a drinking straw) is inserted into the joint through a very small incision. By fiber optics lighting and a camera, there is good visualization of the joint (often viewing the image on a TV screen). This is done without opening the joint up for visualization, which would necessitate making a much larger incision. The advantage of a smaller incision is that there is quicker healing and therefore a shorter rehabilitation process after the procedure. The procedure called arthroscopy was invented in the 1960s by Japanese physician Masaki Watanabe.[5]

The inspiration for arthroscopy was the procedure called cystoscopy that was widely available in the early 1960s. With cystoscopy a rigid, straight cystoscope tube is inserted into the bladder through the urethra (what you urinate through). The procedure is done without opening the bladder

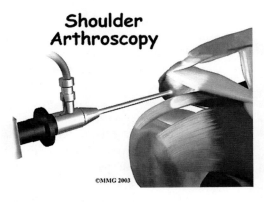

Shoulder Arthroscopy

©MMG 2003

Figure indicates where arthroscope is usually inserted for visualization of rotator cuff of shoulder. A separate scope is inserted into the shoulder if instrumentation repair is needed (used by permission of Medical Multimedia Group LLC).

up through the abdominal wall. With a joint arthroscopy procedure, at least two incisions are made into a joint. One incision is for the visualization tube. The other is for a tube through which very small surgical instruments are inserted to remove or repair damage. Arthroscopy can be used both to diagnose and to repair problems. No matter what joint the scope is inserted into, it is still considered arthroscopy. The two joints most often arthroscoped are the knee and shoulder.

Mark Mulder had his shoulder arthroscoped on Tuesday, September 12, 2006, by New York Mets team orthopedist Dr. David Altchek. A small tear of the rotator cuff was noted. Some damaged tissue was trimmed and the partial tear was repaired (not just cleaned up). He had some slight damage to his labrum which was repaired at the same time.[6]

Once the damage is repaired, the long process of rehabilitation begins. Depending on the severity of the tear, the player may have to have varying degrees of immobilization (maybe the shoulder in a sling for a few days), and then there is a gradual return to normal daily activities. Mulder was supposed to start throwing January 15 and be ready to throw from the mound between March 1 and 15, 2007, almost six months after the initial arthroscopy. He finally made it back to pitching in the major leagues in September 2007. In mid–September 2007, Mulder was found to have to have some scar tissue and unfortunately needed a second arthroscopy. His labrum repair from the previous year looked fine. He ended up only pitching three games in 2007. In 2008 he suffered another setback in his rehab after pitching only three major league games for the Cardinals (one start). He stated that he would just as soon retire rather than have a third arthroscopic evaluation.[7] Mulder did not pitch in the minors or majors in 2009. He worked with former Oakland A's and New York Mets pitching coach Rick Peterson to try and make a comeback. He was a free agent in 2010 but was not signed[8] and did not play in 2011.

PEDRO MARTINEZ

There is a long list of pitchers who have had rotator cuff tears of varying degrees. Recent cases include Pedro Martinez and Bartolo Colon. Pedro Martinez opted for surgery.[9] Martinez returned to action in September 2007, though in a somewhat limited manner and made another comeback near the end of the 2009 season and post-season, pitching well for the Philadelphia Phillies. But he has not pitched in the major leagues since.

BARTOLO COLON

Bartolo Colon decided on doing just rehabilitation, with no rotator cuff surgery.[10] Colon's shoulder was fine until he suffered elbow (disabled list) and back problems in 2007. He has had various health issues ever since. He only had seven starts in 2008 for Boston and 12 starts for the White Sox in 2009. He was a free agent in 2010, but went unsigned.

In 2011 Bartolo Colon was the subject of several articles concerning his medical treatment with stem cells injected into damaged tissue, a treatment given in an attempt to heal Colon's chronic shoulder (rotator cuff) and elbow injuries.[11] Colon's medical care was given at the Clinica Union Medica in Santiago, Dominican Republic, in April of 2010. After receiving the injections from Dr. Joseph Purita, Colon pitched successfully between the 2010 and 2011 seasons in Latin winter ball. Because of his success, he was signed to a contract by the Yankees and subsequently made the team out of spring training.[12]

Colon's stem cells were obtained from his own fat cells and bone marrow. This somatic stem cell use is not to be confused with the more controversial embryonic stem cell use. Stem cell treatment for sports injuries is filled with a lot of hype, and its use is not presently backed by scientific research to evaluate its possible effectiveness.

According to an article at SI.com by C. J. Nitkowski, who also received treatment by Dr. Purita, Colon in all likelihood also received injections of PRP (platelet-rich plasma) isolated from his own blood.[13]

Major League Baseball has looked very closely at Colon's medical records to make sure Colon did not receive human growth hormone (HGH) at the same time as his stem cell injections. HGH use, as previously noted, is banned by Major League Baseball.

BRET SABERHAGEN

Bret Saberhagen pitched in the major leagues for 16 years, eight with the Kansas City Royals. He won two Cy Young Awards, one in 1985 (the year the Royals won their only World Series title) and one in 1989. He pitched a no-hitter for the Royals against the White Sox on August 26, 1991. He won the 1998 Tony Conigliaro Award and *The Sporting News* "Comeback Player of the Year" award in 1987 and 1998. He holds a respectable career record of 167 wins and 117 losses with a career ERA of 3.34. He might have had a better career record if not for major rotator cuff shoulder problems which forced him to miss the entire 1996 and 2000 seasons and ultimately led to his retirement in 2001 at age 37.

Saberhagen started the 1995 season with the New York Mets. He had five wins and five losses when he was traded to the Colorado Rockies on July 31 as the Rockies were trying to make the playoffs.

He did just fine in his first three starts for the Rockies. On August 13 he pitched against the Braves at Atlanta Fulton County Stadium. He threw 115 pitches and held the Braves to six hits and two runs in the seven innings pitched, not a bad day at the ballpark. The very next day his future changed.

"The first ball I picked up and threw, it felt like something exploded in my shoulder," Saberhagen said.[14]

His next start on August 18 against the Cubs was a disaster. He lasted only ⅓ inning in the Rockies' 26–7 loss to the Cubs. He complained that his arm felt dead following the game.

"I normally throw about 92 (mph)," Saberhagen said. "Last night I was probably 86. My ball was up and I couldn't throw a curve or my changeup for strikes. It was ugly. But if I go out there next time and I'm on my game, I'm not concerned about it."[15]

The shoulder didn't get much better the rest of the season, nor did it in his Game 4 start against Atlanta in the NLDS, which the Rockies lost. An MRI on September 16 had showed just some shoulder inflammation and no structural damage, but MRIs don't show everything every time.[16]

After the playoff game against Atlanta, Saberhagen seriously considered having an arthroscopy done to evaluate why he had had so much trouble the last month and a half of the 1995 season. On October 24 in New York, an arthroscopy was done by Dr. David W. Altchek. Some dead tissue was removed from his rotator cuff and a ligament (most likely from the shoulder capsule) had to be re-attached.[17] As usual, aggressive rehabilitation followed. Nothing went right in 1996 despite the previous arthroscope with a rotator cuff cleanup and concomitant ligament re-attachment. Something more aggressive needed to be done, a shoulder reconstruction. There was looseness in the shoulder that had to be addressed. On May 28, Dr. Altchek, who had done the 1995

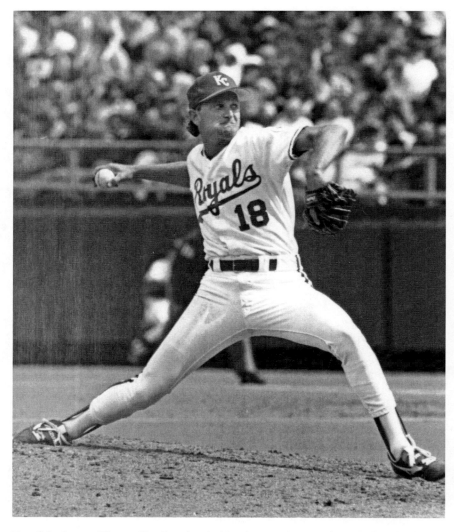

Bret Saberhagen, Kansas City Royals, pitching in 1989 (National Baseball Hall of Fame Library, Cooperstown, New York).

arthroscopy, completed the more extensive surgery. The ligament (in the capsule, most likely) that had previously been re-attached in 1995 had come loose and had to be re-attached. The torn ligament, if not repaired, would have caused continued instability in Saberhagen's shoulder. Two tears in Saberhagen's rotator cuff needed to be repaired as well.[18]

The Colorado Rockies, Saberhagen's team in 1996, declined the 1997 $5 million option they had on Saberhagen. The Boston Red Sox decided to take a risk on Saberhagen even though he would not be available until June of 1997 at the earliest.[19] Rehabilitation went slowly, as expected, maybe even slower. He pitched five rehab games at three different minor league levels before finally appearing at the major league level on August 23, 1997, a span of 685 days since his last major league game pitched. His results weren't pretty. In the first inning he gave up four runs on four hits, a walk, a hit batsman, and his own throwing error. He settled down after that, pitching three more innings without a score for an 83-pitch outing.[20]

Saberhagen ended up making six starts over the last two months of the season, totaling 26 innings with a 0–1 record and a very high ERA of 6.58.[21]

The 1998 season was much better for Saberhagen, who pitched 31 games with a 15–8 record and a good ERA of 3.96. He pitched 175 innings while giving up 181 hits and only 29 walks. This was good enough to win *The Sporting News* American League "Comeback Player of the Year" award and the Tony Conigliaro award for 1998.[22]

In 1999 things went well for Saberhagen except for two trips to the DL for ... shoulder problems. He won ten games with six losses and a fine ERA of 2.95 in 21 starts. He did pitch three games in the post-season with fair to poor results, earning him two losses.

When Saberhagen continued to have trouble with his shoulder after the playoffs, he again went under the knife. Dr. Altchek again did arthroscopy on Saberhagen's right shoulder, this time on November 2, 1999. A preliminary MRI had shown only fraying of the rotator cuff, but the arthroscope revealed that the rotator cuff was torn. It had to be repaired. At age 35 Saberhagen had to start the whole rehab process on his shoulder all over again.[23]

Saberhagen did not pitch at all at the major league level in 2000. He pitched seven games at various levels in the Boston minor league system before he had to be shut down in early September because of severe shoulder pain.[24]

After a period of rest, the rehab process started all over in the 2000-2001 off-season. Saberhagen again worked his way through four levels of the minor league system of the Red Sox in 2001. He finally pitched at the major league level for the Red Sox on July 28, 2001— 21 months after his last major league start. He made three starts for the Red Sox before being shut down again on August 8 because of tightness in his shoulder. He would never pitch again in a major league game.[25]

Saberhagen was elected to the Kansas City Royals Hall of Fame in August 2005. He might have had even a greater career if not for rotator cuff injuries.[26]

DON DRYSDALE

In the past, before arthroscopic surgery, there were many pitching careers cut short by rotator cuff tears at the major league or amateur level. Look at the example of Don Drysdale, whose career was cut short in 1969 at age 32 with a rotator cuff tear.[27]

Unfortunately, Drysdale's condition brought a clinical diagnosis of rotator cuff tear by Los Angeles Dodgers team physician Dr. Robert Kerlan and well-known orthopedic surgeon Dr. Frank Jobe. Since MRI technology was not available at the time, he could very well have had some labrum issues as well. No reference was found that mentioned tests later in Drysdale's life to confirm the diagnosis.

Drysdale's career was good enough to get him in the Hall of Fame. In 14 seasons with the Dodgers he finished with 209 victories and 166 defeats, with a very fine career ERA of 2.95.

MARK FIDRYCH

Mark Fidrych, who died in an accident on his farm in 2009, barely started his career before his rotator cuff injury ruined his career.

Fidrych burst on the scene in 1976 in Detroit at age 21. He did not start the year in the Tigers' rotation, but once he got in the rotation he did well, as he finished with 24 complete games in 29 starts and a 19–9 record in 250 innings pitched. He was also a very popular, somewhat zany player who drew large crowds to see him pitch whether at home in Tiger Stadium or on the road. He won Rookie of the Year honors in the American League in 1976.

Early 1977 did not go as well. He injured his knee shagging flies in the outfield during spring training. He landed awkwardly on a sprinkler, tearing cartilage. The injury required open knee surgery (they weren't doing arthroscopy in Detroit in 1976). When Fidrych returned from knee surgery, he noticed his arm simply went "dead" while he was pitching against Baltimore It is uncertain if the knee injury could have led to the development of Fidrych's shoulder problems.[28]

After 1976 Fidrych only won 11 more games, six of these in 1977. He struggled because of shoulder pain and decreased effectiveness. He was done after 1980 at the age of 25. Contrary to the information obtained on Drysdale, Fidrych later in life had tests to diagnose his rotator cuff tear.

Fidrych, even after he quit baseball, continued to have "pain in his shoulder (that) kept him awake and that hurt him to close the car door or lift a can of beer." He was motivated by his pain to have a procedure when one was available. At the Hughston Clinic in Columbus, Georgia, in 1985, Dr. James Andrews arthroscoped Fidrych's shoulder, both diagnosing his rotator cuff tear and repairing it. Fidrych did not go back into pitching, but he did get considerable relief of his pain.[29]

Even with modern medicine and the advent of arthroscopic surgery, some injuries simply do not result in full recovery. Any pitcher, no matter how good he was at any time in his career, may have a career-ending injury. Statistics show that the worse the rotator cuff tear, the more likely the injury is career-ending. A tear of the labrum in addition to a rotator cuff tear is even worse.

Labral Tear

The humerus (the upper arm bone) is held in place by strong muscles, tendons, and ligaments. The head (top that is shaped like a ball) sits in a small cartilage cup called the labrum. The labrum is shallower than the deep hip joint socket, but still important for the stability of the shoulder. It provides support to allow smooth movement about the shoulder. Damage to the labrum and the head of the humerus doesn't sit well; it is unstable. When damage is severe enough, surgery must be done to sew or tack the labrum back in place and hope that it heals correctly. This surgery can be done with an arthroscope. Damage to the labrum can occur in two fashions, by overuse or by trauma. Jason Schmidt and Chris Carpenter both experienced overuse damage to the labrum.

Torn labrums and/or rotator cuffs carry a worse prognosis than torn medial collateral ligaments in the elbow. The latter's success rate is 85 percent for Tommy John surgery (ulnar collateral ligament reconstruction at the elbow, see Chapter 3) for pitchers, whereas shoulder issues carry a much lower success rate with treatment. Exact statistics for recovery from torn labrums and rotator cuffs are difficult to cite. The success rate depends on the severity of the injury. With torn ulnar collateral ligaments with significant symptoms, the treatment is very similar — Tommy John surgery. Surgery for rotator cuff/labrum injuries often depends on how severe the injury is, and even with significant symptoms is a tough call.

Repair of torn labrums is common. In an article in the *Los*

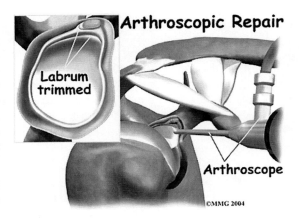

A cross-section (end on) view of the inside of the shoulder joint, showing labral tear and possible arthroscope visualization, is pictured. A separate scope is inserted for instrumentation repair of labral tear. Treatment would be dependent on severity of tear. This could range from just trimming frayed tissue to removing torn ends, or suturing together of torn ends (used by permission of Medical Multimedia Group LLC).

Angeles Times in 2007, Stan Conte, the Dodgers' director of medical services, estimated that there are 180 labral repairs in the major or minor leagues in any given season. He didn't cite the exact percentage who recovered, simply that the prognosis is much worse than with elbow surgery. Even if a pitcher does recover from surgery, can he ever return to his previous level of performance? Most of the literature is full of individual cases — those who never come back and those who continue to pitch though with decreased performance.[30]

The severity of the tears needs to be considered in assessment of recovery, though very few articles that specifically address the recovery rate based on the severity of the problem are found. Most group all rotator cuff tears in one basket no matter how severe. Most ignore a common co-existing problem — labral tears — these occurring at the same time as the rotator cuff tears. The combination of the two, as previously mentioned, is even worse than having just the labrum tear.

JASON SCHMIDT

Jason Schmidt has had two shoulder arthroscopies. The first, as a Pittsburgh Pirate, was August 17, 2000, performed by Dr. James Andrews of the famous clinic in Birmingham, Alabama. Compared to some procedures, damage noted was rather minor. Some fraying of the labrum and rotator cuff with tears was noted. He recovered nicely, winning 84 games over six seasons for the Pirates and Giants.[31]

During the off-season between 2006 and 2007, Schmidt signed a $47 million, three-year contract with the Los Angeles Dodgers. He started poorly in April of 2007 with a 1–2 record and a high ERA after three games pitched. Shoulder bursitis was found to be the culprit, and Schmidt was placed on the DL.

After a 51-day absence he returned and pitched well for one start, throwing six shutout innings and reaching velocities of 89 to 91 miles per hour on his fastball. In the next two starts after his return from the DL, his velocity was down in the mid–80s and his performance was poor, giving up six runs and three runs in starts lasting only four innings and four and two-thirds innings respectively. Once again Schmidt's shoulder did not feel right. With the lack of improvement with conservative treatment, it was time for an arthroscopy.

The findings were a scarred bursa sac (this is a sac in the shoulder lubricating between bone and tendons), a frayed biceps tendon (a big tendon attached to the biceps muscle), and a torn labrum. The torn labrum was the most serious of these injuries and contributed the most to the decrease in velocity on Schmidt's fastball. The tear prevents the shoulder from getting into a stable cocking position as the pitcher initiates the throwing motion. The labrum and other injuries were repaired.[32]

Schmidt did not pitch at the major league level in 2008.[33] In 2009 he made four starts and his ERA was a poor 5.60. He was a free agent in 2010 but went unsigned,[34] and has not pitched since 2009.

Chris Carpenter

Another pitcher having a labral tear was Chris Carpenter. Shoulder problems shortened his season in 2002. He only had 13 starts when he was put on the DL in September, retroactive to August 15. He had arthroscopic surgery to repair the frayed labrum in September of that year. That winter he was signed by the St. Louis Cardinals. His rehab didn't go well and he needed a second arthroscopic surgery on July 29, 2003, to clean up scar tissue. The result: he missed the entire 2003 season.[35]

In 2004 he returned in a big way. He finished with 15 wins and five losses for the Cardinals and was voted "Comeback Player of the Year" in the National League. Unfortunately some shoulder nerve irritation developed at the end of the regular season which forced Carpenter to miss the 2004 post-season.[36]

He came back again in 2005, winning the Cy Young Award with 21 wins and five losses, an ERA of 2.83, and 213 strikeouts in 241⅔ innings.

Since 2005 Carpenter has had issues with his elbow, but he has experienced no further significant problems directly related to the repaired labrum. Not everyone's recovery from a torn labrum goes as well as Carpenter's.

Roger Clemens

Also doing well after labrum surgery was Roger Clemens. In fact, Clemens is probably the most successful pitcher ever following arthroscopic shoulder surgery. This might lead one to suspect Clemens' problems prior to surgery were minor, but certainly his symptoms were not minor.

Clemens pitched college ball at the University of Texas. He was the 19th player chosen in the 1983 amateur draft, taken by the Boston Red Sox. He made it to the major leagues the year after the draft. His career has to be considered one of the most successful of any modern pitcher. He won seven Cy Young Awards and one MVP (1986). His career record was 354–184 with an ERA of 3.12. He recorded 4,672 strikeouts, third only to Nolan Ryan and Randy Johnson. There is some controversy about his possible use of steroids after 1998. But even if one discounts a potential area of concern from 1998 to 2004, one cannot ignore the four Cy Young Awards before 1998 as well as his MVP Award. Without the controversy over steroid use, he would be a shoo-in first-round Hall of Fame candidate. Despite the controversy, which may never be proven one way or another, he probably will still eventually make it into the Hall of Fame.

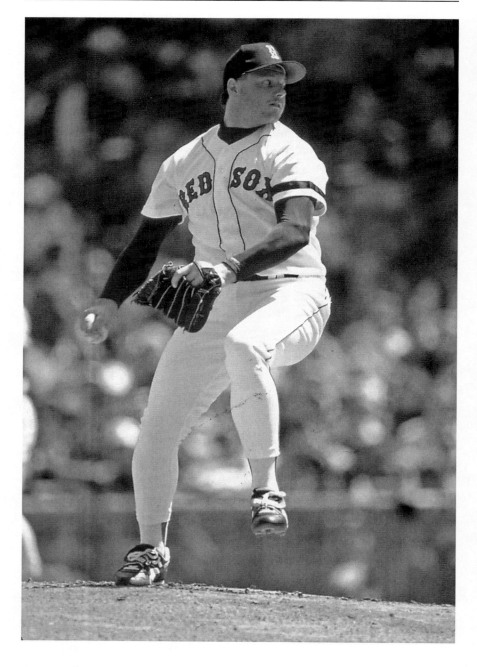

Roger Clemens, Boston Red Sox, pitching in April 1990 (National Baseball Hall of Fame Library, Cooperstown, New York).

Clemens' career had a major bump in the road during his first and second years in the majors, 1984 and 1985. The problems with his shoulder are best described in his book *Rocket Man: The Roger Clemens Story*, co-authored with Peter Gammons, and in several articles appearing in the *Boston Globe* in 1985.[37]

Clemens, as one would figure from the title of his book, *Rocket Man*, possessed a blazing fastball. Because of it he spent very little time in the minors, appearing in 11 games in the minors in 1983 and only seven games in 1984 before being called up from the AAA affiliate in Pawtucket. His minor league record at that point was only 7–5, but his ERA was less than 2.00.

He finished his 1984 rookie season with a 9–4 record and one of the highest ERAs of his career, 4.32. But his 126 strikeouts against 29 walks in 133⅓ innings indicated future success. His stats would have been even better had he not suffered from blisters on his pitching hand and some forearm and shoulder pain.

In his book, Clemens discussed a game in early August of 1984 where he tried to put extra speed on some of his pitches. He was hitting 97 mph on the radar gun and tried to give a little extra kick on the fastball to hit 98 or 99 mph. In doing so he felt a stinging pain in his shoulder unlike any he had felt before.[38]

He had had pain with shoulder tendonitis in college and got over it. Could he pitch through this pain like he had done before?

Something was different this time. In addition to having the pain, the velocity on his fastball slipped down to the 92–93 mph range, and quite often he even had trouble maintaining that velocity during an entire game.

He did extensive workouts in the winter between the 1984 and 1985 seasons but his shoulder kept getting worse. By late May he was lucky to hit 90 mph, and on occasion he could not even hit 85 mph on the radar gun. While warming up for a game on July 7 he felt a very intense, sharp pain in his shoulder, as if "someone stuck a knife in the back of my shoulder."[39]

It was soon after a game on August 11 that Clemens was put on the DL.

Why? True, during this game Clemens could only hit 88 mph on the radar gun with his best stuff. True, he was having significant pain. But in addition to those problems it was now apparent that he was altering his motion to compensate for his discomfort. His mechanics were off, a bad sign.

He had been seeing Dr. Arthur Pappas, the Red Sox team physician, in consultation. Dr. Pappas' initial diagnosis was shoulder tendonitis. When Clemens continued to have problems later in August, not responding to rest and physical therapy, an arthroscopic procedure was recommended. Before getting this procedure, Clemens decided to get a second opinion from Dr. James Andrews of the Hughston Clinic in Columbus, Georgia. The recommendation was the same. Clemens needed arthroscopy.

Initial tests at Massachusetts Medical Center in August had revealed a triceps muscle tear (the muscle in the back of the upper arm). That tear would heal by itself but the tear noted within his shoulder would not.

In two articles appearing in the *Boston Globe* by Larry Whiteside, one on August 24 and one on August 25, Clemens was described as having what is called a SLAP tear (superior lateral anterior posterior tear of the labrum). The location of the tear was likely close to the attachment of the long head of the biceps muscle to the top part of the labrum.[40]

The exact date of Roger Clemens' surgery by Dr. Andrews is not given in his book, nor is it told in articles in the *Boston Globe*. In an article in the *Boston Globe* on September 4, the date of Clemens shoulder surgery is simply listed as the "previous week."[41]

In Clemens' book he describes the labrum tear in somewhat generic terms. He was awake during the 20-minute procedure. A loose piece of cartilage was "zipped in with a little Pac-Man, scooped out," and the area around the rotator cuff was "vacuumed."[42]

Clemens' post-op recovery was made easier because he had started a rehab program prior to surgery. Clemens had been instructed by Nolan Ryan as to the specific exercises for his rotator cuff, and he had instituted them well before his surgery. Dr. Andrews told Clemens that his recovery would depend considerably on how well he did his rehabilitation.

The rest is history. In 1986, the year after his surgery, Clemens had his best season ever. He finished with a record of 24–4 and won both the Cy Young Award and the American League MVP Award. Boston made it to the World Series, though they lost to the New York Mets. Clemens pitched two games in the World Series, giving up four earned runs in 11⅓ with no decisions. He had previously recorded a win and a loss in three games pitched in Boston's victory over the California Angels in the ALCS.

Clemens went on to pitch 24 seasons in the major leagues, recording over 300 victories after his labrum surgery and minor rotator cuff clean-up. One would have to call Clemens' recovery from the labrum surgery very successful, much better than most. Clemens also learned rehab techniques to keep his shoulder in good condition. He continued to use those exercises successfully throughout the rest of his career.

Isolated Shoulder Capsule Damage

OREL HERSHISER

There are three main problems with a pitcher's shoulder that can jeopardize his career: labral injuries, rotator cuff injuries, and capsule injuries. The latter is the most unusual and probably the most career-threatening of the three. Orel Hershiser, then of the Los Angeles Dodgers, had a capsule injury (and labral injury) and it was a miracle that he was ever able to pitch again after his surgery to fix these problems.

Orel "Bulldog" Hershiser pitched 18 years in the majors, mostly for the Dodgers (13 years) and Cleveland Indians (three years). He won 204 games and lost 150 with a fine career 3.48 ERA. He is best known for breaking Don Drysdale's scoreless streak record when he pitched 59 consecutive scoreless innings in 1988. That season he led the National League in wins (23), complete games (15), and innings pitched (267). It should not be surprising that in 1988 he also won the Cy Young Award. That year he was the MVP of the playoffs against the New York Mets and MVP of the World Series. For his effort in 1988, Hershiser was named the top National League pitcher by *The Sporting News* and "Sportsman of the Year" by *Sports Illustrated* magazine.

In 1990 Hershiser came down with his career-threatening injury. The injury illustrates one reason current major league managers are unwilling to let their pitchers pitch excessive innings and complete games. Hershiser led the league in innings pitched for three consecutive years (1987 to 1989) with 264, 267, and 256 innings respectively, and 1989 marked the fifth straight year Hershiser had pitched more than 230 innings.

Spring training in 1990 was abbreviated by three weeks due to an owners' lockout, but this lockout probably had no bearing on the development of Hershiser's injury. Hershiser's damaged shoulder did not develop overnight. Rather, the damage had developed over a long period of time.

From the beginning of 1990 spring training, Hershiser noticed a dull ache and stiffness in his shoulder. He did not report this problem to anyone except to mention it briefly to the Dodgers' team physician, Dr. Frank Jobe. From the very start of the regular season, Hershiser also noticed significant arm fatigue. He was having difficulty getting past the fifth inning, something very unusual for a pitcher who was used to throwing complete games. After his fourth start of the season, a 6⅓-inning, 5–1 loss to the St. Louis Cardinals on April 25, it was obvious he had a significant issue with his shoulder, though at the time its severity wasn't clear.

An MRI done on April 26 revealed the worst: Hershiser's had damage to his shoulder capsule and labrum; it was a career-threatening injury.[43]

What to do? In 1990 the procedure deemed necessary to correct Hershiser's injury would be the first procedure of its kind performed on a major league pitcher. Previous to Hershiser only a few minor league pitchers, NFL quarterback Jim McMahon, and pro golfer Jerry Pate had had the procedure done. If Hershiser wanted to continue to pitch, the surgery was necessary, and who better to do it than Dr. Jobe, the physician who did the first Tommy John surgery?

Dr. Jobe performed the surgery on Hershiser on April 27, 1990. First, a

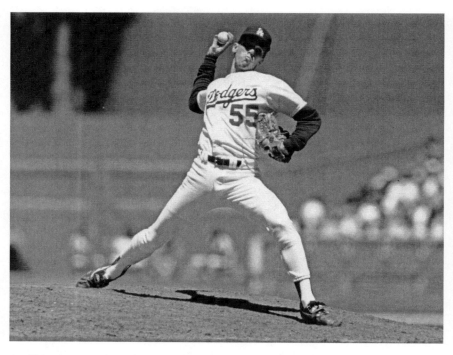

Orel Hershiser pitching for the Los Angeles Dodgers, date unknown (National Baseball Hall of Fame Library, Cooperstown, New York).

pre-surgery arthrogram was done; dye was injected into the shoulder and x-rays were taken. Results noted were as bad as the MRI had indicated. Thus, an open surgery (bigger hole) was deemed necessary. No arthroscopic procedure was going to help here. To keep the ball of the humerus bone from slipping out of the socket, an anterior (front of shoulder) repair of the capsule and ligaments within the shoulder, as well as the anterior labrum (where the ligaments and capsule attach), had to be done. Before this radical procedure, some frayed portions of the posterior labrum were trimmed. Slight tears in the rotator cuff were not repaired. The ligaments within the capsule were carefully stretched back into place, as close to the correct anatomic position as possible.[44]

An article by David Falkner in *The Sporting News* in May of 1996 outlines Hershiser's treatment with long rehabilitation after surgery.[45] Just out of surgery, Hershiser was place in a removable cast with the arm pushed out laterally. The cast was designed so the arm could be taken out of the cast and put through passive range-of-motion exercises three times a day for the first few weeks. After the cast was removed, more and more movement of the arm became possible unassisted, by active range-of-motion exercises. Pain was Hershiser's constant companion.

Initially the recovery was estimated to take two years, but Hershiser progressed much quicker than this schedule. There had been little thought of his pitching effectively at the major league level in 1991, but he surpassed these estimates, a credit to his determination and faith.

Falkner describes Hershiser's comeback well.

> He [Hershiser] threw first in simulated games, then in extended spring training, finally with the big team. None of it was "pretty," Hershiser says. Adrenaline was absent in the simulated games, pain was constant in real games. Even when he made it back, the pain was so searing, any sense of accomplishment was missing. On the mound, he says, he hurt so much he had to fight back tears. Between innings he withdrew to a corner of the empty clubhouse and broke down.[46]

In the rehab process, arm strength to throw the ball harder needs to increase. Along with arm strength, command of the pitches has to improve, including the ability to locate pitches within the strike zone. The ability to locate pitches is partly related to proper mechanics, including correct arm angle and release point. In the article by Falkner, Hershiser states that ultimately these abilities did not come back until the two-year point originally set for his rehab to last.[47]

Statistics for the 1991 season do not necessarily agree with the two-year rehab. In 1991 Hershiser made 21 starts, pitched 112 innings, and had a 7–2 record with an ERA of 3.46. He walked only 32 batters in 112 innings, not a stat that would indicate a loss of command.

Hershiser's record in 1992 and 1993 was fair, with records of 10–15 and 12–14 respectively, though he had respectable ERAs of 3.67 and 3.59.

Post major surgery Hershiser pitched ten more years, eventually retiring at age 42. He did not perform as well as before his surgery. He had 105 wins and 85 losses after surgery as opposed to a record of 99–65 before surgery. His ERA often went above 4.00 in his last five seasons. He never pitched more than 216 innings in any one season after surgery. But not all of this can be attributed to decreased ability that came from his shoulder injury and subsequent surgery. Simple advancing age could explain much of Hershiser's declining statistics.

MARK PRIOR

Orel Hershiser's capsule injury repair and recovery are rather remarkable. More typical of a capsule injury is the career of Mark Prior, who has not pitched in the major leagues since 2006.

Prior was the second overall pick by the Chicago Cubs in the 2001 amateur draft. He had just finished his junior year at USC, where he had a record of 15–1 and a 1.70 ERA.[48]

Prior pitched only nine games in the minors before being promoted to

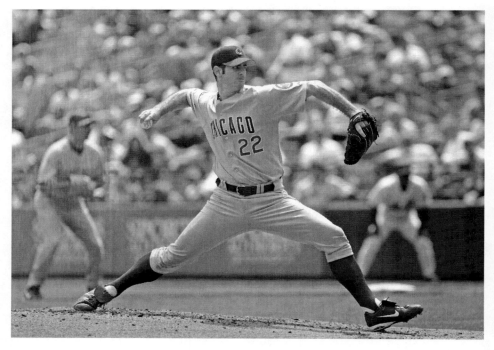

Chicago Cub Mark Prior delivers against the New York Mets at Shea Stadium, Wednesday, July 26, 2006, in New York. Note inverted "W" pitching form (AP Photo/Mary Altaffer).

the majors at age 21 by the Chicago Cubs. He started 19 games in 2002, finishing with six wins and six losses, an ERA of 3.32, and 147 strikeouts in only 116⅔ innings. In only his second year in the majors, in 2003 Prior went 18–6 with an ERA of 2.43 and 245 strikeouts in 211⅓ innings, despite a brief visit to the DL because of a shoulder contusion. He would never pitch that many games in a season again.

In 2004 he had some problems with Achilles tendonitis, landing him on the DL from March 26 until June 4. In 2005 he was on the DL twice, first with right elbow inflammation (March 25–April 12) and a right elbow fracture. In 2006 he was on the DL for a shoulder strain and tendonitis (March 27–June 18) and twice for left oblique muscle strains (July 5–21 and August 11–October 2). But it was the shoulder injury in 2007 that permanently set his career back.[49]

Prior had had some problems with his shoulder in 2006 as previously stated. In fact, he had seen Dr. Andrews in the fall of 2006. Andrews stated that Prior had no structural damage and just had "genetic looseness." But Prior's poor performance in spring training in 2007 mirrored his poor performance in 2006, when he had only one win and six losses with an ERA of 7.21 before being demoted to AAA Iowa. When Prior reported significant pain during a game on March 28, 2007, he was once again off to be evaluated by Dr. Andrews.

Dr. Andrews did an arthroscopy on Prior's shoulder on April 24, 2007. Reports on exactly what was done on Prior's shoulder vary. It would appear he had a split in his capsule, a slight 180-degree tear in his labrum, and some minor damage to his rotator cuff that needed some debridement (surgical removal of damaged tissue). Cubs general manager Jim Hendry called the procedure "touch ups."[50]

Prior signed with the San Diego Padres as a free agent during the off-season of 2007–2008. He was warming up in extended spring training in Peoria, Arizona, when his life took a dramatic turn for the worse. Prior states while throwing a pitch, it "felt like a firecracker went off in the back of my shoulder." Padres team physician Dr. Jan Fronek reported that Prior had a tear of the anterior capsule, with the capsule pulling off the front of the humerus bone, tearing ligaments within the capsule (called an avulsion injury). It was an injury more typically seen with a "traumatic event," such as falling with one's arm extended, than with an overuse injury from throwing a baseball. Getting hit hard in the shoulder from a hard collision with another player could also cause the injury. Surgery to correct the tear was done by Drs. Jan Fronek and Heinz Hoenecke on June 4, 2008.[51]

Prior signed a minor league contract with the Padres in January of 2009. Well into the season, Prior reported soreness in his shoulder while rehabbing in Arizona. At that point the Padres decided enough was enough and cut ties with him on August 1, 2009.[52]

He was not signed in 2010 and it appeared as though Prior's career was over at age 30 due to his history of shoulder injuries, the last of which was an extremely bad capsule tear. Then, in a change of events, Prior signed a minor league contract with the Yankees for 2011.[53] He was trying to convert to being a relief pitcher.

Why did Mark Prior's career come to an abrupt stop for so long (and maybe an end)? There is much debate. There have been questions about Prior's delivery. He achieved the position of an inverted "w" prior to the acceleration phase of throwing. There is some opinion that this type of pitching motion puts excessive stress on the arm and shoulder, making them more vulnerable to injury, more so than with other pitching motions.[54]

Peter Gammons agrees. In a recent article discussing the 2010 amateur baseball draft, Peter Gammons said, "Prior had a flawed delivery."[55]

Some disagree. The Jeff Passan article at yahoo.com quotes Padres' manager and former major league pitcher Bud Black as saying, "I think he's (Prior) got a good delivery. Good mechanics. Good fundamentally. Sound thrower."

Others apparently agree, as there were no apparent attempts to change Prior's mechanics.

A final opinion: Surgeon Frank Jobe drops his own two cents in when referring to the possible premature end to Prior's career saying, "everybody's got a finite amount of pitches [in his arm]," and maybe he (Prior) hit his.[56]

Biceps Tendon Injury in Pitcher

MILT WILCOX

In addition to damage to the rotator cuff muscles mentioned, there can be damage to the tendon of the long head of the biceps tendon which moves along the top of the humerus bone and inserts into the scapula at the top of the glenoid socket (also labrum). It attaches to the top part of the labrum and can be involved in damage to the labrum (called SLAP tears). The biceps tendon provides support to shoulder movement in addition to the stability given by muscles of the rotator cuff.

Tendonitis of the shoulder can be localized to the biceps tendon, and there can be impingement of this tendon with shoulder movement from the acromium and clavicle bone superior (above) the humerus. Bursitis of the shoulder can also involve this tendon, as it runs through the bursa lubricating sac.

Milt Wilcox, a pitcher with Detroit, had a biceps tendon injury at the shoulder. His medical problems give yet another example of potential problems from excessive cortisone shots. Wilcox's second shoulder surgery was a relatively new procedure, shaving off the bone of the acromium and/or clavicle to increase room for the shoulder to move (decreasing impingement).

Wilcox was drafted by the Cincinnati Reds in the second round of the 1968 amateur draft. He made his debut in the major leagues at the young age of 20. Expectations were high, but great performance did not follow. From age 20 till 27 Wilcox bounced around from team to team, moving from being a starter to the bullpen until finally establishing himself as a starter for the Detroit Tigers in 1977. Wilcox had come up initially as a power pitcher, but by his early 30s he came to rely on a split finger fastball and a pitch called a "Yack-adoo," a parabolic curve ball.[57]

Wilcox spent nine years as a starting pitcher for the Tigers, winning 11 to 13 games per year before his career peaked at the same time as the Tigers in 1984, when he won 17 games against eight losses. The Tigers made the playoffs and the won the World Series in 1984. Wilcox recorded a win in the American League Championship Series against the Kansas City Royals and won Game 3 in the World Series against the San Diego Padres.

His stats in 1984 do not tell the whole story. He pitched the whole year with considerable shoulder pain. He tried just about everything short of surgery to deal with his pain. He used a relatively new pain killer, DSMO, and took Motrin and Ascriptin up to 12 in a day. He also received cortisone shots, many cortisone shots. At first his shots were every two months, then every month, and then finally toward the end of 1984 season every week, just to be able to get some relief of his shoulder pain in order to continue to pitch.[58]

Because of all his shoulder difficulty, he was examined by Dr. James Andrews at the Hughston Clinic in Columbus, Georgia. It didn't take much to convince Wilcox that he needed to have a shoulder arthroscopy, and he had this done by Dr. Andrews on October 19, 1984.

It is difficult to find a clear report of the final diagnosis noted on the arthroscopy. An article in the *Seattle Times* on February 11, 1986, states that this arthroscopy did reveal that a "biceps tendon had frayed like a rope down to its last strand. It literally was hanging there." Wilcox reported much later that he was convinced that some of the damage detected on his arthroscopy in 1984 was a result of all the cortisone shots he received in 1984.[59]

Wilcox attempted to come back in 1985 after his shoulder difficulties and 1984 surgery. He once again had shoulder pain. He had two cortisone shots before succumbing to yet another surgery for shoulder impingement caused by the structure of the bones surrounding his shoulder socket. The acromium and clavicle bones above (superior to) the biceps tendon and rotator cuff were wearing on these structures underneath. His surgery included what at the time was thought to be a "relatively new procedure primarily used (previously) on weight-lifters and those involved in muscle sports." Bone was shaved underneath the acromium and clavicle bones (A/C joint) to increase space for the humerus bone and supporting structures. The procedure was performed in June of 1985.[60]

Wilcox spent the rest of 1985 on the disabled list. When he was not offered a contract in 1986 by the Detroit Tigers, he was signed by the Seattle Mariners. This signing followed successful pitching by Wilcox in the Dominican Republic Winter League.[61]

It just wasn't to be. Wilcox started off the year with no wins and eight losses with an ERA of 5.50 for a bad Mariners team that would go on to finish last in the American League West. Wilcox, 36 years old, was released by the Mariners on June 14, 1986. He never pitched again at the major league level.[62]

Nerve Injuries to Shoulder

BRUCE SUTTER

In addition to rotator cuff, capsule injuries, biceps tendon injuries, and labrum damage, pitchers and sometimes position players can have damage to the nerves in the neck and shoulder. Two frequent forms of nerve damage can come from thoracic outlet syndrome and from disc problems from the cervical (neck) spine. (See discussion later.)

Less frequent and more poorly understood is injury to nerves in the shoulder and upper arm. One possible cause is simply overuse; repetitive traction by movement is applied to the nerves, causing damage.

Another reason for nerve problems is nerve compression from enlargement of neck muscles due to overuse. There have been cases where small muscles (scalenes for instance) in the neck and upper shoulder have been surgically divided to make room for the nerve. This surgical procedure is usually a last resort when all conservative measures fail.

A rare complication from ligament impingement and overuse is suprascapular nerve compression and entrapment near the scapula (shoulder blade). The suprascapular nerve and blood vessels go through a space surrounded by the bone (spine of the scapula) on one side and a ligament on the other. The condition is very similar to carpal tunnel syndrome at the wrist; a nerve is compressed in a very small space. Overuse problems at the wrist are much more common than at the shoulder scapula bone. Carpal tunnel problems are very common. Almost everyone knows someone who has carpal tunnel issues. Often you can see people in normal work places wearing a wrist splint. Rarely does a pitcher or position player develop suprascapular nerve entrapment from overuse of his shoulder.

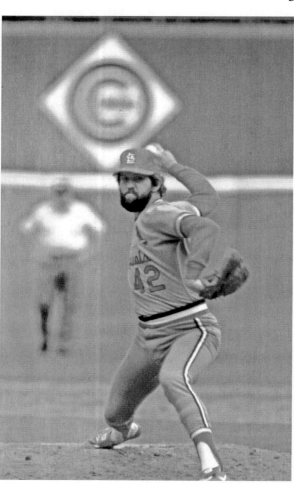

St. Louis Cardinal Bruce Sutter throwing a split-finger pitch in 1983 (National Baseball Hall of Fame Library, Cooperstown, New York).

Hall of Fame pitcher Bruce Sutter had suprascapular nerve entrapment in his right pitching shoulder. He had to have surgery twice to correct this problem. It is not clear that muscle atrophy from nerve damage was ever completely resolved, and it is quite possible that muscle weakness created by the nerve entrapment caused instability in his shoulder leading to two rotator cuff tears, the last tear ending Sutter's career.

Bruce Sutter pitched 12 years in the majors, recording 300 saves for three teams. He pitched for the Cubs (five years), the Cardinals (four years), and finally the Braves (three years). He was an undrafted player and signed as a free agent for the Cubs in 1971. He did not make it to the majors until 1976, helped considerably when Cubs coach Fred Martin taught Sutter the split-finger pitch in the minor leagues. Many players have learned the split-finger fastball, but few have thrown it as well with as much movement on the ball as Sutter. Quite often batters knew exactly what Sutter was going to pitch, and they still couldn't hit it.

Sutter finished with a very fine career ERA of 2.83 in 661 games (all in relief). He was the premier relief pitcher in the National League in the 1970s and early 1980s, leading the league in saves five times. He won a Cy Young Award in 1979. As opposed to the brief one-inning appearances by present day closers, it was not unusual for Sutter to pitch two innings to get his saves. He was elected to the Hall of Fame in 2006.

Sutter pitched his last game for the St Louis Cardinals in 1984. He became a free agent and signed a six-year, $10 million record contract with the Atlanta Braves in the off-season. Very soon after he began to pitch for the Braves, his injuries started, one right after another. Where has that been heard before — big contract, big injuries?

In Sutter's first year with Atlanta, he began having problems with his shoulder, mainly after the All-Star break. He went 2–3 with a 9.00 ERA in 32 innings the remainder of the season. In late August he had two cortisone injections within a week's time, the last on August 31. Apparently he had only mild pain relief, as on September 26 he had an arthrogram, tomograms, and a bone scan. The arthrogram revealed no rotator cuff tears.[63]

With continued problems, Sutter had surgery on December 12 for a nerve and blood vessel entrapment near his shoulder blade. This required a ligament be cut in a 90-minute procedure done by Dr. Robert Wells in Atlanta. It is fairly easy for a medical professional to conclude from newspaper articles that he had a suprascapular nerve and blood vessel entrapment. (Blood vessels and nerves quite often travel throughout the body in close proximity. Damage to one often involves damage to the other.) In 1987, when Sutter had further shoulder nerve problems, the specific nerve identified was the suprascapular nerve.[64] Harold Klawans, in his book *Why Michael Couldn't Hit and Other Tales of the Neurology of Sports*, also identifies the nerve causing Sutter's problems as the suprascapular nerve.[65]

Suprascapular nerve entrapment is similar to carpal tunnel syndrome of the wrist (an entrapment of the nerve).[66] The median nerve at the wrist is compressed and irritated by repetitive motion, though not everyone who has repetitive motion of the wrist gets carpal tunnel syndrome. Similarly, not everyone who has repetitive motion of the shoulder blade gets suprascapular entrapment. It had been noted rarely in volleyball players, but never before in a baseball pitcher.[67]

Sutter's final stats for 1985 were very uncharacteristic for him. He had seven wins and seven losses with an ERA of 4.48 and only 23 saves.

Sutter's 1986 season ended rather early. Possibly he tried to come back too soon after his 1985 surgery, as he had further surgery on his same right shoulder only eight months after his first surgery. Sutter only pitched 18 games with three saves in the regular season before ending up on the DL because of shoulder pain. He did not pitch after May 27. Shoulder arthroscopy was done on August 13, 1986, by Dr. Lanny Johnson in East Lansing, Michigan. Sutter had a slight rotator cuff tear and fraying of the anterior and posterior glenoid labrum. In addition he was found to have loose pieces of cartilage in both the shoulder and acromial-clavicular joints. Possibly some of these findings had been present when the previous arthrograms were done, as arthrograms often do not show the whole picture, especially when damage is not severe.[68]

A comeback in 1987 did not happen. Sutter did not pitch a single inning at the major league level in 1987. In fact he needed to have more surgery on February 10, 1987, at the University of Colorado Health Sciences Center in Denver, Colorado. He had persistent shoulder pain despite his arthroscopic treatment in August. Muscles in his shoulder were noted to have atrophied (gotten smaller in size) and weak, causing continued instability in his shoulder. The pre-surgery diagnosis was continued damage to his suprascapular nerve, for whatever reason. Post-surgery diagnosis was damage to the nerve (possibly permanent) and scar tissue around the nerve. The scar tissue had formed since the original nerve surgery, causing recurrent entrapment (pressure) of the nerve. This cleanup surgery on the suprascapular nerve, as opposed to his first surgery, lasted much longer, taking three and one-half hours to complete.

Dr. Steven Ringel, a neurologist, the spokesman for the surgical team, stated he was pessimistic about Sutter's chances for recovery of nerve function after surgery. He thought Sutter may have come back too soon after the first nerve surgery.[69]

Sutter did come back in 1988. He pitched in 38 games with an ERA of 4.76 and only 14 saves. He experienced two trips to the DL in 1988, but they were unrelated to his shoulder. He was on the DL from July 18 to August 19 with Bell's palsy, a nerve condition which causes drooping of the facial muscles. This is unrelated to pitching a baseball. Then he experienced right knee pain which resulted in arthroscopic surgery on September 26. The surgery was done by Dr. Joe Chandler in Atlanta at Piedmont Hospital.[70]

Sutter did rehab and appeared for spring training in 1989. He had some trouble with the knee and received an injection of cortisone on March 9. He made six appearances in spring training and then contacted Dave Pursley, the Atlanta Braves trainer, complaining he had had an ache in his shoulder for over a week. The pain at that point was so severe it was waking Sutter up from his sleep. Pursley talked to Braves manager Bobby Cox, who encouraged Sutter to see Dr. Joseph Chandler, the team's orthopedic doctor.[71]

Dr. Chandler ordered an MRI (already we are seeing the transition from ordering arthrograms to MRIs on shoulders just from 1985 to 1989 in Sutter's case). Dr. Chandler suspected a rotator cuff tear, and that is exactly what the MRI confirmed, a tear much worse than his previous partial tear for which Sutter had surgery in 1986. Whether Sutter had some residual muscle weakness from his nerve problems that led up to this recurrent rotator cuff tear was not discussed.[72] Muscle weakness of shoulder begets instability, which begets shoulder damage.

Sutter announced he was "99.9 percent" sure he would never pitch in the majors again. Dr. Chandler urged Sutter to give himself three to four months of complete rest to let the pain in the shoulder subside. If the pain did not improve, Sutter should consider further surgery.[73]

Sutter was placed on the 21-day DL and later transferred to the 60-day DL. The Braves released Sutter on November 14, 1989, and he never pitched in the major leagues again. Sutter had one year left on his original six-year contract, and the Braves were obligated to pay the last year of his salary.[74]

An article by Ray Ratto appearing in the *San Francisco Chronicle* in 1989 speculated that throwing the split-finger fastball might be hard on the shoulder. The pitch might be the culprit in the development of so many shoulder problems in Giants pitchers, who threw the split-finger pitch at the urging of their manager Roger Craig. The conclusion was that the split-finger pitch was not the culprit, as the presented evidence did not support that conclusion. The stated culprit: throwing the ball is simply an unnatural act and "the human arm wasn't designed to go through the tortures pitchers put theirs through."[75]

An unidentified pitcher's history discussed in a medical article edited by Dr. Steven P. Ringel of the University of Colorado in 1990 is strikingly similar to Bruce Sutter's story both in age and history.

A 34-year-old right-handed veteran pitcher developed an incapacitating shoulder pain during cocking [arm farthest back in throwing motion], muscle weakness of external rotation [position of arm in cocking phase], and atrophy [loss of muscle mass] of the infraspinatus muscle [the muscle supplied by the supraspinatus nerve in the lower half of the scapula/shoulder blade in one's upper back].[76]

The article says that the pitcher underwent two procedures on the suprascapular nerve (just like Sutter). The first was cutting a ligament that the nerve went under near the top of the shoulder blade. The second required neurolysis (freeing scar tissue around the nerve and/or freeing up nerve at a different location). Each time, nerve conduction tests showed improved nerve conduction post surgery. But weakness in the infraspinatus muscle (one of the rotator cuff muscles) persisted. This persistent rotator muscle weakness could cause a somewhat unstable shoulder joint and make it prone to further injury (rotator cuff tears).

Biceps (Musculocutaneous) Nerve Injury

CHRIS CARPENTER and BRAD PENNY

The next section on nerve injuries is largely based on a medical article that appeared in *The American Journal of Sports Medicine* in 2007. The discussion of the injuries of two pitchers sounds strikingly similar to Chris Carpenter's and Brad Penny's nerve injuries that occurred in 2004.[77]

Studies are "possibly" about Chris Carpenter and Brad Penny as the history, age of pitchers, and career statistics fit the pitchers mentioned even though their names aren't given. Both pitchers gave permission to be discussed in the medical article.

A rare nerve injury occurred to 29-year-old Chris Carpenter (his career was previously discussed here under shoulder injuries). Pitching during the last month of the 2004 season, Carpenter began to have problems with flexion in his right biceps tendon (contraction of the muscle was impaired). He had muscle weakness. The nerve to the biceps (probably a branch of the musculocutaneous nerve) in the upper arm was the suspected culprit. He was completely shut down from pitching on September 19. Tests revealed no structural damage to neck, shoulder, or arm; rest appeared to be the major option. Brad Penny of the Los Angeles Dodgers apparently had suffered a similar rare injury in August of 2004. Carpenter missed the 2004 playoffs and World Series but experienced no difficulty with the nerve and the biceps muscle during spring training or the 2005 season. Nothing would indicate this nerve injury has ever recurred.[78]

The medical article gives more detail about two pitchers of similar age with similar career statistics, a right-handed 29-year-old pitcher and a 26-year-old right-handed pitcher having nerve problems in the upper right arm. The 29-year-old starting pitcher felt a "sharp pain in the mid portion of his upper right arm, in the region of the right biceps, during a game in September of 2004." He had felt a "pull in the region in the right arm" during warm-ups that gradually worsened as the game went on. He had previously had two arthroscopic procedures, one two years before for labral damage and one ten months before for debridement.[79]

Initially the exam was normal. The pitcher was diagnosed with a biceps muscle strain. Soon thereafter the pitcher complained of weakness in the right biceps area, and exam confirmed this. The patient did not pitch again that year. Nerve and muscle conduction tests were slightly abnormal in two muscles, the biceps and the coracobrachialis, the latter a lesser-known, smaller muscle right next to the biceps in the upper arm.

The patient was treated with anti-inflammatory meds and given a short course of methylprednisolone, an oral cortisone-like medicine. Rest was recommended. Repeat nerve conduction tests done in January were improved. Slight decreased strength noted previously had gone away. Spring training went fine and this pitcher did fine in 2005, pitching 241⅔ innings with an ERA of 2.83 and a 21–5 record. In 2006, the pitcher went 15–8.

In the article, a 26-year-old starting pitcher had a similar history. The second pitcher's symptoms started with a sharp pain on the follow-through on a pitch to the plate. He was removed from the game "because of the severity of the pain."[80] Interestingly, he had a slight elbow contracture, an old injury, which improved with the pitch.

An MRI of the patient's shoulder was normal except for some tendonosis noted. The patient was diagnosed with a brachial plexus stretch injury (an injury to the nerve complex in the neck). Rest for six and one-half weeks was followed by a return to the mound. Seventy-five pitches into the game, he had a recurrence of his pain in his upper arm. He also now had both weakness in his upper arm and numbness in his right forearm. An MRI with neurogram was done which showed slightly unusual anatomy at his C5 and C6 nerve roots. Nerve conduction tests of the musculocutaneous nerve in the upper arm and biceps muscle were abnormal. Another exam soon after (17 days) showed some decreased muscle mass in the "lateral muscle belly of the right biceps."[81]

The patient was shut down for the season with rest and anti-inflammatory medication given. By spring training the pitcher was fine. A repeat nerve conduction test was not done, at the pitcher's request. The pitcher started 29 games in the 2005 season with an ERA of 3.90 and a record of 7–9 losses. In 2006 he improved to 16–9.

Is the last pitcher mentioned in the article Brad Penny? Is the first pitcher mentioned Chris Carpenter? Draw your own conclusions.

Chapter 2

Blood Vessel Injuries Including Blood Clots of Shoulder Area

The shoulder has structures other than the muscles, tendons, bones, ligaments, and labrum. There are blood vessels and nerves that run through it from the heart and spinal column respectively. A rare injury to the shoulder happens to the blood vessels that move from the body to the arm (the subclavian and axillary arteries and veins). The vein or artery can develop blood clots from compression damage to the vessels through the repetitious and often violent movements involved in throwing a baseball.

The arteries and veins travel through a small hole in the shoulder to get to the arm as they travel to and from the heart. (Arteries carry blood from the heart to the arm, and veins carry blood from the arm back to the heart.) The vessels travel through what is called the thoracic outlet. The outlet has three sides: the scapula, clavicle and first thoracic rib. Of these the clavicle (or collar bone) and the first rib are the most important.

The subclavian artery runs right over the top of the first thoracic rib. In certain individuals, because of their unique anatomy, there can be (cocking, phase-abducted and externally rotated) compression of the arteries, veins, and nerves as they travel through the thoracic outlet during the throwing motion.[1] This compression, partly from the torque exerted by the humerus, occurs every time the pitcher cocks his arm and throws the ball, especially with the effort professional baseball players use to throw the baseball. Individuals may have varying degrees of compression present with movement of the arm, some worse than others. No study, as of yet, has directly linked the degree of compression with a prediction of future damage. Logic would indicate that with more severe compression while throwing, more damage should result. This just hasn't been proven.[2]

Also, logically over time (overuse) compression leads to damage to the veins and arteries which can lead to clots. In the case of arteries, damage can also manifest in what is called an aneurysm (both an abnormal weakening and bulging in the artery). Blood clots and aneurysms are serious matters. Blood clots in veins can lead to the complication of a pulmonary embolus, a life-threatening event. Blood clots in arteries can impair circulation to the arms, and if on the right side of the body can lead to a stroke.

Clots in the main artery usually cause a "dead arm" feeling, and there can be coldness in the arm, decreased pulses noted at the wrist, weakness, and occasionally numbness. Because blood is not flowing to the arm as needed, the arm may fatigue earlier than it normally would. Clots in the vein can give rise to swelling in the arm. The blood is not returning from the arm to the heart as well as it should because of the blockage.

A subclavian/axillary vein clot in the shoulder is called effort thrombosis and PSS — Paget Schroetter Syndrome.[3] It is treated acutely with a clot buster (urokinase, streptokinase, or the expensive tPA) instilled into the vein through a catheter. This is followed by a blood thinner that is administered in intra-venous fluid. If there is narrowing of the vein, a balloon at the end of a catheter is inflated to widen the vein. If the narrowing can't be maintained open, a small stent, which holds open the narrowing, is inserted.

Venous thrombosis, or clots of the upper extremity, are supposed to be more common in the throwing athlete than arterial clots.[4] Yet research done for this book found only two clear-cut cases of venous thrombosis in specific major league pitchers — Aaron Cook of the Colorado Rockies (2004) and Jeremy Bonderman of the Detroit Tigers (2008). Research revealed several major league pitchers stricken with arterial thrombosis (see text to follow). Based on this information it would appear anecdotally that upper extremity arterial clots are more common in throwing athletes (pitchers) than venous clots. In arterial and venous clots, if there is an anatomic problem causing compression of a blood vessel (e.g., a thoracic outlet narrowing), this needs to be addressed with surgery to relieve the compression.

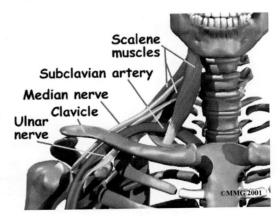

Figure indicating structures of thoracic outlet, mainly clavicle (collar bone), first thoracic rib, and scalene muscles. Structures, blood vessels and nerves pass between scalene muscles and the clavicle and first rib. Conservative treatment is recommended first, but sometimes the first rib needs to be removed to widen the opening. Sometimes the scalene muscles are cut if compression is caused there. The clavicle cannot be removed without significant impairment of shoulder function (used by permission of Medical Multimedia Group LLC).

Research revealed no cases of a pitcher choosing to retire instead of having surgery to correct the blood vessel compression. Why? This could be because of the considerable financial gain pitchers get from pitching at the major league level. For others it may simply be reluctance to give up their life profession and to move onto other goals. Pitching in the major leagues is often part of the competitive spirit they possess, and they are unwilling to give that up. Lastly, pitchers develop friends (teammates) and are reluctant to deal with this loss. This may not be as important as it has been in the past because of free agency. Players just don't develop ties to particular teams as much as players did before free agency.

Some people are born with an extra rib called a cervical rib, and it must be removed if it is causing problems. This condition is very rare. Where there is not a cervical rib noted, and the problem is thoracic outlet compression, the upper first thoracic rib on the affected side is often surgically removed to make more room for the vessels and nerves. The upper border of the thoracic outlet, the clavicle, cannot be removed as this would present significant impairment in the functioning of the shoulder. If muscles in the neck (scalene muscles) are compressing the vein or artery, these less essential muscles sometimes can be cut in half. More rarely, compression of an artery by the pectoralis minor muscle (upper chest) indicates surgery to make more room. Not everyone needs these types of surgeries, especially if thoracic outlet compression is not noted or if compression is only mild in nature. Some patients with a mild anatomic problem can get by with taking a blood thinner on a regular basis, getting surgery only if the problem becomes recurrent or severe.[5]

Artery blood clots, like venous clots, can be treated with a blood thinner (streptokinase, urokinase, or tPA) instilled into the artery by a catheter in the blood vessel. If this is not helpful and the artery is severely occluded, cutting down circulation to the arm, the obstructed artery may need the clot surgically removed and the artery bypassed by a graft. If there is damage to the artery (such as an aneurysm), this is also an indication for resection of the damaged artery and a bypass graft. The blood vessels in the arm, because of the high mobility of arm and narrow lumen (when compared to the arteries in the legs) cannot be bypassed by a *synthetic* graft (tube), but must be bypassed with a vein or artery taken from another site in the patient's body (called an autograph).

Vein Problems in the Shoulder

AARON COOK

As previously stated, only two clear-cut cases of venous upper extremity blood clots in a major league pitcher were found. Aaron Cook of the Colorado

Rockies was one of these. Keep in mind that veins carry blood to the heart and lungs, and arteries carry blood away from the heart. Because of the risk of a pulmonary (lung) embolus, as in Aaron Cook's case, venous clots have more serious ramifications than artery clots. True artery clots can lead to a stroke, a bad outcome, but clots to the lungs carry an even higher risk of death.

Aaron Cook has been in the Colorado Rockies organization his entire career. He was drafted in the second round of the 1997 amateur draft. He made his major league debut in 2002. His statistics are not outstanding. He pitched in 2002 and 2003 as a part-time starter/reliever. His 2003 ERA of 6.02 with four wins and six losses in 43 appearances and 16 starts was nothing to write home about. In 2004 he started off better. As of August 7 he was 6–4 with an ERA of 4.28 in 16 starts, when difficulties developed.

In his start on August 7 he experienced problems. Just before the game, while warming up, he experienced dizziness. At the start of the game his fastball, which was usually noted to be 95 mph, was only 87 mph. Soon he began to experience shortness of breath and continued dizziness. After only 30 pitches and after allowing a single to the Cincinnati leadoff batter, Ryan Freel, in the third inning, he was taken out of the game because of the shortness of breath.

Rockies team physician Dr. Allen Schreiber, in conjunction with Rockies trainer Tom Probst, insisted Cook be taken to Rose Medical Center in Denver just after the game as a precaution. At two o'clock the next morning Cook learned he had a pulmonary embolus in both lungs. He was hospitalized from August 7 until August 17, treated with blood thinners and oxygen.[6]

In retrospect, Cook had had some shortness of breath between his August 7 start and his previous start on August 1 in Arizona, but he had attributed the symptoms to the change in altitude.

The next step after treatment for Cook's pulmonary embolus was to determine the origin. It was found to be a vein in his right shoulder that had compression from thoracic outlet syndrome. On September 10, 2004, he underwent surgery in St. Louis to remove the first thoracic rib on the right side.[7]

When blood flow did not return to normal, he underwent a second surgery on December 27, 2004, to address that though the specific surgery is not known.[8] He could have had a balloon angioplasty where a balloon at the end of a catheter is inserted into the vein and then inflated to widen the lumen. He could have had a stent put in the vein via the catheter. (A stent is a device inserted into the vein to hold it open. It is left in place after the catheter in the vein is removed). Or he could have had the diseased portion of the vein excised and a graft from some other vein put in its place. No newspaper articles on the specifics of the second surgery were found, and no medical research articles were found discussing the second surgery that matched Cook's age or history.

Aaron Cook continued on blood thinners for at least six months after his pulmonary embolus. That is standard of care for such an event. He didn't make a pitching start until a minor-league game for the Rockies' Tri-City affiliate on June 26, 2005. This followed extended spring training. He finally started a major league game the end of July 2005. He has not been noted to have any problems with blood clots since.[9]

JEREMY BONDERMAN

Jeremy Bonderman suffered a clot in his axillary vein in June 2008. He was only 25 and already had five complete seasons in the majors, averaging 30 starts per season with 56 victories. Detroit felt so positive about the young pitcher's future that they signed him to a four-year, $38 million contract prior to the 2007 season.[10]

Bonderman did not pitch in 2008 after the June 1 game in Seattle. He had gone seven innings with no decision in a 7–5 Detroit victory. On Friday, June 6, he told Detroit Tigers trainer Kevin Rand that he didn't feel right. His pitching arm felt heavy, and on examination there was swelling under his armpit.[11]

He was sent immediately to Detroit Medical Center, where he was admitted to the Intensive Care unit. He underwent thrombolysis of the clot in his right axillary vein and a balloon angioplasty to open up the vein to get better circulation. He was discharged the next day.[12]

Bonderman was found to have thoracic outlet syndrome and had surgery on June 30 performed by Dr. Greg Pearl in Dallas, Texas. Bonderman had the first rib removed on the right side and had a bypass of the damaged vein in the shoulder.[13]

Bonderman had three wins and four losses in 12 starts at the time he went on the DL in June. He did not pitch another major league game in 2008.

In 2009, Bonderman continued to have issues with his throwing shoulder. His recovery from thoracic outlet surgery had progressed slower than expected. He lost velocity on his fastball and had issues with shoulder weakness and inflammation despite ongoing rehabilitation. He missed most of 2009, pitching only eight games at the major league level, only one of those a starting assignment, with a high ERA of 8.71. In 2010 Bonderman went 8–10 with a high ERA of 5.53.[14] Bonderman has not pitched at the major league level since 2010.

Artery Circulation Problems and Clots

J. R. RICHARD

The most famous case of a major league baseball pitcher with an arterial blood clot is J. R. Richard of the Houston Astros. His case was discussed in detail in Harold Klawans' book, *Why Michael Couldn't Hit and Other Tales of the Neurology of Sports*.[15] A medical journal, the *American Journal of Roentgenology*, in 1986 presented a strikingly similar case of an unnamed major league pitcher.[16] The history presented in the article followed Klawans' book presentation very closely.

In 1980, J. R. Richard was one of the best pitchers in baseball, with a fastball approaching 100 mph. In 1979 he finished third in the Cy Young Award voting with a National league-leading ERA (2.71), 18 wins and 13 losses, and a league-leading 313 strikeouts. He had also struck out over 300 batters in 1978.

He started the season of 1980 with 10 wins and 4 losses and was named starting pitcher for the National League in the All-star Game. He had an ERA of 1.90. Well before the All-Star Game, however, he began to complain of the sensation of a "dead arm," citing discomfort in his shoulder and forearm starting around the fifth or sixth inning of each game. In 1979 he had completed 19 of

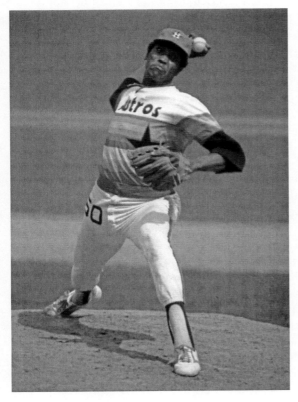

his 38 starts. In 1980, his endurance was definitely reduced, as he completed only four out of 17 starts. In a game just after the All-Star break (July 14), he was pitching against the Atlanta Braves when he had to depart in only the fourth inning, noting that his arm felt dead. In addition, he had numbness in the first three digits of his right hand and could not grasp the baseball well. He simply could not continue to pitch. He was placed on the disabled list. Nine days later he checked into Methodist Hospital in Houston for testing. On July 25 an angiogram was done which revealed a complete obstruction (blood clot) in the

J. R. Richard pitching for the Houston Astros in 1979 (National Baseball Hall of Fame Library, Cooperstown, New York).

right subclavian artery.[17] (An angiogram is an x-ray procedure in which pictures are taken after dye is injected into the artery.)

It is difficult to exactly say what plan of treatment was begun at this time. One would think that some specific treatment, be it surgery or a clot-buster IV drug, would have been initiated. Maybe the angiogram showed sufficient circulation around the clot that there wasn't much concern. There is no mention of any attempt to instill a blood thinner into the artery. No information exists as to whether a bypass was considered. It would appear the decision was made just to wait and see.

Five days later, on July 30, Richard's condition took a turn for the worse. He had some manipulation done that morning by his chiropractor.[18] He then went to the ballpark, following his normal routine. As he was taking some warm-up tosses before a game, his symptoms suddenly became much worse. He first developed a headache which progressed to visual problems and paralysis of the left side. Richard had had a stroke. He was taken to the hospital and had another angiogram done. The test revealed that his previous clot had worsened and now involved the more proximal innominate artery (an artery that gives rise to the right common carotid artery in the neck, the artery that goes to his brain) and subclavian artery.[19] Only now did J. R. Richard have emergency surgery to remove the clot from the arm and neck arteries to save his life. A large amount of clot was removed from the innominate and subclavian arteries, and a small amount from the proximal segment of the right common carotid.

A CT scan in September of 1980 revealed infarcts in right basal ganglia, right occipital lobe, and right cerebellar hemisphere, confirming that Richard had had a stroke.[20] By then he was walking with only minimal difficulty, with mild right upper extremity and left facial weakness. A significant finding at the time was left visual inattentiveness (he had trouble paying attention to objects in his left visual field). (Note that strokes on the right side of the brain affect the left side of the body, because in the brainstem, the nerves of the right side of the brain cross over to the left side.)

In early October of 1980, his chances for rehabilitation and a return to baseball were assessed. He had a repeat arteriogram which still showed poor circulation of the subclavian artery. Noted was collateral blood to his arm flowing around this subclavian blockage. Films of the contrast dye returning to the heart from the arm showed narrowing of the venous flow at the first thoracic rib (he had thoracic outlet syndrome with narrowing in the opening at the first thoracic rib). Because of angiogram findings, a bypass of the subclavian artery to the brachial artery (closer to the arm) was thought necessary. Because of his 6-foot, 8-inch height, an adequate bypass was thought difficult. Thus a graft from the external iliac arteries from his lower abdomen (this provides blood to his thighs) was used to bypass the blockage in his arm. The arteries from his lower abdomen were replaced with synthetic grafts.

On October 14, 1980, the surgery to bypass Richard's blocked arm artery was done. At the same time, because he was assessed to have thoracic outlet syndrome, his first thoracic rib on the right side was removed, the scalene muscles in his right lower neck were cut, and he had an upper thoracic sympathectomy done.[21]

By January of 1981, Richard had almost complete strength back, but persisted in having a left eye visual perception defect from the stroke. He continued his rehabilitation in 1981 and even pitched batting practice near the end of the year. He went to spring training with the Astros in 1982 and pitched minor league ball. He did well at the Double-A minor league level, but had control problems at the Triple-A level. He did not pitch in the major leagues in 1982.

During the off-season of 1982–1983, as he continued his rehab, Richard suffered a setback. He developed a clot in the left iliac synthetic graft.[22] This blockage had to be bypassed with yet another synthetic graft. This set Richard back on his rehab until June of 1983. When his contract expired with the Astros in 1984, he was put on waivers, giving him his release. When no other teams gave him a contract, he retired from baseball. He did not pitch in the major leagues after his stroke in 1980. This was a very sad end to a promising career, a career cut short by thoracic outlet syndrome, by clots in an artery in his arm, and by a stroke he developed as a result of his artery clots.

WHITEY FORD

Another pitcher having blood clots in the subclavian/brachial artery in his shoulder was Whitey Ford of the Yankees. As he is left-handed, it is not surprising that his blood clots were in his left shoulder from wear and tear to the blood vessel caused by the pitching motion of the dominant arm.

An article by Tullos, et al. in *Clinical Orthopedics* in 1972 is strikingly similar to the sequence of events in Whitey Ford's case as presented in *Whitey Ford*, by Miles Coverdale, Jr.,[23] so the article is probably about Ford.

At age 36 Whitey Ford was admitted to a hospital on November 8, 1964, for evaluation of a two-year history of easy fatigability of his left arm. His symptoms had taken a turn for the worse three weeks prior to admission. He reported severe tiring and muscle aches while pitching in first game of the 1964 World Series (Yankees vs. Cardinals).[24]

On his initial exam, he had an unobtainable blood pressure in his left arm. He had a pulse above the clavicle of his left shoulder but not below the clavicle. The fingers on his left hand were cool and moist, especially when compared to the fingers on his right hand. An arteriogram revealed complete blockage of the left axillary artery just below (distal) the pectoralis minor muscle. The arteriogram revealed some circulation in smaller blood vessels around this blockage.

Noted vascular surgeon Dr. Denton Cooley was seeing the patient. He recommended a vein graft (a vein taken from his leg) to bypass this blockage. An alternative plan of transthoracic cervical dorsal sympathectomy was presented. Cutting the sympathetic ganglion near the left upper thoracic spine would cause dilation and increased blood flow around the blockage (loss of blood vessel-constricting sympathetic input). This latter plan was chosen. On November 9, 1964, the sympathetic ganglion was cut.[25]

In 1965 Whitey Ford again had a good season, though not up to his usual standards. Ford finished with a 16–13 record and was able to pitch 244⅓ innings. He pitched without difficulty on warm days but experienced fatigue and other symptoms related to a lack of blood to his arm on cold days and night games.[26]

In 1966, he pitched more in relief with only nine starts. He had to be readmitted for evaluation on August 4. His symptoms had worsened. He was once again experiencing fatigue, tiredness, and cramping in his left arm and hand.

A subclavian arteriogram (also called an angiogram) revealed a continued obstruction of his axillary artery. More aggressive therapy in the form of a saphenous vein bypass was now thought to be necessary (taking a vein from the leg to bypass the obstruction). This was performed on August 25, 1966. On August 31, the date of his discharge, he was noted with excellent circulation in his left arm.[27]

He was able to pitch in 1967, starting seven games before retiring. He had an ERA of 1.64 for 1967 when he retired. His retirement was not due to any pre-existing circulatory problem. The circulation in his arm had improved considerably. In 1967, he was having trouble with his elbow. In his last two starts, he lasted only three innings and one inning, respectively, each time exiting because of elbow pain.

Dr. Sidney Gaynor, long-time team physician for the New York Yankees, determined that Ford had a bone spur in his elbow. Surgery was recommended. Ford declined at age 38. He stated, "I won't have another operation. If I were 33 or 34 years old, I definitely would, and try again. But not now."[28] Whitey Ford, with his career record of 236 wins and 106 losses, retired on May 30, 1967. He was elected to the Hall of Fame in 1974.

DENNIS "OIL CAN" BOYD

Right-hander Dennis "Oil Can" Boyd suffered arterial blood clots in his right shoulder. Boyd, from Meridian, Mississippi, is the son of former Negro leagues star Willie James Boyd. He was drafted by the Boston Red Sox in the 16th round of the 1980 amateur draft. He managed to progress quickly through the Red Sox farm system, arriving at the major league level in 1982. From 1984 to 1986 he averaged 30 starts a year and had 12, 15, and 16 wins respectively, helping the Red Sox to the World Series in 1986. He came down with a shoulder injury in 1987, spending much of his time on the DL until he ultimately had arthroscopic surgery in August for a slightly torn ligament pressing on a tendon. No other specifics concerning the particular surgery have been found.[29]

The problems with his clots in his right shoulder didn't start until 1988, and it appears to be Boyd's case that is discussed in a scientific article, "Axillary Arterial Compression and Thrombosis in Throwing Athletes," in the *Journal of Vascular Surgery* in 1990.[30] From the description of the player in the article, his course of treatment, and one of the authors named, Dr. Arthur Pappas (Boston Red Sox team physician), there is a high probability the article is about Boyd.

The article identifies three places where compression of the axillary/brachial artery can occur: the thoracic outlet, the pectoralis minor muscle, and the head of the humerus. The latter would occur when Boyd pulled back his arm in the cocked position, ready to throw. The article identified the player as having two types of compression, by the thoracic outlet and the head of the humerus bone. Yet Boyd never received a strong recommendation that thoracic outlet surgery would be helpful, and he received several opinions from well-known circulation specialists who would be familiar with that problem.[31]

Thus it would appear that the compression of the artery by the humeral head during Boyd's overhand pitching motion was the single most important factor leading to the blood clots.

Another possible cause of arterial clots is an aneurysm of the artery (an abnormal bulge in an artery — see later discussion). An arteriogram done after Boyd's clot had been dissolved by the enzyme urokinase revealed no structural abnormalities in his shoulder arteries and no evidence of an aneurysm.

Oil Can Boyd first experienced problems with a blood clot near the end of July 1988. Following urokinase treatment to dissolve the clot, he was started on aspirin three times a day plus the medicine dipyrimdole daily (a blood vessel dilator). Boyd was on the DL from July 29 until August 19, when it was deemed safe for him to resume pitching.[32]

During his second start for Boston after returning from the DL, Boyd had a recurrence of the clot and went back on the disabled list on August 27, missing the rest of the season.[33]

After the second clot was lysed Boyd received a different medication; he was treated with a three-month course of coumadin, an oral blood thinner, after which this medicine was gradually tapered off with decreasing dosage over several weeks. Finally it was stopped.

There was some controversy as to how to treat Boyd's clot problems after the coumadin was stopped. It was deemed too dangerous for Boyd to take while he actively pitched. The medicine carried the risk of external or internal bleeding if Boyd should sustain any traumatic injury. To continue on coumadin, Boyd would have to stop pitching, an unacceptable option.

Boyd did well until he suffered yet another setback in 1989. No medication is mentioned, but he probably was taking daily aspirin when he had yet another clot in his right shoulder immediately after his start on May 1. He was on the DL once again starting May 5. He received blood thinner medicine to dissolve the clot.

Then came the question of what to do next. Surgery was considered. Boyd saw at least seven specialists, the top vascular surgeons in the country. What were their recommendations?

One recommendation: no surgery, a blood thinner, and calcium heparin injected subcutaneously three or four times during the 36 hours after each of Boyd's starts. This he agreed to do.[34]

A second recommendation: Boston Red Sox team physician Dr. Pappas recommended that Boyd throw sidearm to lessen the compression caused by the head of the humerus bone against the artery in Boyd's shoulder. But when Boyd started throwing again, after his third trip to the DL for clots, he apparently had paid little attention to this recommendation as he was once again throwing overhand. There is no indication he ever took Dr. Pappas' advice on this matter.[35]

After becoming a free agent following the 1989 season, Boyd pitched for Montreal in 1990 and for Montreal and Texas in 1991. He received no major league contracts after that. After 1991 he pitched in the minor leagues, Mexico, and Puerto Rico.

After being on the DL from May till August of 1989, Boyd didn't experience any more clots in his shoulder until late July 1994, while pitching for the Sioux City Explorers of the Class A Northern League. He admitted he was no longer taking the subcutaneous heparin injections after his starts. He reported he took the heparin for three years after 1989, and then quit. It didn't take much to convince him to restart the medication with the fourth recurrent clot. No sources were found that indicated Boyd ever had any clots after 1994.[36]

Oil Can Boyd's career was not spectacular. In his ten-year major league career his record was 78–77 with an ERA of 4.04. Yet his career does demonstrate a clear point: The pitching motion can result in clots in the arteries in the shoulder due to repetitive compression of the arteries by movement of the head of the humerus bone. Boyd is one of the few pitchers with arterial or venous clots who did not require surgery to correct an anatomic problem that contributed to the formation of these blood clots.

KIP WELLS

Kip Wells has always been described as having great stuff, but has never lived up to this billing. The former first round pick (16th overall) of the Chicago

White Sox in the 1998, he has bounced from team to team, with a lifetime record of 67–99.

Wells' circulation problems started in 2006. He initially complained of arm fatigue in the February. He was noted to have a decreased pulse in his right pitching arm. Dr. Robert Thompson, a vascular surgeon at Washington University in St. Louis, did an angiogram. He detected a completely blocked artery in Wells' right shoulder. There was some concern that Wells might need the first rib removed from the right side of his chest due to possible thoracic outlet syndrome, but that was not found. A replacement of the artery in his armpit using a vein graft from his leg resolved the blockage problem. It would appear the replacement was done because thrombolytic therapy was not successful in dissolving the artery clot. No articles indicating Wells had an aneurysm in this blocked artery were found. An aneurysm would also indicate a need for a graft replacement.[37]

Wells had no further problems with his right arm until May 2008, when he experienced numbness in his fingers on his right hand. Another arteriogram was done and clots were found, though only in Wells' right hand. Surgery to remove the clots was performed once again by Dr. Thompson. No problems with his previous vein graft were mentioned.[38]

Wells was on the DL in 2008 from April 9 to July 20. When he finally pitched, he pitched ineffectively. This led to his release by the Colorado Rockies in August 2008. He was picked up by the Kansas City Royals, for whom he also pitched ineffectively. They released him on October 24, 2008. He pitched for Washington and Cincinnati in 2009, but has not pitched at the major league level since then.[39]

Artery Circulation Problems and Aneurysms

ANEURYSM

David Cone

Compression of the arteries of the shoulder can also lead to damage to the arteries and formation of an aneurysm (bulge in the artery), as illustrated in the case of David Cone. An article in the *Journal of Vascular Surgery* in 1998 called "Aneurysms of the mid axillary artery in major league pitchers: A report of two cases" presents a case very similar to David Cone's aneurysm history,[40] even though the pitcher's name is not mentioned.

David Cone had a very good 17-year pitching career in the major leagues. He won 194 games against 126 losses, a .606 winning percentage. His career ERA was a very respectable 3.46 and he recorded 2,668 strikeouts in 2,898⅔ innings. He won a Cy Young Award in 1994, was an All-Star five times and pitched a perfect game on July 18, 1999, for the New York Yankees against the Montreal Expos. He also struck out 19 batters in one game on October 6, 1991.

His career almost ended in 1996. He had started off the year in fine fashion and had a 4–1 record with a league-leading 2.03 after his start on May 2. Then he began to notice numbness in his right hand, cyanosis of his fingers (bluish discoloration), and decreased temperature in his fingers. His symptoms were particularly intense after pitching and especially in cold weather. Prior to this he had a history of pain in his shoulder and arm.

On physical exam, all his palpable pulses were normal. A chest x-ray didn't reveal a cervical rib (an uncommon extra rib problem that can appear at birth and cause problems later in life). Punctuate bruising lesions of his second, third, and fourth fingers were noted. An arteriogram revealed evidence of incomplete filling of some of the small arteries of his hand, evidence of occlusion

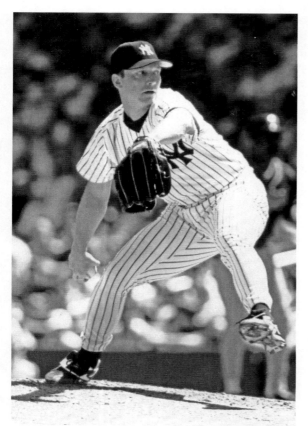

(possibly from small emboli that were being released from somewhere). On the arteriogram there was an aneurysm noted of the right axillary, anterior circumflex artery, and posterior circumflex artery (circumflex arteries go around the upper part of the humerus). The conclusion at the time: David Cone had an aneurysm which was causing small clots to form which were moving downstream to the digits of his hand, causing occlusion of the small blood vessels in the hand and impairing circulation to his fingers.[41]

Intra-arterial urokinase improved color and temperature of his fingers by dissolving many of the clots present in his hands. Something had to done about the source of the clots (the aneurysm). Sur-

David Cone, New York Yankees, pitching in 1996 (National Baseball Hall of Fame Library, Cooperstown, New York).

gery was performed on the aneurysm on May 10, 1996. The aneurysm was surgically removed and replaced by a graft from the expendable saphenous vein of his left thigh.[42] (There is considerable circulation in the thigh that goes around this large vein.)

Once David Cone's surgery was done, recovery and rehabilitation followed. He started range of motion exercises at six weeks, soft tossing of the baseball at eight weeks, and throwing from the mound at 12 weeks after surgery. He was able to return to pitching in the major leagues in September 1996. His return was successful, and in his first game four months after his surgery, he pitched seven innings of no-hit ball. Unfortunately, the reliever, Mariano Rivera, gave up a single that broke up the no-hitter. Cone would have pitched the eighth and ninth innings except he was on a pitch count restriction.[43]

Five and one-half months after his surgery Cone pitched Game 3 of the 1996 World Series for the Yankees, in which he was the winning pitcher (the Yankees won that World Series four games to two over the Atlanta Braves). The next year, David Cone won 12 games and lost six in 29 starts, and pitched 195 innings. He went on to pitch six more years after his aneurysm surgery, finally retiring in 2003 because of chronic hip problems. It would have to be said that his aneurysm surgery in 1996 was a success.

Kenny Rogers

Kenny Rogers, a left-hander, had a long career spanning 20 years with 219 wins against 156 losses. His lifetime ERA wasn't fantastic at 4.27, he never won 20 games in any single season, and he never won a Cy Young Award, but most would say he had a long, successful career.

Kenny Rogers had circulation problems in his left shoulder twice. The first episode happened in 2001. Rogers, age 36 at the time, was evaluated for complaints of tingling and numbness in his left arm in July. He had been ineffective with a record of 2–4 and an ERA of 6.98 after June 1. There is no indication he had a complete blockage of the artery in his left shoulder, but he was diagnosed as having thoracic outlet syndrome causing compression of the axillary artery. This needed to be fixed. He had surgery to remove his first rib and clean up some scar tissue on July 30, 2001, performed by Dr. Gregory Pearl, a vascular surgeon at Baylor University in Dallas, Texas. Rogers missed the rest of the 2001 season, but came back to record five straight winning seasons.[44]

During spring training with the Detroit Tigers in 2007, Rogers began experiencing problems with arm fatigue and numbness. He was found to have a clot in his axillary and brachial arteries (in the left shoulder). Dr. Pearl determined that Rogers once again needed surgery. This time Rogers was found to have an aneurysm leading to a blood clot and blockage. This was the same artery (axillary) that had bothered Rogers in 2001. This aneurysm and clot was removed and replaced (bypassed) by a vein graft taken from Rogers' thigh on

March 30, 2007. He was out three months, finally pitching on June 22, throwing six shutout innings against Atlanta to become the winning pitcher.[45]

Rogers, at age 43, pitched with mixed results for the Detroit Tigers in 2008 (9–13 with a high ERA of 5.70) before retiring after the season.

Roberto Hernandez

Roberto Hernandez's aneurysm problems predated those of both Kenny Rogers and David Cone. His problems began at age 26 while pitching in his rookie year for the Chicago White Sox. The surgery he had to correct the problem was a success, as he went on to pitch 17 seasons as a middle relief and a closer. He recorded 326 career saves, retiring at age 42 in 2007. In six years he had more than 30 saves and in 1999 for the Tampa Bay Devil Rays he had a career-high 43 saves, all after his surgery in 1991 for an aneurysm.

Hernandez noted soreness and numbness in his throwing (right) hand at the beginning of spring training in 1991. It was cooler than normal in Florida that March, but once the cool spell went away, Hernandez's soreness also went away.

Hernandez did not make the team out of spring training and was sent back to the minor leagues. In cooler weather he again began to have problems. Often he had a pale discoloration in his middle two fingers. During one game in Edmonton, Alberta, his thumb "turned violet, close to purple."[46]

After complaining for some time, he was evaluated by a vascular surgeon at the University of British Columbia Hospital and diagnosed as having blood clots in his hand. From there Hernandez was referred to a vascular surgeon in Chicago, Dr. James Yao. He had surgery on June 4, 1991.

The surgery was not without complications. As is typical in these cases, a vein from the leg was grafted into the place where the aneurysm was. The aneurysm was removed. Apparently there were bleeding complications from the surgery, and Hernandez had to have a second operation on June 5. The first surgery took ten and one-half hours and the second operation took five hours.

Initially there was doubt Hernandez would ever pitch again. But three weeks after his procedure he was given the green light to resume training. He started playing catch around the All-Star Game. Two weeks later he pitched his first minor league game. He pitched several games at Double A, and then was called up to the White Sox on August 29, less than three months after his major surgery.

His final major league stats in 1991 were not good; he pitched in nine games with three starts and an inflated ERA of 7.80. But from then on his major league career took off. In 1992 he pitched 43 games in relief for the White Sox, with 12 saves and an ERA of 1.65. The following year he had 38 saves for the White Sox in 70 games pitched.

OTHERS WITH ANEURYSMS

Other pitchers having aneurysms in the shoulders include Derek Wallace of the New York Mets in 1997, Felix Heredia of the Mets in 2005, and more recently Ian Kennedy of the New York Yankees in 2009. A 1997 article about Derek Wallace's aneurysm mentioned minor leaguers Ethan McEntire, Kevin Rodgers, and Steve Soderstrom as having had aneurysms.[47]

Derek Wallace

Expectations for Derek Wallace's baseball career were very high. He was the 11th overall pick in the 1992 amateur draft by the Chicago Cubs. After some minor setbacks, he ended up with the Mets in 1995. The 24-year-old rookie pitched in 19 games for the Mets in 1996 with 3 saves and an ERA of 4.01. There was some speculation that Wallace was the Mets' closer of the future, the likely successor to John Franco. This was not to be.[48]

In March 1997, Wallace was complaining of intermittent coldness in the two middle fingers of his pitching right hand. When the Mets staff learned he had had this problem off and on for three years, tests were quickly ordered. These tests revealed an aneurysm in his right shoulder which required surgery.

Thereafter Wallace never played for the Mets, though he did pitch in the minor leagues, mostly for the Mets' Triple-A affiliate, Norfolk. The Kansas City Royals obtained him in a trade in 1999 and he appeared in eight games in relief with a respectable 3.24 ERA. The following year he was cut in spring training by the Royals and optioned to Omaha, but decided to retire instead.[49]

He might have had some post-op complications after his aneurysm surgery. He was quoted as saying, "There was weakness in the back of the shoulder that led to bursitis. After the surgery, the muscles atrophied in the back." Maybe the muscle strength never came back completely.[50]

Felix Heredia

Felix Heredia, a left-hander, pitched ten seasons in the major leagues, starting his career at age 21. He was signed as a free agent originally by the Florida Marlins. He mainly pitched for the Florida Marlins (2½ seasons), Chicago Cubs (3½ seasons), and New York Yankees (1½ seasons). He pitched one season for Toronto and most of one season for Cincinnati. In his last season he pitched three games for the New York Mets. He started only two games in his major league career. Heredia mainly pitched in middle relief, though he did record six saves in his career.

His career can't be classified as outstanding as he posted a career record of only 28 wins and 19 losses with a fair ERA of 4.42.

In spring training of 2005, he complained of some numbness and coldness in his throwing hand. Apparently this was resolved, only to recur during the regular season on April 18. After throwing three pitches in one inning all the way to the backstop, two of which went over the head of batter Bobby Abreu, he was escorted off the field. Heredia admitted to having weakness in his thumb resulting in difficulty locating his pitches. Later on, Heredia admitted to having had numbness in his left hand off and on for over five years.[51]

Tests revealed an aneurysm in Heredia's shoulder for which he needed surgery. He never pitched in the major leagues again. During rehab after his surgery, he tested positive for steroids and faced a ten-game suspension at the beginning of the 2006 season. The Mets subsequently did not pick up his option. He pitched briefly for Cleveland's Triple-A Team in 2006 and briefly for Veracruz, Mexico, in 2009.[52]

Ian Kennedy

Ian Kennedy was chosen in the first round of the 2006 amateur draft by the New York Yankees out of the University of Southern California (21st overall pick). His history isn't typical for an aneurysm as he mainly experienced some numbness in his right hand during the four starts he made for the Yankees' Triple-A affiliate Scranton in early 2009. Initially it appeared he might have thoracic outlet syndrome, but in early May the aneurysm was found. He had surgery on May 12 by noted vascular surgeon Dr. George Todd, who had also done aneurysm surgery on David Cone.[53]

Kennedy made a nice comeback from the surgery and was called up by the Yankees in September after a successful rehab at Scranton. He was part of a three-way trade that sent him from the Yankees to the Arizona Diamondbacks in December 2009. In 2010 Kennedy pitched well for Arizona, starting 32 games and going 9–10 with a respectable 3.80 ERA for a team with a losing record. The 2011 season was far better. He went 21–4 with a 2.88 ERA, which helped the Diamondbacks get into the playoffs, and earned him fourth place in the 2011 Cy Young Award vote.

Rich DeLucia

In 1997 Anaheim Angels relief pitcher Rich DeLucia developed an aneurysm in his pitching shoulder. It occurred during the eighth year of his ten-year major league career (1990–1999), and he was having one of his better seasons. At the time he went on the DL he had a record of six wins with three losses, three saves, and an ERA of 2.41 in 29 appearances.

What were the presenting symptoms? During a game on July 10, DeLucia noticed coolness and numbness in the middle finger of his right hand. These are not symptoms to be taken lightly. Tests were done. An arteriogram done on July 18 at St. Joseph's Hospital in Orange, California, revealed an aneurysm in DeLucia's right shoulder.[54]

Three days later and following a second opinion, Delucia had surgery performed by Dr. James Yao at Northwestern University Medical Center in Chicago. The exact details of the surgery, other than noting that the aneurysm was removed, were not given. More than likely the diseased blood vessel segment (aneurysm) of the shoulder was removed and replaced by a vein from the lower leg.[55]

DeLucia did come back before the end of the 1997 season, though his results were not as good as he had before the surgery. He pitched 61 games for the Angels in 1998 but only six games for the Cleveland Indians in 1999. He pitched most of 1999, 2000, and 2001 in the minors, not pitching again at the major league level after 1999.

OTHERS

Research revealed no position players having aneurysms in their shoulders, the usual location of these dilated arteries. John Olerud had an aneurysm in his head, but that was not caused by baseball activity. Those types of aneurysms (bulging arteries) are usually congenital (called Berry aneurysms). One is born with it, and if lucky nothing ever happens. If unlucky, it ruptures.[56]

Chapter 3

Elbow Injuries

The elbow is just as important in throwing a baseball as the shoulder. The elbow is a unique joint, actually two joints in one. First, it is a hinge joint similar to the knee. The hinge extends and flexes the elbow joint. This is the humerus moving against the one of the bones in the forearm, the ulna bone. There is another joint where the other bone in the forearm, the radius, moves against the elbow. It rotates, thus the name radius (part of a circle).

The ulna-humerus joint is rigid, allowing only motions of flexion and extension. The radius-humerus joint allows for more flexible movement called supination-pronation (palm up–palm down).

When throwing a baseball, the shoulder and elbow pull the arm through the throwing motion, helped tremendously by the muscles in the lower extremities and back. The elbow remains pronated throughout much of the motion (palm pointed down). Initially, in what is called the cocked position, the elbow is at a right angle. As the arm moves through the throwing motion to release the ball, the elbow moves towards an almost completely extended, straight position.

The elbow, like the shoulder joint, is enclosed within a capsule (a flexible, fibrous material). The capsule has cells that line the inside of the joint and secrete slippery synovial fluid that lubricates the joint, allowing for free movement. In the elbow joint there are rigid ligaments, allowing only a certain amount of movement of the two joints. Side to side movement of the elbow is more restrictive than extension and flexion. It should be noted, though, that when the elbow reaches full extension the ligaments and bones put a quick halt to further extension. The ligaments are much more restrictive on movement of the elbow than the shoulder.

The elbow ligaments add a lot of stability to the throwing motion but many things that can go wrong in the elbow with repetitious hard throwing. One of the most common problems is damage to the medial ulnar collateral ligaments on the inside of the elbow (often abbreviated UCL). This ligament

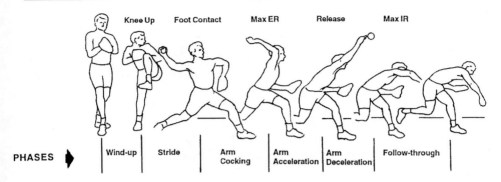

PHASES ▶ | Wind-up | Stride | Arm Cocking | Arm Acceleration | Arm Deceleration | Follow-through |

The six phases of the pitching motion are indicated. (This is a modification of an image appearing in Fleisig, et al., "Biomechanics of Overhand Throwing with Implications for Injuries," *Sports Medicine* 21, 6 (1996): 421–437, Fig. 1. Reproduced by the permission of the publisher, Wolters Kluwer, and the author.)

is literally responsible for pulling the forearm, hand, and baseball through the throwing motion initiated by the shoulder. The acceleration motion in pitching occurs in a very small amount of time, 0.05 seconds, exerting a tremendous amount of stress on the inner aspect of the elbow.

It is not difficult to see that this motion causes considerable strain on the elbow, causing possible damage to the medial ulnar collateral ligament.

Ligaments are very strong. But, as with the shoulder, stresses put on the elbow over a long period of time at excessive speed and force, stress these ligaments to their limit and they become damaged. Even though a large tear in the ligament may occur rather suddenly, and the pitcher may feel a sudden pop at the time of the tear, ultimately the tear would not happen if the ligaments hadn't been weakened over a long period of time by repetitive motion. The sudden (acute) tear of a ligament is classic, but it must be understood that many complete tears are gradual in onset, a small tear followed by another and yet another until the performance in the elbow is significantly impaired. At this point arthritis may form inside the elbow, with wearing down of the joint surface. Bone fragments float around inside the joint, and bone spurs may form near the joint line.

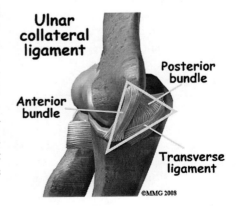

View of inside of right elbow with muscles, tendons, and blood vessels, and nerves not visualized. Tears with significant damage would mainly be through anterior bundle (ligament) and transverse ligament (used by permission of Medical Multimedia Group LLC).

It should be noted that in addition to damage to ligaments, the nerves, muscles, tendons, and bones can become damaged. The player can have ulnar nerve problems at the elbow, flexor muscle tears, stress fractures, and arthritis.

It should not be surprising — as hard and as often as baseball pitchers throw compared to other position players — that pitchers suffer by far more injuries to their medial collateral ligaments, nerves, muscles, tendons, and bones than any other position player.

Before there was a method to repair the UCL ligament, this was a career-ending injury. If you tear your medial ulnar collateral ligament and cannot throw effectively, speed and accuracy are impaired. There is also considerable pain. The elbow develops arthritis, and instability impairs function. The ulnar collateral ligament is important in many ways. If torn, it needs to be repaired for the player to continue to play baseball. The procedure to correct a tear of the medial collateral ligament is named after the first player to have a successful repair, Tommy John.

Previously, to repair the ulnar collateral ligament, the ligament was simply sewn together. This did not work very well, quite often because the ligament's connective tissue fibers were damaged throughout and the ligament had been stretched out of shape. Sewing the ligament back together simply didn't return normal function. The alternative procedure, replacement of the ligament with a tendon graft from some other part of the body, was introduced by Dr. Frank Jobe in 1974. Tommy John, the first pitcher to have the procedure done, had a graft of a relatively unimportant tendon from the wrist and forearm used to repair the injury. The tendon, called the palmaris longus tendon (tendons connect muscles to bone, whereas ligaments connect bone to bone, mostly around joints), attaches to the palm of the hand. This tendon simply tightens the skin of the palm during contraction, a process most individuals can function perfectly well without. The tendon is expendable. This is great to use, except for the small percentage of people born without the palmaris longus tendon and muscle. In their case a small part of the hamstring tendon (a large tendon belonging to the muscles in the back of the thigh that run to the back of the knee) is usually used instead.

The tendon of the palmaris longus, as previously stated, is removed from the wrist and forearm and used in the elbow. The tendon is often made into a "figure-of-eight" loop attached through holes drilled in the bones of the ulna and the humerus with the tendon placed in the same anatomic position as the torn ulnar collateral ligaments (see illustration on page 61). In the alternate "docking technique" the tendon is looped in the ulna bone as in the figure-of-eight technique, but ends of the tendon are threaded (not looped) through and then anchored at the ends of the longitudinal holes in the humerus bone.

The graft is a tendon, not a ligament. The body has to convert the weaker tendon into the stronger ligament. This takes time and is the main reason that a return to pitching at the major league level takes a long time, a year or longer.

Typically, after surgery, the elbow is immobilized in a hard cast for a week. Normal activities are resumed by the second or third week. Light tossing of the baseball doesn't begin till four to six months. During rehab of the elbow, strengthening of the shoulder needs to occur; otherwise when the elbow is ready, the shoulder won't be ready, and the shoulder will become damaged, causing yet another problem.

Tommy John

Tommy John was the first major league player to have elbow ligament replacement surgery.

It is significant to note how Tommy John's performance actually improved after his elbow injury and subsequent elbow replacement procedure. John's major league pitching career was exceedingly long compared to most major league pitchers lasting 26 years, until age 46. He started out with the Cleveland

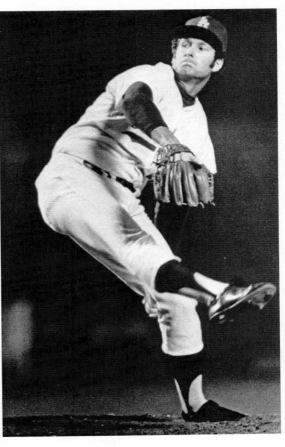

Figure-of-eight technique

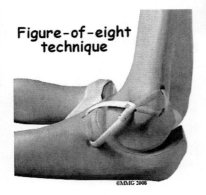

Above: Left-hander Tommy John of the Los Angeles Dodgers throwing a pitch, date unknown (National Baseball Hall of Fame Library, Cooperstown, New York). *Left:* Illustration shows one very common method of Tommy John surgery showing tendon placed in "figure-of-eight fashion" through holes drilling in adjacent bones of injured elbow. Damaged ligaments are not seen. Not pictured is the alternative "docking technique" for doing Tommy John surgery (used by permission of Medical MultiMedia Group).

Indians before moving onto the Chicago White Sox, Los Angeles Dodgers, New York Yankees, California Angels, Oakland A's, and then back to the Yankees. His lifetime record was 288 wins and 231 losses. The number of wins sounds impressive until you realize it was spread out over 26 years and only comes out to 11 wins per season. Tommy John did have three 20-win seasons, but only four times was he an All-Star, and he never won a Cy Young Award (he finished second in the balloting twice). He is not in the Baseball Hall of Fame.

His claim to fame is the elbow replacement surgery that has been named for him — "Tommy John surgery." His book, *TJ: My Twenty-Six Years in Baseball*, chronicles his elbow problems well, both before and after his famous surgery.[1]

John's elbow problems started in 1972 while pitching for the Los Angeles Dodgers. He does not note a particular date for onset of the elbow soreness he suffered; he simply noted difficulty for most of the 1972 season. X-rays obtained early in 1972 by Dr. Frank Jobe showed a couple of floating bone fragments within the elbow joint. As surgery to remove the fragments would have ended John's season, conservative non-surgical treatment was tried which included frequent cortisone shots, sometimes as often as every five days.

John's elbow problems took a turn for the worse on September 23, 1972. Sliding into home plate, attempting to score from second base on a single, he jammed his elbow, making it much worse. On x-ray the fragments appeared to have shifted from their previous position to a more compromising position. This increased John's soreness and pain significantly. After this injury, John couldn't throw the baseball with much velocity and couldn't locate his pitches. With the 1972 baseball season almost over, the decision to have surgery to remove the bone fragments was a fairly easy one to make.

John recovered well by 1973, and that year finished with 16 wins and seven losses. The 1974 season started well, and at one point just before the All-Star Game he led the league in wins with 13 and had only three losses. Despite this fine record, John was not named to the All-Star squad.

Then came "The Pitch."[2] It was thrown on July 17, 1974, John's last start before the All-Star break. In the third inning, he was leading 4–0 against the Montreal Expos and was well on his way to victory number 14. The first two runners got on via a single and a walk. Up came Montreal's Hal Breeden. John was hoping his best pitch, a sinking fastball, would result in a double play, blunting the Expos' threat. In John's autobiography he expressed what happened that July 17 well.

> My first pitch to Breeden was ... strange. As I came forward and released the ball, I felt a kind of nothingness, as if my arm weren't there, then I heard a "pop" from inside my arm, and the ball just blooped up to the plate.
> I didn't feel soreness or pain at this point, but just the strange sensation that my arm wasn't there. It was the oddest thing I'd ever felt while pitching. I shook my left arm, more baffled then concerned. My next pitch would be the last I threw in a big league game for the next twenty-one months.

I released the ball, and this time I heard a slamming sound, like a collision from inside my elbow. I felt as if my arm had come off. I immediately called time and started walking off the mound.[3]

After an examination of this injury, Dr. Jobe's initial opinion was that John had torn a ligament in his elbow. He advised three weeks of rest and then a re-evaluation.

John denied having any pain for the three weeks following the injury, after which he tested his elbow by throwing batting practice. He not only couldn't throw a strike, he couldn't even get the ball over the plate. Also, to add insult to injury, he now had pain.

Dr. Jobe's re-evaluation was the same as it was before, a torn elbow ligament. A colleague, Dr. Herb Stark, gave a second opinion. He concurred that John had a torn ligament in the elbow (no MRIs existed in 1974 to confirm the diagnosis).[4]

Dr. Jobe explained to John that without surgery he had no chance of ever pitching again. Even with surgery his chances of pitching again were one in a hundred and involved a long rehabilitation period. Jobe went over possible different tears that could be present in the ligament. The worst case scenario was that the ligament was torn completely through in the middle. In that case, he would have to do an experimental procedure to replace the ligament using a tendon from a muscle at the wrist, the palmaris longus. A similar tendon graft procedure had been done before on some polio victims, but it had never been attempted on a baseball pitcher.

The surgery was performed in early September of 1974. Additional damage to the ulnar collateral ligament and some torn muscles/tendons was noted, which also had to be fixed. The arm was put in an inflexible cast for a few weeks.[5]

After the cast was removed and John began using the arm, it became apparent that he had developed a complication of the surgery. John had no feeling in the little finger on his left hand. Movement in his hand was limited, and he had what appeared to be a claw hand. He had developed damage to the ulnar nerve, probably secondary to scar tissue that had formed around the ulnar nerve from the elbow transplant surgery.[6]

Another surgical procedure was needed or John probably would have permanent damage to this nerve. John would need scar tissue around the nerve removed and the nerve moved to the front of the elbow. Even with surgery, there was no guarantee the nerve function would ever come back. Without surgery, there was no chance of a return of function. With surgery, because of the length of the nerve distal to the elbow (18 inches), it could take up to 18 months for the nerve to regenerate through its nerve sheath, the length of the nerve from the elbow to the hand (one inch per month).

The nerve-sparing surgery was done in December 15, 1974. Surgery confirmed the build-up of scar tissue around the nerve. This scar tissue was removed and the nerve, which is normally positioned on the inside of the elbow behind the ulnar bone, was moved to the front of the elbow and put into some local fatty tissue, thus taking some pressure off the nerve. The nerve was transposed.[7]

It didn't take 18 months for the function of John's nerve to come back. By June of 1975, John was able to open and close his hand. By August 1975, almost 12 months after his ligament surgery and nine months after his nerve repair surgery, he was able to throw batting practice. By late September 1975, he was able to pitch to live batters in a game during the Fall Instructional League.[8]

Spring training in 1976 was interrupted by an owner's lockout from March 1 until March 17. The players had reported in February, but because of the lockout Tommy John was limited to three games and fifteen innings pitched in preparation for the season, the last game six innings pitched against the Angels just before the start of the season.

In spring training John was hitting 85 miles an hour on the radar gun, not fast by most major league standards, but ok for John as during his major league career he never threw faster than 85 to 87 mph. His success depended on movement on his sinking fastball and good location on his pitches.

Not all were optimistic about his recovery. He was given a short leash once the season started. His scheduled start at the beginning of the season was rained out and he was skipped over for his next start. So his first start of the regular season was not until April 16 against Atlanta. He did ok, pitching five innings and giving up three runs in a 3 to 1 Dodger loss. The bad thing, his sinker didn't sink much. Tommy John was given just one more chance to prove himself. Alston, the Dodger manager, told him, "We're giving you one more shot, then we've got to decide what we are going to do with you. We've got to see if you can pitch. You still haven't shown us."[9]

Fortunately for Tommy John that one more game went very well. He pitched seven innings of shutout ball against the Houston Astros on April 21, his sinking fast ball working very well. He came away with a no-decision as J.R. Richard was also pitching shutout ball for the Astros. With this fine performance Tommy John earned a reprieve.

John next pitched on April 26, 1976, and came away with his first win since July 7, 1974. He gave up one run in seven innings in a 7 to 1 victory over the Pirates at Dodger Stadium, a victory some twenty-one months after his initial elbow ligament injury. This victory was just icing on the cake as Tommy John had cemented his return in his previous start five days before.

Tommy John passed the test. He went on to pitch 207 innings in 1976 with ten wins and ten losses and a good ERA of 3.09. With better run support he might have done better in the win/loss column.

Then the remarkable happened. In 1977, 1978, 1979, and 1980 he won 20, 17, 21, and 22 games respectively, the best four-year total of his career, and the only times he won 20 games in a year during his long career.

Tommy John's career actually improved after his elbow ligament surgery. He went on to pitch 14 more years after his surgery, his career ultimately one of the longest ever.

FURTHER DISCUSSION OF TOMMY JOHN SURGERY

Tommy John was the first person to have "Tommy John" surgery. The total number of pitchers and position players since then having the torn ulnar collateral ligament (UCL) replacement surgery is staggering.

James Andrews, the Birmingham, Alabama, physician, estimated he performed 1,169 Tommy John surgeries from 1994 to 2005 — about 100 per year.[10]

Dr. Timothy Kremchek, the Cincinnati Reds' team physician, stated he does about 120 UCL replacements per year.[11]

Dr. Lewis Yocum, Frank Jobe's partner, averages about 100 surgeries per year.[12]

Dr. Frank Jobe, in an article appearing in the Long Beach, CA, *Press-Telegram*, estimated in 2001 that he had done 2,000 Tommy John surgeries (1974–2001).[13]

Who gets Tommy John surgery? Dr. Andrews estimates that 20 percent are major league players, 20–25 percent are minor leaguers, and the rest are college or high school players.

What percentages of active major leaguer players have had Tommy John surgery? An article in *Baseball Digest* in 2004 estimated that during 2002 and 2003, more than 75 active pitchers had had Tommy John surgery. This is close to one in every nine pitchers pitching at the major league level during this time.[14]

Why do the procedure? First, it is virtually impossible to perform at the major league level with a torn UCL. Second, the success rate the first time the procedure is done is very high, 85 percent. Many of the failures are not at the major league level. At the non–major league level rehab isn't supervised as closely as it needs to be, and many of these failures occur when the pitcher simply tries to do too much too soon.

With a failed first procedure, the statistics for a successful second procedure are much worse. The chance of success with a second procedure is only 20 percent. Thus, it is best to get the rehab right the first time, not taking many chances, not pushing progress too fast. A full rehab takes a minimum of 12 months and for many 15 months. Sometimes the pitcher isn't back to pre-injury major league performance until 24 months after the procedure.

Some of the pitchers who have been very successful after Tommy John surgery are Tom Candiotti, David Wells, and Jason Isringhausen. Those who were not successful after surgery for UCL replacement include Jose Rijo, Darren Dreifort, and Brian Anderson.

TOM CANDIOTTI

Tom Candiotti was a right-handed knuckleball pitcher who played for 16 seasons, mainly for the Cleveland Indians (seven seasons) and Los Angeles Dodgers (six seasons). His record was not fantastic at 151 wins and 164 losses, but he was often victimized with poor run support, especially in the first two years he pitched for Dodgers. His career ERA of 3.73 indicates he might have had a better record with a few more runs scored behind him.

Then again, he might never have pitched in the major leagues if it had not been for the "Tommy John" surgery he had in 1981, performed by Dr. Frank Jobe.

Candiotti, then in the minor leagues with the Milwaukee Brewers' Double-A team in El Paso, had to convince Dr. Jobe that he was major league material (a prospect) to get Dr. Jobe to do the procedure. Jobe had only done eight previous procedures. In 1981, "Tommy John" surgery was not a routine procedure.[15]

Candiotti missed the entire 1982 season, but made his debut the following year for Milwaukee. His career lasted till he was age 41 (16 seasons). He last pitched in the majors on July 24, 1999.

DAVID WELLS

David Wells also had his Tommy John procedure (1985) before he made it to the majors. Later he was on the DL for elbow pain in 1993 and subsequently had some bone chips removed from his elbow in 1994, but from his autobiography, *Perfect I'm Not*, there is no indication he had any other significant problems with his elbow, at least as of his book's publication in 2003.

David Wells' career at the major league level spanned 1987 to 2007, 21 seasons with nine franchises. He pitched the most seasons for the Toronto Blue Jays (eight) and the New York Yankees (four). His career ERA of 4.13 is worse than Tom Candiotti's, but Wells won more games with an impressive career record of 239–157, a winning percentage of .604. He never won a Cy Young Award, but he did finished in the top three twice. He recorded 2201 strikeouts in 3439 innings pitched, but striking out batters was not his forte. He exhibited very good control, only walking 719 batters.

If David Wells is remembered for anything other than winning ball games with his arm, it was his controversial behavior and colorful metaphors, both of which are spelled out clearly in his autobiography.

He was never short of colorful language to describe his problems. The following is from his book about his elbow problems in June of 1984.

> Tossing a simple curveball, down and away, towards home plate, I suddenly felt
> a sharp burning pain, sort of like someone had run a lawnmower over my elbow,

then scraped a fork around inside the open wound, then poured molten lead on the top to seal it up. I saw stars. I tried to shake it off, but that just sent a wave of agony up my arm. Tears welled in my eyes. A knot clamped in my stomach. I was fucked and I knew it. By the time the trainers got to me, I was already sure my season was over. My career seemed to be on life support as well.[16]

At this point Wells in all probability had only a partial tear of his collateral ligament. Preferring to avoid surgery if at all possible, Wells stopped throwing the rest of the minor league season. Over the winter he slowly prepared for spring training. In spring training of 1985, after finally throwing nine pitches at full speed (95 mph), Wells tore his UCL completely: if pain the previous year was "rated a 7 on a scale of 1 to 10, this one's maybe a 49."[17] That ended Wells' season; the pitch never even made it to home plate.

Wells saw Dr. Andrews in Birmingham, Alabama. An MRI confirmed that the medial collateral ligament was torn. Tommy John surgery was needed. Surgery revealed, in addition to a torn UCL, torn muscles (flexor muscles more than likely) and loose bone fragments in the joint.

Wells did just fine with his elbow. In 1986 he had a setback with his shoulder problems and had to have a shoulder arthroscopy. The shoulder injury probably occurred because he was overcompensating for his elbow injury, a common problem for pitchers recovering from Tommy John surgery. Despite this setback, Wells finally made the Toronto Blue Jays' major league squad as a rookie in 1987.

He did well at the major league level, staying relatively injury-free until June of 1993 while he was pitching for the Detroit Tigers. He began to experience elbow pain once again and pitched the rest of the 1993 in pain.

The off-season did wonders for Wells' elbow pain. Then he recalled, "very shortly into the (1994) season, the same elbow that nagged me at the second half of last season came roaring back, this time bigger and more bad-assed than before.... MRIs revealed a little squadron of bone chips floating near the elbow."[18] Surgery, once again performed by Dr. Andrews, relieved the problem, and fortunately no other significant damage in the elbow was noted.

Wells' 21-year career was very long by major league standards. He was relatively healthy compared to many other major league players. In *Perfect I'm Not*, he relates no further elbow problems from 1994 to 2003. His major problems were more related to his back. He had back surgery in July 2001, surgery which revealed a herniated disc and loose bone fragment, but back injuries are discussed in a different section of this book.

JASON ISRINGHAUSEN

Jason Isringhausen has had two Tommy John surgeries, one in 1998 and one in 2009. The one done in 1998 would have to be deemed a success.

Initially, Isringhausen was not thought of as a great prospect, as he was not selected until the Mets picked him in the 44th round of the 1991 amateur draft. But Isringhausen quickly made himself into a top prospect within the Mets organization.

Isringhausen, then age 22, arrived at the major league level in 1995 with the Mets as a starter, starting 14 games in 1995 and 27 games in 1996. He had a minor setback late in the 1996 season as he required arthroscopic surgery on September 28 on both his shoulder and elbow, performed by Dr. Altchek. On his shoulder he had only some fraying of his labrum that needed to be cleaned up. On his elbow he had four bone chips removed.[19]

The surgery in 1996 delayed his return to the majors. That he had tuberculosis and broke his hand punching a garbage can in 1997 didn't help his return (for the latter, see article on bizarre injuries) and in six late-season starts he experienced significant elbow pain.[20]

He pitched well in winter league ball in San Juan, Puerto Rico, but with continued elbow pain he required Tommy John surgery, which was done on January 13, 1998, by Dr. David Altchek, the Mets' team physician. Surgery revealed a 90 percent tear of the right UCL, much worse than initially suspected. He missed all of the 1998 season.[21]

The Mets, frustrated with Isringhausen's ineffectiveness as a starter, traded him to the Oakland A's on July 31, 1999. Oakland decided to convert him to a reliever and started grooming him as their closer of the future.[22]

The rest is history. Isringhausen saved 33 games for the A's in 2000 and 34 games in 2001 before signing a free agent contract with the St. Louis Cardinals. Presently he is the Cardinals' all-time saves leader with 217 over seven years. At the end of 2009 he had 293 career saves.[23]

It is bad to get older. Isringhausen had a series of injuries the last few years with the Cardinals. He had recurrent hip problems requiring surgery (see article on hip injuries) and more recently a torn flexor muscle in his left elbow repaired in September of 2008. He signed in 2009 with Tampa Bay, but once again suffered a torn medial collateral ligament in his right elbow, requiring a second Tommy John surgery in June of 2009. In May of 2010, at age 37 Isringhausen was thought to be at the end of his career.[24]

But, Isringhausen did recover from his second surgery and was signed by the Mets in 2011. He was able to pitch in 53 games in relief for the Mets, pitching 46 innings and finishing with an ERA of 4.05. And, Isringhausen even recorded 7 more saves in 2011 to bring his career total to the 300 save mark. He signed with the Los Angeles Angels in 2012.

Between Tommy John surgeries Irsinghausen with his 293 saves recorded would have to be called a big success following his first ulnar collateral ligament repair. He came back at age 38 to pitch for the Mets in 2011 and record 7 more saves.

JOSE RIJO

Jose Rijo, formerly of the Cincinnati Reds, is one of the greatest failures of Tommy John surgery, though this failure is not directly related to the specific procedure itself. Through 1995 he had a major league record of 111–87 with an extremely good ERA of 3.16. While playing for the Cincinnati Reds from 1988 to 1995, he had 92 wins and 57 losses and an ERA of 2.71. Rijo was the 1990 World Series MVP for the Reds, winning both Game 1 and Game 4 in the Series sweep over the Oakland A's. He only gave up one run in his two World Series starts.[25]

Rijo did not display the classical history of an acutely torn UCL. There was no ligament popping suddenly, leading to his initial Tommy John surgery. His symptoms came on gradually. (Chronic UCL tears with chronic and episodic symptoms are more common than acute onset of symptoms with classical acute UCL tears, as noted by at least one medical source.)[26] Even if there is an acute tear, often there is a history of prior medial elbow pain symptoms.

In an article in the *Dayton* (OH) *Daily News* in 1995, Rijo said he had had pain in the elbow ever since he was 17, when he was pitching in the Yankees' minor league system. An x-ray taken on Rijo's elbow in 1982 by his family doctor in the Dominican Republic showed a bone abnormality in the elbow, possibly a bone spur. Rijo's pain got worse over the years, then better, but the pain was never as severe as the pain Rijo experienced in 1995.[27]

It should be noted that Rijo saw Dr. Andrews, the noted sports medicine specialist, several times for elbow pain over the years. In 1995, while he was pitching for the Reds, the frequency of these visits would dramatically increase.

Rijo's 1995 season represents the classic dilemma of how to deal with your ace's injury. It is difficult to face the possibility of season-ending surgery. The tendency is to do whatever necessary to hang on to hope for some degree of recovery. Maybe the ace pitcher could be used in some capacity, if not during the season, then maybe in a crucial playoff game. Surgery, especially Tommy John surgery, would end any such hope.

When Rijo began having increased pain in June of 1995, more tests were ordered. The bone spur that had been present since Rijo was 17 had grown two and one-half times bigger. Still, despite this finding, surgery was not recommended, a course of action chosen under careful consultation with Dr. Andrews in Alabama. As is often the case, initial treatment included a cortisone shot, given on June 19, and it should be noted Rijo did experience some pain relief following the shot.[28]

After a short period of rest, Rijo resumed pitching, but when Rijo experienced severe pain after throwing a slider in the third inning on July 18, so severe he had to be quickly removed from the game, his pitching was shut down completely, and a re-evaluation was made.[29]

A repeat MRI showed a partially torn UCL ligament as well as some bone formation within the ligament. Because of some bleeding seen within the ligament on the MRI, there was some hope the ligament might heal on its own without surgery. Further rest was prescribed.[30]

But Rijo continued to have pain, even a month later, without even throwing a single pitch in a game. By then, whatever tear was noted was not going to heal on its own. Further rest wasn't going to help. The possibility of Rijo helping lead the Cincinnati Reds into the playoffs in 1995 was simply not going to happen. Rijo's season was over. Surgery was necessary. It was time to look ahead to 1996.

Rijo's surgery was performed on August 22, 1995, by Dr. Andrews in Birmingham, Alabama. Three procedures were done. First, the ulnar collateral ligament was repaired. There was enough of the right forearm tendon present to make three loops of the tendon graft to replace the ligament (usually only two loops are possible). An unnamed tendon also had to be repaired; more often than not this is a flexor tendon that is torn and needs repairing. Finally, the ulnar nerve was moved and fitted snugly in a different location, out of harm's way.[31]

Spring training in 1996 went well initially; Rijo's recovery was a full two months ahead of schedule. Initially he was throwing 90 mph fastballs, but as spring training went along his velocity dropped off and he once again experienced elbow pain, excruciating in nature, before an intrasquad game on April 4. Tests revealed a small bone formation in the elbow. When the pain became much worse, Rijo again had surgery, this time an arthroscopic procedure to remove elbow calcification, bone formation, and scar tissue on April 8, 1996.[32] Rijo's progress through the rest of 1996 was marked by rest, rehab, and setbacks because of pain.[33]

There had been hope on Rijo's part, after he had missed the entire 1996 season, that he would be able to pitch winter ball in the Dominican Republic. But it wasn't to be. Recurrence of pain during rehab resulted in a third operation on November 20, 1996. The exploratory surgery revealed a ruptured flexor tendon that needed repair. Scar tissue and loose material were also removed from the elbow. This operation was more invasive than the one done in April and certainly threatened any possibility of Rijo's pitching at the major league level in 1997.[34]

Things got worse for Rijo in 1997, much worse than he could imagine. His comeback was stalled in April. A procedure to remove some sutures and scar tissue from Rijo's elbow on April 7 was the least of Rijo's worries; he again severely injured the flexor tendon in his right elbow in August. The tendon, which was completely torn off the bone, was repaired on August 14, 1997, in a procedure once again done by Dr. Andrews in Alabama.[35]

Obviously by the end of 1997 season, retirement was becoming a serious consideration by Rijo, but he would eventually make one more attempt at a comeback. He sat out the 1998, 1999, and 2000 seasons before attempting a comeback in 2001 at age 36. He pitched at three levels in the Cincinnati Reds' minor league system before pitching 13 games for the Reds in the second half of the 2001 season, all in relief. He finished with a very fine 2.12 ERA in 17 innings pitched.

In 2002 Rijo pitched 31 games for the Reds, 22 in relief and nine starts. He finished with a high 5.14 ERA with five wins and four losses in 77 innings pitched, the most innings he had pitched since he originally suffered his torn UCL in 1995. He won the Tony Conigliaro Award in 2002 for his efforts.

Rijo's elbow became a problem again in spring training of 2003 after pitching only five innings. He underwent the sixth surgical procedure on his right elbow on March 11, 2003, to remove a single bone chip. When he continued to have elbow pain, he received a cortisone shot by Dr. Andrews around the first of June. It didn't help. The 37-year-old never again pitched at the minor or major league level.[36]

Contrary to many references cited on the internet, Jose Rijo had only one Tommy John surgery, this on August 22, 1995.[37] Three times Rijo tore his elbow flexor tendon. He had six procedures on his elbow during his major league career.

DARREN DREIFORT

Expectations for Darren Dreifort's career were great. He was drafted in the first round of the 1993 amateur draft out of Wichita State University by the Los Angeles Dodgers. He was the second player picked overall, taken just after the Seattle Mariners' pick, Alex Rodriguez.

He made the Dodgers' staff in 1994 without pitching a minute in the minor leagues. There is a distinct possibility he was overutilized at the beginning of the 1994 season by the Dodgers. He pitched in relief in 17 of their first 35 games, and in one stretch nine times in 13 days.

Dreifort cannot remember exactly when his elbow started to bother him. But in 1994, as his pain got worse, so did his performance. With decreasing performance he was sent down to the Dodgers' Double-A affiliate, San Antonio, where instead of pitching in relief he started eight games. He then pitched one game in August for the Dodgers' Triple-A affiliate before being shut down for the season.[38]

When he continued to have elbow pain in the off-season, an MRI was done in November which revealed a partially torn medial collateral ligament in his right elbow. Rehab followed which was unsuccessful. When spring training started and Dreifort continued to have elbow pain, he was examined by Dr. Frank Jobe. Tommy John surgery was recommended. Subsequently, the surgery was performed on March 14, 1995, by Dr. Jobe at Centinela Medical Center in Inglewood, CA. A tendon from a muscle in Dreifort's left forearm (palmaris longus) was used to replace the torn ligament. Dreifort missed the entire 1995 season.[39]

Dreifort bounced between the majors and minors in 1996 and 1997 before establishing himself as a major league starter from 1998 to 2000, though during that time his ERA never got below 4.00 and he won only 33 games against 34 losses.

For whatever reason the Dodgers decided to sign the 28-year-old pitcher to a $55 million, five-year contract on December 11, 2000. The signing looked to be based more on potential than on past results. That Dreifort's agent was Scott Boras didn't help the Dodgers in negotiating a reasonable contract. The day Dreifort signed his contract was the same day Alex Rodriguez, whose agent was also Scott Boras, signed his record ten-year $252 million contract with the Texas Rangers.[40]

In light of Dreifort's history of health problems (elbow, shoulder, and knees) the Dodgers were smart enough to take out an insurance policy on his contract. Unfortunately benefits did not cover the first year of the policy, and Dreifort had a major injury during that season.

The 2001 season didn't go well for Dreifort. He struggled from the get-go. He had an ERA of 5.13 and a 4–7 record when he went on the DL on June 29. Almost from the start of the season, he had stiffness in the elbow. The elbow problems took a sharp turn for the worse in a game on June 29 against the Padres. He had to be removed rather suddenly in the sixth inning because of difficulties with his elbow, though his catcher indicated Dreifort might have actually injured the elbow the inning before. Dreifort denied feeling any sensation of a pop in his elbow. Such would be rather typical of an acute UCL tear.[41]

Dreifort had an MRI two days after his injury. It revealed that the previously repaired UCL was now almost completely torn (90 percent). To make matters worse, the flexor muscle at the elbow had completely torn off the bone. Dr. Jobe once again repaired Dreifort's elbow on July 10, 2001. The palmaris tendon, this time from the right wrist area, was used to repair the torn UCL.[42]

Dreifort would go on to miss the rest of 2001 and all of the 2002 season, a long time out even for recovery from Tommy John surgery. He finally made it back in 2003, starting ten games for the Dodgers with four wins and four losses and a respectable 4.03 ERA.

In 2004 Dreifort was moved to the bullpen and appeared in 60 games before going on the DL in mid–August because of his right knee. He would never again pitch at the major league level.

An article in the *Kansas City Star* in 2005 notes that from August 2004 until May 2005 Dreifort had four surgeries: on his right hip, right knee, left knee, and right shoulder.[43]

Why so many injuries? All along there was speculation that Dreifort might be prone to shoulder and elbow problems because of his flawed mechanics. He threw with a slingshot-type release. Maybe his mechanics could have been changed early on, though at least one source noted that Dreifort's delivery put extra movement on the ball. The delivery was what got him to the major leagues. Maybe altering his throwing mechanics would have made him even less successful than he actually was.[44]

One source suggests that Dreifort's assortment of injuries, including his elbow ligament problems, may have been from bad connective tissue (quoting Dr. Jobe). In other words, he had bad genetics. There are no tests to check for that at present, but certainly an early personal history of injuries could point towards potential future problems; Dreifort did have arthroscopy on both knees even before his first Tommy John surgery.[45]

Dreifort has to be called a failure of Tommy John surgery. The most significant point is that he had to have the procedure repeated, in itself a bad sign. The prognosis for continuing to pitch at the major league level after a second Tommy John procedure is much worse than after one procedure. With the surgeries he missed two and a half seasons rehabbing, seasons lost during a pitcher's usual prime. It is pure speculation whether having to have repeat Tommy John surgeries had anything to do with the assortment of other injuries that hastened the end of Dreifort's career.

BRIAN JAMES ANDERSON

Why use a pitcher of minor reputation such as Brian Anderson as an example of Tommy John surgery failure? He represents the worst possible outcome. Jose Rijo's demise was mainly due to recurrent flexor muscle tears, not another torn UCL. Rijo *did not* have repeat Tommy John surgery despite what some Internet and newspaper references might say. That is not the case with Brian Anderson. He ruptured his ulnar collateral ligament three times, the last time ending his career.

There was optimism initially for Anderson's career. He was selected in the first round of the 1993 amateur draft out of Wright State University by the California Angels, the third pick overall. He pitched at the major league level the same year he was drafted at age 21 (after only four games in the minor leagues). His results in his major league career thereafter have to be called mixed.

His longest tenure at the major league level was the five years he spent with the Arizona Diamondbacks, which included pitching for the World Series champions in 2001. His career ERA was only 4.74 with a mediocre win/loss record of 82–83. His best season was actually 2003, which he split between the Cleveland Indians and Kansas City Royals. He finished the year with 14 wins and 11 losses. The most innings he pitched was 213⅓ for Arizona in 2000, making 32 starts with an 11–7 record.

Anderson, a left-hander, started six games for the Kansas City Royals in 2005 before going on the DL with elbow inflammation. It was during his first rehab start in July at the Royals' Triple-A affiliate that his elbow pain became much worse. Shortly after this start he saw Dr. Timothy Kremcheck, the Cincinnati Reds' team physician. Surgery on July 21 revealed a mess; Anderson had two bone fragments removed, a torn elbow flexor muscle repaired, and Tommy John surgery to repair his torn ulnar collateral ligament (UCL).[46]

Rehab went well. The Royals did not sign him in 2006, but the Texas Rangers did. Maybe he returned too fast from his surgery, as during an extended spring training game he once again began having significant elbow pain. An MRI on June 6, 2006, revealed he had torn the previously repaired UCL and needed a second procedure if he wanted to continue to pitch. He took his time making a decision as he did not have the repeat surgery by Dr. Kremcheck until July 14, 2006.[47]

Anderson sat out the 2007 season, working as a broadcaster. He got the urge to pitch again during the off-season. He tried out for several scouts in late January of 2008, was signed by the Tampa Bay Rays to a minor league contract, and was to report to spring training.

Well, it just wasn't to be. Anderson had taken much longer to come back after his second Tommy John surgery, but it made no difference. He left the mound suddenly while pitching to Bobby Abreu on March 11. He was pitching in only his third game of spring training. An MRI the following day revealed that he had once again torn his UCL and flexor muscles in his elbow.[48]

The 35-year-old Anderson had not pitched at the major league level since May 8, 2005. He had suffered three torn ulnar collateral ligaments. His career was over. Anderson had what could be called the worst possible outcome from an initial repair of a torn UCL.

Flexor Muscle/Tendon Tears

Flexor muscle/tendon tears are at least as common as ulnar collateral ligament tears. The flexor muscle/tendon attaches to the inside, medial side, of the elbow, the area of maximum stress when the elbow is accelerated, or dragged, through the arc of the throwing motion. One of the muscles, the pronator muscle, is especially prone to injury though most references simply say flexor muscles when reporting this type of muscle tear. When Tommy John had his initial UCL surgery, he had torn flexor muscles repaired at the same time.

Occasionally a pitcher is reported to have had Tommy John surgery when in fact he had only a flexor muscle repaired. That was the case with Jose Rijo, who had one Tommy John surgery. He had three repairs of torn elbow flexor tendons, one occurring at the same time as his Tommy John surgery.

Research revealed no source trying to estimate the total occurrences of flexor muscle tears in any given year in the major leagues. The subject apparently is just not as interesting a subject as the Tommy John surgery. Thus the amount of time devoted here in no way reflects the frequency of this injury.

With flexor muscle tears, the diagnosis is made either by an MRI or during surgery. Who knows if someone like Hall of Fame Yankees pitcher Lefty Gomez (1930 to 1942), who was simply reported in most sources as having had a "bad arm," could not have had a partially torn flexor muscle, or a partially torn ulnar collateral ligament for that matter? Gomez, who started out as a power pitcher early in his career, ended up as a finesse pitcher later because of his bad arm. Before modern surgery to repair flexor muscle tears and before MRIs, who knows how many other pitchers' careers simply ended because of flexor muscle tears?[49]

TOM GLAVINE

Tom Glavine pitched 22 seasons for the Atlanta Braves and New York Mets, retiring in 2008. His career record of 305–203 with two Cy Young Awards makes him almost a shoo-in for the Hall of Fame when he becomes eligible.

Glavine's career was marked by very few injuries and he went from 1997 to 2006 without going on the DL. In 2006 he had some clots in his hands, determined to be from scar tissue in an artery in his shoulder. No surgery was necessary as the injury was treatable with blood thinners only.[50] (It was not an aneurysm.)

At age 42, Glavine suffered a flexor muscle/tendon tear confirmed by MRI on August 20, 2008. He had surgery on August 21 done by Dr. James Andrews in Birmingham, Alabama. At the same time Glavine had a shoulder arthroscopy to clean up some minor wear on his labrum.[51]

Glavine was supposed to be ready for spring training in 2009, but it wasn't to be, as he did not pitch again after 2008.

BRAD LIDGE

Brad Lidge is a relief pitcher who has had a successful major league career. Taken in the first round of the 1998 amateur draft by the Houston Astros, "Lights Out" Lidge has pitched in the majors since 2002 for the Astros and Phillies. He was part of the 2008 World Series champion Philadelphia Phillies, recording 41 saves in 41 opportunities during the regular season. He had an ERA of 1.95 with 92 strikeouts in 69⅓ innings pitched.

However, 2009 was a bad season for Lidge. Even though he saved 31 games, he had eight losses against no wins and an ERA of 7.21. It was apparent something was wrong. Tests revealed damage, and Lidge had surgery to fix a tear in his flexor/pronator muscle, performed by Dr. Michael Ciccotti on November 11, 2009. He also had a loose body removed from his elbow.[52]

Results of surgery were very good. Lidge saved fewer games in 2010 than in 2009, 27, but with a more respectable ERA of 2.96 in 45⅔ innings.

The beginning of 2011 did not go well for Brad Lidge. In spring training he was down for two weeks with biceps tendonitis. When he finally was able to pitch, he experienced shoulder discomfort in a March 24 game against Minnesota in Clearwater. An MRI revealed a small tear in the posterior rotator cuff. For the third time in the four years he had been with the Phillies, Lidge started the season on the disabled list.

It was initially hoped Lidge would miss only three to six weeks, just long enough to rehabilitate his shoulder, but elbow pain prolonged the need for rehab to four months.

He finally made his first big league appearance for the season on July 25 recording three outs to prevent a 5–4 deficit from getting any worse.

For the rest of the 2011 season Lidge made 25 appearances with a fine 1.40 ERA in only 19 and ⅓ innings pitched. As Ryan Madson had become the Phillies closer in Lidge's absence, Lidge only recorded 1 save in the remainder of 2011.

Not willing to take another chance on a pitcher having such frequent injuries the Phillies did not pick up the $12.5 million option on Lidge for 2012, making him a free agent. He signed a $1 million contract with the Washington Nationals for 2012.

BILLY WAGNER

In 2010 Billy Wagner pitched his 16th and final year in the majors. The 12th pick overall by the Houston Astros in the 1993 amateur draft, Billy "The Kid" Wagner had 422 career saves with a fine ERA of 2.31. Even more impressive, he had 1196 strikeouts in only 903 innings.

In 2000 Wagner, then with the Houston Astros, tore the flexor tendon in his left elbow. He had problems throughout 2000, with nine blown saves in 15 opportunities before tests revealed the injury. His ERA at the time was an uncharacteristic 6.18. He had surgery on June 27 and was done for the season.[53]

In 2008 he again had trouble with the pronator/flexor tendon in his left forearm. Tests had revealed a partially torn tendon. At age 37, Wagner and the Mets decided to rehab the elbow instead of having surgery. But during rehab on Sunday, September 7, while throwing in the bullpen, Wagner was suddenly forced to quit on only the 13th pitch. The result: not only did Wagner further injure the flexor muscle but he also tore out his medial collateral ligament. Wagner joined the group who have had both Tommy John surgery and surgery to correct a flexor muscle tear in his elbow.[54]

Wagner recovered well and actually came back to pitch 17 games in 2009 for the Mets and Boston Red Sox. In 2010 he had one of his better years for the Atlanta Braves when, at age 38, he won 7 games against 2 losses with a 1.48 ERA. He had 37 saves with an impressive 104 strikeouts in only 69⅓ innings. Unfortunately Wagner suffered an oblique injury in the second game of the first round of the 2010 National League Divisional playoffs against the San Francisco Giants causing him to miss the last two games. San Francisco won that series three games to one.

Wagner announced early in the 2010 season he was going to retire after the 2010 season despite the Braves having a $6.5 million option on Wagner's contract for 2011. The Braves released Wagner from his contract in March of 2011. Wagner did not pitch again in the major leagues after 2010.

Ulnar Nerve

At the medial side of the elbow is the ulnar nerve (see previous discussion of Tommy John). This is probably the most often injured nerve in baseball as it is slightly mobile within the cubital canal and is near the medial elbow, the part of the elbow that is stressed to extremes during the late cocking phase and acceleration phase of pitching. Irritation injury can occur to this nerve with local pain and numbness, tingling, and loss of muscle strength in the hand as a result. The numbness and tingling are usually localized to the fourth and fifth fingers. The same forces that cause irritation and medial collateral ligament injury at the elbow can also cause damage to this important nerve. Tommy John surgery can also lead to the build-up of scar tissue which can irritate the nerve, especially if the nerve is moved by older techniques. With newer surgical techniques involving Tommy John surgery, though, risk of damage of the ulnar nerve has lessened considerably, especially since the nerve is rarely moved with the Tommy John surgery anymore unless there are symptoms of ulnar nerve dysfunction pre-op. The newer technique rarely leads to the build-up of harmful scar tissue.[55]

The nerve, when moved, can be tacked down by several means, but the most common method is to use subcutaneous connective tissue (fascia) to tack down the nerve anteriorly so it is not moving back and forth in front of the elbow (instead of the normal behind the elbow). In the past the nerve was often moved to a position underneath the elbow flexor muscles after the muscles were split and sewn back together.[56]

Tommy John had his nerve moved with a separate surgery after the initial UCL repair because scar tissue had formed where the surgery had been done and he was having significant symptoms of ulnar nerve dysfunction, numbness in the fourth and fifth fingers and muscle weakness in the hand.

As with Tommy John surgery, the vast majority of ulnar nerve transposition patients are pitchers.

DENNY NEAGLE

A disastrous signing by the Colorado Rockies was the five-year $51 million contract given to Denny Neagle in 2001. He finished with only 19 wins and 23 losses for the Rockies in the three years after the signing. His career record of 124–92 looks better than those stats, though.

In October 2002 he had bone chips removed from his elbow. Then, on July 30, 2003, he had Tommy John surgery as well as an ulnar nerve transposition.[57]

Neagle never pitched in the major leagues again.

CHRIS CARPENTER

Having ulnar nerve transposition *after* Tommy John surgery was Chris Carpenter, a miracle of modern science. Much of Carpenter's history is mentioned under the article about his shoulder surgery.

After Tommy John surgery in 2007, the nerve problem started during rehab in May of 2008. Symptoms improved only to return near the end of the 2008 season and into the off-season. Initial treatment was for Carpenter to pitch through the nerve irritation, but when the problem persisted he and the Cardinals gave in and he had the ulnar nerve transposition done. Dr. George Paletta, the Cardinals' team physician, performed the surgery on November 4, 2008.[58]

The result was a 17–4 record in 2009, a "Comeback Player of the Year" Award, and runner-up in the Cy Young Award voting.

RAFAEL SORIANO

Seattle Mariner Rafael Soriano had Tommy John surgery in 2004. While pitching for the Atlanta Braves, Rafael Soriano had another elbow surgery on August 27, 2008. He had a small bone spur removed and had ulnar nerve transposition. He was shut down for the rest of the 2008 season, finishing with a 0–1 record with three saves and a 2.57 ERA in 14 games.[59]

The rest is history. Soriano finished with 27 saves in 77 games for the Braves in 2009. After a trade to the Tampa Bay Rays, he finished 2010 with a

3–2 record, and a sparkling 1.73 ERA and led the American League with 45 saves.

ALBERT PUJOLS

A position player having ulnar nerve transposition without Tommy John surgery was Albert Pujols, a three-time MVP player.

There was concern that Pujols had ulnar collateral ligament damage and might need Tommy John surgery in 2008. He suffered from ulnar nerve problems much of 2008. His symptoms: the nerve would pop out of its groove whenever he straightened out his elbow, and he had discomfort in the elbow and tingling in his "right pinky and ring finger."[60]

Elbow surgery was done by Dr. George Paletta on October 13, 2008, and the ulnar nerve was moved (transposed). During the surgery it was determined that Pujols did not need the Tommy John surgery.

Despite the ulnar nerve symptoms, Pujols won the MVP Award in 2008 and when he recovered from the off-season surgery he again won the MVP Award in 2009.

Pujols' elbow pain problems recurred during the 2009 season, though this time with no ulnar nerve symptoms. After the 2009 season he had an arthroscopic surgery done by Dr. James Andrews on October 21. This involved removal of six bone spurs and some bone chips. Though the medial collateral ligament in Pujols was partially torn, Tommy John surgery was again not necessary.[61]

Pujols recovered and did fine in 2010, finishing second in the MVP voting and extending his major league record of ten consecutive years of hitting more than 30 home runs with 100 RBI to start a major league career

There have been many other players who had ulnar nerve transpositions.

Bone Chips in the Elbow: Bone Spurs

Arthritis is the end result in damage to a joint like the elbow. One could make a strong case that simple overuse can lead to arthritis. In addition, bad genetics can make one more likely to get arthritis if there is a family history of arthritis, especially osteoarthritis. A less stable joint is more prone to get arthritis than a stable one. With the elbow, a completely torn or even a partially torn ulnar collateral ligament can hasten the onset of arthritis, especially in a pitcher, as the elbow joint is less stable because of the tear.

Early signs of arthritis include swelling of the joint and pain. An MRI can show wearing out of the cartilage in a joint. An MRI, CT scan, or even a plain X-ray can show bone spurs or loose bone chips and cartilage fragments within the joint. The bone spurs are a reaction of the bone around the joint to excessive wear. The cartilage fragments or bone chips get into the joint from damage to the bones and cartilage within the joint.

Loose fragments present in the elbow joint of a pitcher, in addition to causing further pain and swelling, can impede the throwing of a baseball. Both speed and location can be affected. Certainly the ability to spin a nice breaking ball can be impaired. Loose fragments, in addition to impairing function, can actually hasten damage to the joint if not removed. Damage begets more damage.

Loose fragments in the elbow and bone spurs are very common in baseball players. One medical journal noted that these problems are the most common diagnoses in baseball leading to surgery. The brief discussion here of loose fragments and bone spurs in the elbow does not reflect the magnitude of the problem.[62]

ALLIE REYNOLDS

Many players have had bone chips or loose cartilage fragments removed form the elbow. Today this is most often done with arthroscopy. Before the advent of the arthroscope, the joint had to be opened up. Allie Reynolds, who pitched eight years for the Yankees, had his elbow joint surgically opened to look for bone chips.

Reynolds, also known as Superchief or simply Chief, had what most would call a very successful professional baseball career. He pitched 13 years in the major leagues from 1942 to 1954. His best years came with the Yankees from 1947 through 1954. He was part of six Yankees World Series Championship teams, including five straight from 1949 to 1953. His career record was 182 wins against 107 losses, with a fine 3.30 ERA. In the post-season he had a record of 7–2 with an ERA of 2.79.

He is not in the Hall of Fame. This may be the case because he started pitching rather late in life compared to most. He originally went to Oklahoma Agricultural and Mechanical College (now named Oklahoma State) on a track scholarship in 1936. After he was spotted throwing the javelin, he was asked to try out for baseball, and he made the team. After leaving college in 1938 he spent four seasons in the minors before making it with the Cleveland Indians in 1942 at the age of 25.[63]

His career was cut short at age 37 after the 1954 season because of complications of a back injury he suffered in 1953 when the Yankees' team bus crashed into an overpass in Philadelphia.[64] Still, his career record is very similar to the Yankees' Lefty Gomez, who is in the Hall of Fame.

His career might have been cut short earlier because of bone chips in his elbow. His worst year for the Yankees, 1950, resulted in 16 wins and 12 losses.

This record was a tribute to his fortitude. "He's (Reynolds) got lumps in his elbow the size of tangerines," said Yankees manager Casey Stengel. "But he's ready every time I call on him."[65]

The bone chips got so bad that Reynolds acquiesced to having the open surgical procedure, one that might end his career if not performed correctly. "During the winter a surgeon was to cut open Allie's elbow to relieve the thickened membranes in the joint and remove a few bone chips which lodged in the thickening and gave the pitcher a restriction in his arm movement."[66]

The surgery caused Reynolds to miss all of spring training. The rest is history. Reynolds went 17–8 in 1951, including two no-hitters — one on July 13 and one on September 28. In 1952, Reynolds finished even better at 20–8 with the best ERA of his career at 2.06, finishing second in the league MVP voting. Reynolds' open elbow procedure was a success.[67]

Arthritis in Elbow

SANDY KOUFAX

Sandy Koufax probably had the most famous elbow injury other than maybe Tommy John. Koufax's problematic elbow ended what could have been an even brighter career than the one Koufax had. It is very easy to speculate. If Koufax's elbow injury had occurred in modern times, he might have pitched a few more years. It is also quite possible that a partial ulnar collateral elbow ligament tear preceded the arthritis, the ligament damage significantly contributing to the arthritis development in the elbow. The ligaments being stretched to their limits is also a possibility. An MRI might have revealed Koufax's ligament problem but MRIs were not available in the early 1960s. But even if a ligament problem was diagnosed, there was no treatment to correct the problem until 1974, the year Tommy John had his ligament replacement surgery.

Koufax still had a stellar career. He needs little introduction. Despite his short 12-year career in the majors, he was elected to the Hall of Fame in 1972 mainly due to his performance from 1963 to 1966, one of the greatest stretches in baseball history. During this four-year period he won three Cy Young Awards (1963, 1965, 1966). In those three years he won 25, 26, and 27 games respectively. Unusual for a pitcher, Koufax garnered a National League MVP Award in 1963. His ERA was near 2.00 or lower from 1963–1966.

That it took Koufax 12 seasons to get his 165 wins is misleading. He was signed as a "bonus baby" out of high school, which required him to stay on the team's major league roster. (This is not the case today.) Koufax never played in the minor leagues. Though he started his major league career at age 19, he

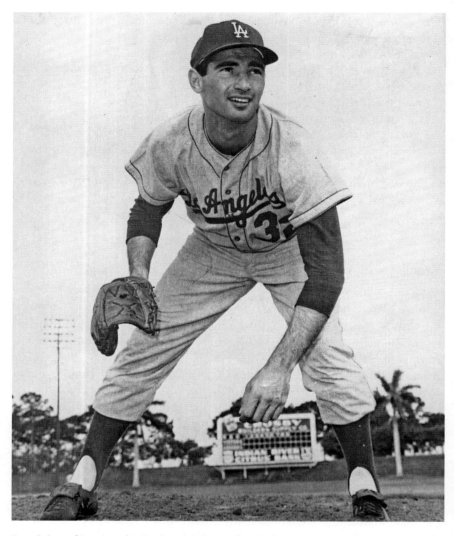

Posed shot of Los Angeles Dodger Sandy Koufax pitching, circa 1963 (National Baseball Hall of Fame Library, Cooperstown, New York).

was seldom used, and thus had very little exposure to major league hitting until 1961. That Koufax had some significant control problems didn't help his progress. During spring training in 1961, catcher Norm Sherry noticed Koufax was trying to throw the ball too hard (overthrowing). By decreasing the effort to throw the baseball and by concentrating instead on hitting spots, Koufax corrected much of his previous control problems. The slight changes made in his delivery had little effect on Koufax's ability to strike out batters.[68]

Effectiveness in pitching is a combination of speed, movement on the ball, and location. Improving location usually makes up for any small drop-off in speed. Both of Koufax's pitches — a wicked curve and a blazing fastball — already had good movement on them. (It should be noted that overthrowing the baseball cuts down on its movement.)

From 1961 to 1966 Koufax won 129 games; from 1963 to 1966 he averaged 24 wins a year.

In his autobiography, *Koufax*, written with Ed Linn, Koufax notes his first significant elbow problems started August 8, 1964.

> On August 8 I had a tough game in Milwaukee. Tougher than I thought. We were behind 2–1 in the fifth inning when I singled off Tony Cloninger (of the Braves) and went to second base on Maury Wills' single. Cloninger tried to pick me off, possibly on the theory that I was a stranger to that part of town. I dove back safely, but I landed hard on my elbow. It stung, as you would expect to sting when you give it a good rap.[69]

Koufax continued to pitch, losing the game 5–4 on a seventh-inning homer by Denis Menke.

The next day, life took a turn for the worse. He woke up with a bump on his elbow. Koufax reported, "It was the kind of swelling you would get when the joint fills up with fluid."[70]

Despite the swelling, Koufax pitched two more games after that and his results were just fine. He won 4–1 over Cincinnati, striking out ten batters. Facing the Cardinals, he pitched a shutout and struck out 13, winning his 19th game of the season. It would be the last major league game he pitched in 1964.

The day after the Cardinals game, the swelling in his elbow became much worse. Koufax reported the whole arm was swollen "all the way from the shoulder to the wrist — inside, outside, and everywhere. The whole elbow was so swollen that the whole arm was locked in a sort of hooked position. I couldn't straighten it out and I couldn't bend it."[71]

X-rays revealed "(bone) spurs and general irregularity." General medical knowledge would indicate these types of changes didn't occur overnight. The injury on August 8, 1964, probably just aggravated a deteriorating condition of the joint that was already present. The swelling revealed an already serious problem.[72]

Were there any signs of trouble prior to August 1964? Yes. In Koufax's third start of 1964 (April 22), he had thrown a curve to Bill White with a two-strike count. After the pitch, "I could feel something tear in the forearm. The ball slipped out of my hand and bounced in front of the plate."[73]

This incident is typical of an injury to the ulnar collateral ligament (though in Koufax's case it was probably only a partial tear). Any tearing and stretching of the ligament makes the elbow more unstable and speeds up the arthritis process.

Koufax did recover from his April 22 start—after taking 12 days off. By May 27 he was only 4–4, not typical for him. He did not attribute this poor record to any elbow problems, but to poor mechanics. He notes that he opened up his delivery subsequently won 15 of his next 16 decisions after May 27, 1964.

After Koufax's marked swelling after his 19th win of the season on August 16, he did not pitch in 1964. An oral medication, Butazoladin (phenylbutazone), a new non-steroidal anti-inflammatory drug (NSAID) was administered. The joint was drained and cortisone injected into it. Two attempts by Koufax to pitch batting practice ended unsuccessfully. The elbow swelled up significantly the day after each trial.

After the second attempt, Koufax again consulted Dr. Kerlan. The decision was made to shut Koufax down completely for the rest of the 1964 season. This decision was not too difficult to make with only ten days left in the season and the Dodgers 14 games behind the first-place team.

In all, Koufax missed the last six weeks of the 1964 season. Despite this he was able to win 19 games, a remarkable feat.

He pitched two complete-game four-hitters at the end of the 1965 spring training. The last start on March 30 was more significant in that it marked the recurrence of pain and swelling in the elbow. Koufax went back to Los Angeles to see Dr. Kerlan, the Dodgers' team physician. He saw him on April 1 for evaluation and therapy.

When the state of Koufax's medical condition was revealed, Dr. Kerlan told *The Sporting News* "Koufax is suffering from traumatic arthritis of his left elbow which tends to flare up under stress. It is too early to tell what the results of the treatment will be, and too early tell when he will be able to pitch."[74]

Events after April 1, 1965, are described well in Koufax's autobiography. He received two cortisone injections outside the joint without much benefit. Finally, the elbow joint itself was drained and cortisone was injected directly into the joint. Butazolidin (phenylbutazone) treatment was resumed about the same time as the first cortisone injection. (Butazolidin at the time was a relatively new non-steroidal anti-inflammatory medication similar to the present-day ibuprofen. It has nasty significant side effects, including blood count suppression and possible aplastic anemia. Those receiving it must have blood counts checked almost every week. Because of this Butazolidin is no longer sold for humans in the U.S.)[75]

Koufax rejoined the Dodgers on April 6, but at this time his future was uncertain. All the while taking Butazolidin, Koufax threw some pitches. He felt good and then tossed two innings in relief against the Washington Senators.

Finally, making his first start of the season on April 18, Koufax pitched a complete game against the Philadelphia Phillies, a 6 to 2 victory. What would be the effect on Koufax's elbow? Many times Koufax would not know till the next day how his elbow would be affected. The result on April 19: the elbow was sore but only a little puffy.

Early in 1965 there was speculation that Koufax would be able to pitch at most once a week during the season. But he managed to pitch the rest of the season, most often every fourth day, not missing a single start. That is not to say he didn't have to do anything to manage the arthritis. He was taking Butazolidin all along. He used ice on the elbow after every game. With a plastic sleeve over his arm, he soaked his arm in ice water at about 36 degrees for 30 to 40 minutes. Even before the 1965 season, he was using Capsolin — a red hot ointment — prior to games, mostly to loosen up his muscles. He continued this in 1965 and required no further cortisone shots in 1965 after April, though at times he was tempted to ask for one.[76]

The result: Koufax pitched 335⅔ innings, setting a record with 382 strikeouts. He won 26 games with 27 complete games. His 336 innings were the most pitched by any left-hander since 1906. Koufax was instrumental in the Dodgers winning the 1965 World Series against Minnesota, giving up only one earned run in 24 innings pitched while recording 29 strikeouts. Because of the excellent results in 1965, it is easy to see why there was some skepticism as to whether Koufax actually had a significant arthritis problem.

The 1966 season was worse for Koufax's elbow. Because of increasing pain and swelling, there was some modification in his treatment. Jane Leavy, in *Sandy Koufax: A Lefty's Legacy*, states that in addition to taking Butazolidin regularly, Koufax was now taking Empirin with codeine (a narcotic), both every night and often in the fifth inning of games he pitched, to manage his pain. He received many more cortisone shots in 1966 than in 1965. Leavy says he had as many cortisone shots as he had complete games in 1966; that would be 27.[77]

He pitched three games with extra innings during the season, and postseason he pitched two games: the October 2 season final and game 7 of the World Series, after only two days of rest.

This number is not an exaggeration. In a November 18, 1966, interview noted in Edward Gruver's biography, *Koufax*, Koufax said, "I don't know if cortisone is good for you or not. But to take a shot every other ballgame is more than I wanted to do, and to walk around with a constant upset stomach because of the pills and to be high half the time during a ballgame because you're taking painkillers, I don't want to have to do that."[78]

Koufax made 41 starts in 1966. Intra-articular cortisone shots every other game would have come to 20–21 shots. Today it is medical opinion that you cannot have more than two or three shots of cortisone in an arthritic joint in a year without suffering significant increased damage to the joint cartilage, thus hastening the process of arthritis formation in a joint. In 1966 this was not known.

Koufax knew early in 1966 that it would be his last year, so he did everything he could to just make it through the year. The end result was 27 wins against 9 losses, 323 innings pitched with 317 strikeouts, an ERA of 1.73, and another Cy Young Award. But it was at a cost to his left elbow. On November 18, Koufax announced his retirement from baseball at the young age of 30. Because of his great performance in 1966, the retirement came as a great surprise to the general public, who knew little of what Koufax had to go through just to survive the season.[79]

Compartment Syndrome

KYLE LOHSE

In 2010 a new, unusual injury occurred in baseball. It had not been noted previously in the literature — chronic exertional compartmental syndrome of the upper extremity in a major league pitcher.

Compartment syndromes are difficult to explain. The muscles and nerves of the extremities are enclosed in compartments surrounded by fascial tissue. For instance, the muscles of the forearm are divided into flexors (bend wrist in) and extensors (straighten wrist out). The flexors attach to the inside of the elbow (medial epicondyle) and the extensors to the outside (lateral epicondyle). Both groups of muscles are separated by fascial tissue (connective tissue) that keeps the compartments separate.[80]

The same applies to the calf muscles. The muscles here are divided mainly into four compartments. There are also compartments of the upper arm and thigh, but they are rarely if ever involved in compartment syndromes because there is much more space for the muscles, blood vessels, and nerves to expand.

A compartment syndrome, in the simplest terms, is an abnormal pressure buildup from swelling within the compartment causing pressure on the structures within the compartment, leading to pain, numbness, and tingling. The structures in a compartment can only expand to a certain extent during activity; blood return from the compartment to the heart is impaired, and this leads to pressure buildup and the lack of oxygen to the muscles, arteries, and nerves within the compartment. The pain one would have is similar to putting a tourniquet on, such as a blood pressure cuff inflated too high, with pressure high enough to allow blood to the arm but not back to the heart. Eventually one is going to have pain.[81]

There are acute compartment and chronic exertional compartment syndromes. The latter is more common. The acute form can develop after severe trauma, as in a fracture, and is an emergency. Blood cannot go into the tissue or return from the tissue. The extremity may swell and die, not from the fracture itself but from the pressure that has built up in the enclosed space, impairing blood to and from the arm or leg. An incision in the skin and fascia around the compartment needs to be made immediately.

The chronic exertional compartment syndrome, the more common form, is not an emergency in which the extremity may die. The pressure, which causes pain, does not build up high enough to warrant an emergency procedure.

The chronic from is exercise-related. When one exercises, pressure builds up in the compartment, and after exercising the pressure decreases. With the compartment syndrome, the pressure is higher than it would be for a normal individual. With exercise the affected individual has pain with impaired muscle function; often numbness or tingling is noted that eventually goes away with rest.

Pressure within the compartments can be measured with a catheter inserted into the compartment. They are checked before, during, and after exercise. The pressures are abnormally high with compartment syndromes, although the numbers are often only one and one-half times to two times the normal pressure.

A classic example of a compartment syndrome can occur with a runner. The runner gets pain in his calf after running a certain amount of time and at certain intensity (sometimes called shin splints). Usually the time period to onset of symptoms is one-half hour. It happens every time.

Why? With training (running), the muscles get bigger, causing increased pressure within the compartment. For the majority of us, the pressure build-up is never severe enough to cause symptoms that persist after running. Everyone gets sore muscles with training, but this is not caused by pressure build-up in the muscles. This pain is due to microtrauma and build-up of lactate in muscles, and these changes lessen with continued training over time.

One way to deal with the chronic exertional pain syndrome is to stop running or run short distances at a slow pace. Often a prolonged period of rest from the offending activity, one or two months, is tried, but this rarely ever corrects the problem. The other treatment is to have surgery to cut a slit in the fascial sheath around the muscles to allow more space for muscle expansion.

Why do people get chronic exertional compartment syndrome? Most often people just seem prone to develop it with particular forms of vigorous exercise. Sometimes there is a minor episode of trauma preceding the development of problems. A case is noted in the literature of a runner, having been hit by a softball in the leg, developing compartment syndrome months later in that same calf.[82]

Chronic exertional compartment syndromes are much more common in the legs than in the forearms. Rarely, weight lifters, motorcycle riders, and field hockey players develop chronic exertional compartment syndromes of the forearms. Now there is also a baseball pitcher.

Kyle Lohse is presently a starting pitcher for St. Louis Cardinals. He is in the middle of a four-year, $41 million dollar contract signed on September 29, 2008. His career record at the time was a mediocre 78–80, but was coming of a career-best year in which he had 15 wins and 6 losses with a career-low ERA of 3.78. His agent was Scott Boras.[83]

Lohse was first injured on May 23, 2009. In the eighth inning of a game, he was hit in the right forearm by a pitch from Kansas City Royals pitcher Ron Mahay. He did not pitch the ninth inning because of the injury but did end up the eventual winner in the 5–0 contest.

He missed his next start when he experienced weakness in his arm during a bullpen session. When he started on June 3, he aggravated the previous injury. The strain of the forearm (possibly a mild tear) occurred as he fielded a bunt attempt and threw awkwardly to first base from his knees.[84]

Apparently Lohse, in addition to the strain, was experiencing some swelling. He ended up on the DL for the first time in his eight-year career, and remained on the DL for 39 days because of forearm discomfort and swelling. To add insult to injury, soon after coming off the DL he landed right back on it with a groin muscle strain which occurred while he was running out a single on August 29, 2009.[85]

When he came back in September, he struggled. He had good velocity but poor command. He denied pain at that point; he just didn't feel right. An MRI of his forearm revealed nothing more than some inflammation in his forearm.[86]

In 2009 he went 6–10 with an ERA of 4.74, close to his career ERA of 4.70. But, likely his high ERA year in 2009 was inflated from 2008 mainly due to his injuries and trips to the DL.

The 2010 season did not go much better for Lohse. After a particularly bad start on May 22, he admitted his right arm was still not doing well. Lohse said, "I can go out there and feel fine, then in the middle of the inning, something happens. That was the case last year and that was what happened Saturday." He had a cramping sensation which got worse as he pitched, and on May 22, it was the worst ever. His stats also reflected a problem; he was 1–4 with an ERA of 5.89.[87]

Dr. Paletta, the Cardinals' team physician, examined Lohse again. Nerve conduction tests were normal. An MRI at rest showed nothing. When the MRI was repeated after exercise, inflammation was noted. A second opinion was given by Dr. Steven Shin at the Kerlan-Jobe Orthopedic clinic in Los Angeles.

The diagnosis: a chronic exertional compartment syndrome of the forearm. Lohse underwent a fascial release procedure on his right forearm by Dr. Shin on May 28, 2010. In the dugout on May 31, he was spotted wearing a wrap around his entire right forearm all the way to his fingers.

After surgery, the time of return from the DL was uncertain — maybe two months, maybe more; since this was thought to be the first time a pitcher had a fascial release of the forearm "the schedule is ultimately murky,"[88] according to an article on MLB.com.

In the end it was 85 days from Lohse's last start before surgery to his next start on August 15. His return was rocky as he gave up seven runs in only three innings, and he was the losing pitcher. On August 23 he defeated the Pirates, 10–2, pitching 5⅔ innings and giving up six hits and two runs.

In 2011 Lohse appeared to have completely recovered from his injury. He finished with 14 wins against 8 losses with a fine 3.39 ERA in 188 innings pitched.

NOAH LOWRY

One other pitcher having surgery for exertional compartment syndrome was Giants pitcher Noah Lowry. Lowry had surgery on his left forearm on March 7, 2008. He had been experiencing numbness when he gripped the ball. Lowry's surgery was not without some controversy as he continued to have problems complicated by pain in the back of his shoulder and neck. He was diagnosed with thoracic outlet syndrome and had surgery May 19, 2010, performed by Dr. Greg Pearl at Baylor University in Dallas. Lowry's first rib was removed. In between those surgeries, he had arthroscopic surgery for bone spurs on his elbow.[89]

Lowry's agent, Damon Lapa, claimed that the original surgery for the exertional compartment syndrome of the left forearm was incorrect and that the forearm numbness was caused by thoracic outlet syndrome, not the compartment syndrome. The Giants' representatives denied that there had been an incorrect initial diagnosis.[90] No information is available on whether the dispute was resolved, but Lowry did not pitch in the major or minor leagues after 2007.

Chapter 4

Wrist and Hand Injuries

Wrist Injuries

The most common reason for a wrist injury, other than trauma from a collision with another player or with a base during a headfirst slide, is overuse from swinging the bat. David Ortiz, Rickie Weeks, Mark DeRosa, Pat Burrell, and Nick Johnson have suffered this injury.

The tendons allow the wrist and hand to move. They have sheaths at the wrist that have two basic functions. First, they supply fluids to lubricate the tendons. Second, they hold the tendon in place so the muscle, tendon, and bone movement is coordinated. The sheath is a little like a pulley allowing the pull of the tendon on the bone. This causes movement with work done to optimal efficiency with the most strength transferred for movement. A disruption of the sheath, if complete, can allow the tendon to move about and not along a fixed path. This reduces strength and causes irritation by the tendon rubbing on adjacent structures, and the snapping sensation that results can be annoying.

A partial tear needs rest and splinting to heal, otherwise it might go on to become a complete tear. After rest, a partial tear can still cause problems. A complete tear more often than not needs surgery to restore the tendon sheath and supporting structures and return anatomical position and functioning. Rarely, with complete tears, if use of the wrist is not severely impaired, the player can tough it out, playing with the tear until the end of the season. Then the sheath surrounding the tendon can be fixed and the player will be just fine and ready for the next season.

DAVID ORTIZ

David Ortiz suffered a partially torn tendon sheath on May 31, 2008, in the Red Sox game against Baltimore, typically while swinging a bat. The tendon called the ECU, or extensor carpi ulnaris tendon, is located on the outside of the wrist extending from the base of the wrist on the side of the fifth finger up the forearm. The muscle then extends up to the elbow. Ortiz had to wear a cast for three weeks after the injury.[1]

Ortiz missed 45 games, returning to the Red Sox lineup on July 25. Over the rest of the season he reported little pain. That doesn't mean he didn't have problems, as he felt a clicking sensation in his wrist. He continued to play, though, taking an occasional day off. His season extended to the ALCS against the Tampa Bay Rays, which the Red Sox lost. Typical of Ortiz's loss of mobility the last part of the season, he struck out twice and grounded into a force out to end his and the Red Sox's season.[2]

Ortiz did not need surgery. By December of 2008, Ortiz was swinging the bat again after a period of rest. He started the 2009 season slow, not hitting his first home run till May 20, but he ended up the year with 28 home runs, knocking in 84 runs after May 20 to end the year with 99 RBI.[3]

Ortiz's stats from 2010 showed a better batting average than 2009 and a few more home runs and RBI, and in 2011 he was just as productive and batted over .300 for the first time since 2007.

RICKIE WEEKS

Rickie Weeks, second baseman for the Milwaukee Brewers, had an injury similar to David Ortiz's in 2009. At the time he was hitting .272 with nine home runs and 24 RBI.[4]

In typical fashion, Weeks completely tore the tendon sheath of the extensor carpi ulnaris tendon at the left wrist while striking out swinging during his first at bat during the game on May 17.[5]

As opposed to a partial tear of the tendon sheath, Weeks' complete tear required surgery. Hand specialist Dr. Don Sheridan performed surgery shortly after the injury. Oddly, Weeks had had the same injury and surgery during the 2006 season, though on the other wrist. Dr. Sheridan commented that he had never seen the injury before on both wrists.

Weeks missed the rest of the 2009 season, but had his best season in 2010.

MARK DEROSA

Mark DeRosa is a versatile player who can play multiple positions, though most often at second base or third base. He has played 14 years in the majors, breaking in with the Atlanta Braves in 1998 after being drafted in the seventh round of the 1996 amateur draft. His best years came from 2006 to 2009, when he played for the Texas Rangers, Chicago Cubs, Cleveland Indians, and St. Louis Cardinals. During that time he averaged 17 home runs and around 78 RBI per season.

On June 30, 2009, he suffered a torn tendon sheath in his left wrist, sustaining the injury while fouling off a ball on a swing in a game between the St. Louis Cardinals and the San Francisco Giants. DeRosa described feeling a "pop" when the injury happened. An article in the *San Jose Mercury News* in early 2010 said the initial injury occurred on a checked swing, not a foul ball. The article noted that DeRosa had no pain at the time of the injury.[6]

In a July 8, 2009, article by Joe Strauss in the *St. Louis Post Dispatch*, the June 30 injury is described:

> Mozeliak [Cardinals GM] insists that DeRosa's injury differs from the tendon sheath injury that sidelined Milwaukee second baseman Rickie Weeks for the season. The club believes it is instead similar to the condition that followed former infielder Juan Encarnacion for several months in 2006. Encarnacion remained active through the World Series before requiring surgery.[7]

DeRosa was on the DL for less than three weeks before returning to play, though he ended up hitting only .228 for the Cardinals. He had surgery for the completely torn tendon sheath in his left wrist on October 26, 2009.[8]

There was optimism for DeRosa's recovery after surgery, so much so that the San Francisco Giants signed him to a two-year contract on December 29, 2009, for $12 million. After spring training for the Giants, DeRosa's stats were poor in the early season, leading up to his being placed on the DL on May 8. At the time he was batting only .194 and had only one home run.[9]

When asked about his wrist, he denied having any pain. "DeRosa reported how his wrist clicks back and forth every time it is rotated, and he said it's unstable when he picks up small objects like the remote control or soda. He says it bothers him during every at-bat, adding that 'sometimes it feels like I have loose change in my batting glove.'"[10]

A second opinion by hand specialist Dr. Thomas Graham confirmed that indeed DeRosa had torn the tendon sheath again. After some failed attempts at rehab, DeRosa underwent surgery on Thursday, July 1, in Cleveland. Because he had some problems with hand numbness, a carpal tunnel release was done at the same time. Yes, major league players who use their wrists constantly, just like the general population, get carpal tunnel issues.[11]

DeRosa sat on the bench while San Francisco played in the World Series in 2010.

DeRosa had more problems in 2011 with his left wrist. He was on the DL in early April for inflammation. Then, on May 18, 2011, he injured his wrist simply cocking his bat getting ready to hit a pitch. DeRosa gripped his left wrist in pain and had to be immediately removed from the game, which he reacted to by slamming his helmet down inside the dugout in disgust.

An MRI a few days later revealed he had not torn the tendon sheath to the ECU tendon as he had in the past, but instead had a partial tear of the ECU tendon.

Before the latest injury he was batting only .162 (6 for 37) in 18 games played, and now he was on the DL for 60 days. He ended up playing in only 47 games total with 97 plate appearances in 2011. DeRosa was able to get his average up to .279 after his very slow start in April and May. DeRosa hit over 20 home runs in 2008 and 2009, but did not hit a single home run in 2011 and only hit 2 doubles in 24 hits. The problems with the left wrist appeared to be greatly affecting his power numbers.

Despite DeRosa's limited play in 2010 (26 games) and 2011 (47 games), the Washington Nationals felt that because of his ability to play multiple positions, the 37-year-old was worth signing for 2012 at a greatly reduced rate of $800,000.

NICK JOHNSON

Often injured Nick Johnson suffered a torn tendon sheath in his right wrist while playing for the Washington Nationals in 2008. In the typical fashion, the injury occurred during an at-bat on May 11. Rehab without surgery was unsuccessful, and he underwent surgery on June 24, missing the rest of the season.[12]

Johnson was able to play 133 games for the Nationals and Marlins in 2009. In 2010, while playing for the Yankees, he again had trouble with the same problematic wrist, in the same location where he had the previous injury.

The inflamed tendon did not respond to a cortisone shot on May 9, and he ended up needing surgery on May 18. When the wrist did not respond, he had a second surgery on August 26, 2010. With the second surgery, one source noted that the tendon was once again unstable. Johnson has not played in the majors since May 8, 2010.[13]

PAT BURRELL

Pat Burrell, then of the Philadelphia Phillies, suffered a torn tendon sheath in his left wrist in 2004 during batting practice. The tear was the ECU tendon sheath. Surgery was initially scheduled but when Burrell responded to rest and a cortisone shot, surgery was avoided.

He was on the DL from August 3 until September 3, and hit a home run, number 19 for the season, in his first game back from rehab. Unlike Nick Johnson, research did not reveal that Burrell had any further problems with the wrist after 2004.[14]

The injury to the tendon sheath is not common, usually occurs while batting, and is an overuse injury from the repeated batting process, both practice and in game situations.

Hamate Fractures

Fractures of the bones of the wrist can occur in baseball or any other sport for that manner. Baseball shares with tennis and golf a rather uncommon fracture of the wrist, a fracture of the hook of the hamate bone.

There are eight small carpal bones in the wrist. Fractures usually occur to only a few of these bones, the exception being severe traumatic injuries where any of the bones can be broken or crushed. With wrist carpal bone fractures, it would seem the same bones are fractured over and over.

The scaphoid bone, a bone at the base of the thumb, is by far the most common carpal bone fracture of the wrist. It accounts for almost 70 percent of all wrist fractures of the carpal bones in the 15- to 30-year-old population.

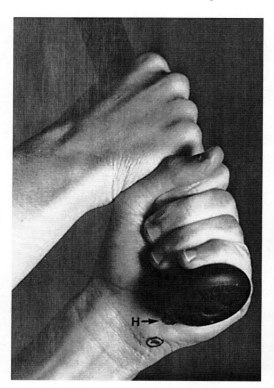

The mechanism of injury is most commonly falling on the wrist with the wrist bent back 90 degrees and the wrist turned slightly inward.[15]

Bob Horner sustained this fracture twice, once while diving for a batted ball while playing third base, and once while sliding into second base.

A rarer fracture of the wrist's carpal bones is a fracture of the hook of the hamate bone. This accounts

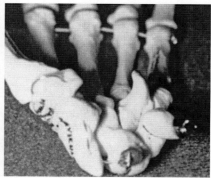

Left: Location of hamate bone hook (H) relative to bat end in non-dominant left hand of a right-handed hitter. (From Richard D. Parker's "Hook of the Hamate Fractures in Athletes" in *The American Journal of Sports Medicine* 14, 6 [1986]: 517. Reproduced by the permission of Sage Science Press.) *Right:* Palmar (palm) view of the left wrist and hand showing the hook of the hamate bone near the base of the fifth metacarpal. The hook part of the bone is what is fractured. (This figure was published in *Hand Clinics* 16 [2000]: 397–403, Figs. 3 and 4. Copyright Elsevier 2000.)

for only two to four percent of all fractures of the wrist. However, it is not uncommon in sports that require the swinging of an object held in the hand, such as a baseball bat, tennis racquet, or golf club. In baseball the wrist most often injured is the non-dominant hand, the one that is closest to the knob of the bat. The mechanism of injury is direct pressure on the hook. This pressure is especially marked on a checked swing, the batter attempting to stop his swing without hitting the ball. The complete fracture often occurs suddenly.

Then there is an incomplete fracture called stress fracture. Repeated stress on the bone day after day can lead to this, thus the name. The symptoms are pain of varying amounts where the bone is located, near the base of the palm of the hand and distal to the ulnar bone at the wrist. X-ray findings of a stress fracture may not be apparent on a plain x-ray and may only be seen on a special x-ray called a bone scan. When the fracture is diagnosed, avoiding the inciting activity is prescribed. Up to six weeks of rest is sometimes recommended. Even rest may not be enough to prevent the incomplete stress fracture from becoming a complete fracture when activity is resumed.[16]

CANSECO TWINS

The Canseco twins give a classic example of hook of the hamate fractures. Both suffered the same fracture of the hamate bone in early 1989.[17]

Jose Canseco, the more successful of the two, was drafted in 1982, and briefly appeared for the Oakland A's first in 1985 at age 21. In 1986 he hit 33 home runs and had 117 RBI, leading to his winning the American League Rookie of the Year (ROY) Award. His peak year was 1988, at age 23, when he hit 42 home runs, had 124 RBI, and stolen 40 bases. He was the first player ever to hit at least 40 home runs and steal at least 40 bases in a year. For his effort, he was selected the American League MVP Award for 1988.

His career spanned 17 seasons for numerous teams including the Oakland A's, Texas Rangers, Boston Red Sox, Toronto Blue Jays, Tampa Bay Devil Rays, New York Yankees, and Chicago White Sox. He had a career .266 average with 462 home runs and 1407 RBI. His last season was 2001, although he continued playing in independent and minor leagues after that.

His chief notoriety has come from his book, *Juiced: Wild Times, Rampant 'Roids, Smash Hits, and How Baseball Got Big*. In it he confesses to using steroids and growth hormones, as well as pointing the finger at many other players using them. He reports experimenting with steroids very early in his career, as early as 1984. Whether the steroids and growth hormones had anything to do with his many injuries is purely speculation at this point.

Canseco's hamate fracture occurred during spring training in 1989. As commonly happens, the injury to the hook of the hamate was to his non-dominant left hand. He had no fracture present on initial exam and x-rays. It is unclear if he had a bone scan at the time, though that would have seemed logical. There was suspicion that he might have a stress fracture, and he was treated appropriately with rest and subsequent rehabilitation. On May 7, while he was taking batting practice, the hook of the hamate broke completely through.[18]

Jose Canseco had surgery to remove the broken hook of the hamate on May 10, 1989. The complex procedure lasted one hour and 45 minutes. It is a complex procedure because the ulnar nerve, which innervates the fourth and fifth fingers, passes very close to the hook of the hamate. It needs to be preserved. Also, there are ligaments and tendons attached to the hook of the hamate that have to be reattached to other fibrous tissue present in the wrist for the wrist to continue to function without problems.[19]

Ozzie Canseco, Jose's twin brother, broke the hook of the hamate during spring training of 1989. In Ozzie's case, there was no preceding stress fracture, and his hamate bone broke acutely. There was no period of pain before the fracture. Ozzie also had to have surgery to remove the broken hook of the hamate bone. As in Jose's case, he returned to playing baseball after a period of rest following surgery with no further reported problems related to the hamate hook. If the surgery is done correctly, one can function fairly well without this piece of bone, the hamate hook.[20]

The surgery to Ozzie's wrist did *not* help his baseball career, though. One inch shorter and over ten pounds lighter than Jose, Ozzie had only a very brief major league career spanning parts of three seasons with the Oakland A's and St. Louis Cardinals. Ozzie was late in developing into a hitter as he spent his first three years in the minor leagues in the New York Yankees' farm system as a pitcher.[21]

CARLOS GOMEZ

More recently, Carlos Gomez of the New York Mets broke the hook of the hamate of his non-dominant left hand. This occurred rather suddenly on a checked swing in a game on July 4, 2007, against the Colorado Rockies. Gomez was on the DL for eight weeks after having surgery to remove the broken hook of the hamate bone.[22]

Carlos Gomez had only played 42 games in the major leagues when the injury occurred. At present he is most famous for being the major part of the trade that sent Johan Santana from the Minnesota Twins to the Mets on February 2, 2008.[23] He played for the Twins in 2009 and then for the Milwaukee Brewers in 2010–2011.

OTHERS

Ryan Zimmerman of the Washington Nationals had surgery for a hamate fracture between in the 2007–2008 off-season after breaking it swinging a bat.[24]

More recently Joe Mather, a right-handed rookie outfielder for the St Louis Cardinals, broke his left hamate bone on a checked swing on August 25, 2008. He saw a hand specialist and had surgery on September 4, 2008.[25]

Canseco's injury after a stress fracture was obviously an overuse injury. The other hamate fractures were acute injuries. It is uncertain if any underlying structural weakening from overuse occurred prior to the acute bone fracture, though it is a distinct possibility.

Hand Injuries

There are many injuries to the hands. Getting a blister of the fingers where the pitcher grips the ball is very common. Sometimes the pitcher even ends up on the disabled list if the blister or skin ulcer does not heal. Nolan Ryan (see later discussion) suffered from finger blisters.

Also, repetitive motion can result in damage to tendon sheaths and tendons in the hands. More often than not the injury to the tendon sheaths occurs to pitchers, and the tear happens while throwing a breaking ball. The tendon sheaths in the hands, like those in the wrists, hold the tendon in place. Disruption of the tendon sheath in the hands, depending on the severity of the injury, does not always result in surgery. In pitchers, flexor tendon sheaths or pulleys, as they are also called, help to grip the ball and are much more frequently injured than extensor tendon sheaths.

Injury to tendon sheaths is from overuse. The damage occurs over time until the tendon sheath partially or completely ruptures because it is in a weakened condition.

ADAM WAINWRIGHT

Adam Wainwright, a right-handed pitcher for the St. Louis Cardinals, was originally drafted by the Atlanta Braves in the first round of the 2000 draft. He was traded to the Cardinals in 2003. In 2006 he pitched in relief and came on as the Cardinals' closer in the 2006 playoffs and World Series when Jason Isringhausen got injured at the end of the regular season. In 2007 Wainwright was converted to a starter and has been very successful since, winning 19 games in 2009 and 20 games in 2010.

In 2008 he suffered a partially torn tendon sheath of the flexor tendon of the middle finger of his right hand. On June 7, he noticed an "awkward snap" while warming up for a game against the Cincinnati Reds at Busch Stadium. In the sixth inning, while throwing a curveball, he heard a "tell-tale pop. The next pitch, a fastball, sailed wide." Wainwright was removed from the game and ended up on the losing end of a 5–1 score.[26]

Soon after that game, Wainwright was diagnosed with a tear of the tendon sheath (pulley) in the middle finger of the right hand. Wainwright was lucky. His injury was not so severe that he needed surgery. Following splinting, rest, and rehab, he was back pitching, though at the minor league level, in August of 2008. He experienced no further problems. He won only 11 games in 2008 but soon became one of the top pitchers in the National League winning 39 games in 2009 and 2010. However, in 2011 he underwent Tommy John surgery.

A *St. Louis Post-Dispatch* article on June 22, 2008, is a great source for information concerning the type of injury Wainwright had. In the article, Wainwright was informed that his type of injury occurs to about one pitcher a year at the major league level.

Other pitchers who have had a similar tendon sheath injury include John Maine of the New York Mets in 2006, Adam Eaton of the San Diego Padres in 2005, Ben Sheets of the Milwaukee Brewers in 2007, and Atlanta's John Thomson in 2005. In almost all cases the injury occurred while throwing a breaking ball. Quite often a popping sensation was felt at the time of the injury.[27]

More recently, pitcher Jorge De La Rosa of the Colorado Rockies suffered the torn tendon pulley of the middle finger of his left hand on April 25, 2010. Articles don't mention how he injured it, only that he was removed in the fifth inning after complaining of finger numbness. He was placed on the DL, started rehab in late June, and didn't pitch again in the majors until July 9.

Of the pitchers noted, Eaton was the only one to require surgery. He missed time in 2005 with a partial tear (strain) of the tendon sheath and then after he completely tore (split) the sheath in spring training of 2006, he had surgery.[28]

CARL CRAWFORD — EXTENSOR TENDON

Carl Crawford, an outfielder, suffered a torn tendon sheath in his right, non-throwing hand on a checked swing in a game against Seattle on August 9, 2008.[29]

As opposed to the pitchers noted with ruptured flexor tendon sheaths (inside of hand), Crawford ruptured the extensor tendon sheath, a tendon used to straighten the middle finger. After the injury, the extensor tendon was subluxing (sliding) out of its groove at the knuckle, impairing the finger's function.

Crawford required surgery on August 14 and missed the rest of the regular season. But he did make it back in time to play in the American League playoffs against the Chicago White Sox and Boston Red Sox and in the World Series, which his Tampa Bay Rays lost to the Philadelphia Phillies in five games.[30]

JOEL ZUMAYA — TENDON RUPTURE

Joel Zumaya, nicknamed Zoom Zoom, is an oft-injured middle reliever for the Detroit Tigers. The talented player, who often hits 100 mph on the radar gun, has been sidelined almost as much as he has pitched since making the major leagues in 2006 at the age of 21. His first season was his best with a 1.94 ERA and 97 strikeouts in 83⅓ innings.

In 2007 he suffered an unusual injury where he completely tore the flexor tendon off the end of the bone of his right middle finger. Called an avulsion injury, this is much more common in football, where it is often called a "jersey finger"[31] (tendon torn while grabbing an opposing player by the jersey).

How did this occur? The injury did not happen under any unusual circumstances. Zumaya was simply warming up, throwing in the bullpen, getting ready to come into a game on Saturday, May 5. He felt a pop on two pitches as he threw. Initially he thought he had dislocated the finger, but when the rather severe pain persisted into Sunday, further tests were ordered (MRI) and the torn tendon was found.[32]

The flexor tendon allows the pitcher to grip the ball and apply pressure on the ball up until the release point. Surgery was necessary to fix the injury. Dr. Charles Melone of New York, an orthopedic hand surgeon, operated on Zumaya's middle finger, re-attaching the tendon on May 10. Zumaya missed the next three months.[33]

Later in 2007, Zumaya suffered second injury, a freak off-the-field injury on October 27. While he was moving two boxes for his father, the heavier top box slipped, falling on Zumaya's right pitching shoulder. The box tore the ligaments in the acromioclavicular joint (AC joint), and the injury was severe enough that once again Zumaya had to have a surgery, performed on October 31. Happy Halloween![34]

In 2008, Zumaya suffered a stress fracture of his shoulder, and in 2010 he suffered a stress fracture of his elbow (see section on stress fractures).

SANDY KOUFAX — CLOTS IN HAND

Sandy Koufax's career was discussed under overuse elbow injuries. He also suffered a hand problem, a circulatory issue with his left index finger on his pitching hand. Edward Gruver, in his book *Koufax*, addresses this issue very well.[35]

In 1961 Koufax finished with 18 wins and 13 losses and the league's lowest ERA of 2.54. In light of this there was considerable optimism concerning his projected performance for 1962. In fact, in his first 18 decisions in 1962 Koufax was 14–4. At this point there was some speculation that Koufax might even win 30 games.

In mid–May, Koufax had begun to experience problems with numbness in his left index finger. Normally this should interfere with a left-hander's grip, but Koufax continued to pitch effectively without consequence.

However, on July 8, just before the All-Star Game, the course of events changed. The finger changed color from its normal pink to a reddish color. Just as significant, Koufax began to experience pain, very sharp in nature.

This change in symptoms prompted a visit to Dr. Robert Kerlan, the Dodgers' team physician. A wise physician, he recommended that Koufax see a vascular specialist to evaluate a possible circulatory problem in Koufax's hand. Koufax apparently didn't follow through with this plan right away. He waited until after the All-Star Game (in which he didn't pitch). In fact he didn't see a vascular specialist until after he had pitched in two more games following the All-Star Game.

During the first game, Koufax's symptoms changed once again. The problematic finger changed to a bluish-red color. If that wasn't bad enough, Koufax developed a blood blister at the end of the finger that broke open. As a consequence of the blister, Koufax was removed from the game after seven innings.[36]

Why Koufax was allowed to make another start is not clear. On July 17, he lasted only one inning before being removed, as the blood blister on the index finger once again broke open and the skin around it split.

Finally, after this abbreviated start, Koufax saw a vascular specialist, Dr. Travis Winsor. He suspected a vascular difficulty and ordered an arteriogram of Koufax's left shoulder and arm (pictures by X-ray taken after dye is injected into the arteries leading to the arm). The X-rays revealed decreased blood circulation in the left palm. Gruver makes no mention of a possible aneurysm present in the left shoulder which could send clots downstream to the hand, causing very similar symptoms to what Koufax was having (aneurysm was discussed previously under overuse injuries of the shoulder). There was no mention of an aneurysm. Only after the arteriogram was done did Koufax remember a possible traumatic event that could have led to his vascular problem.

Virtually 100 percent of the time, Koufax, a left-hander, batted right-handed. In major league history there have been very few left-handed throwers who bat right-handed exclusively. The opposite, a right-handed dominant player batting exclusively left-handed, is very common. Koufax, the left-hander, sustained his injury in one rare instance where he indeed switched over and batted left-handed. He did so against Pirates pitcher Earl Francis in a game in late April.[37]

Why Koufax decided to bat left-handed in this one particular instance is not clear. Maybe he was concerned that his batting right-handed was exposing his pitching arm to getting hit by a pitch. Koufax was a poor hitter, so maybe his decision was motivated by his poor right-handed batting average. Batting almost exclusively right-handed, Koufax ended up his career with a dismal .097 lifetime batting average with only 75 hits in 776 at-bats. He struck out almost half the times he came to bat, so he couldn't bat much worse left-handed than he batted right-handed. In fact, in this rare left-handed at bat Koufax got a hit.

Koufax was not hit by a pitch during this rare left-handed at-bat, but he was jammed by a pitch and hit the ball off the handle of the bat. In doing so, the bat pinched his left palm.[38] He recalled much later that he was concerned about the palm the rest of the game, but soon forgot about this slight injury in the many games that followed. Koufax was treated with shots and blood thinners for his circulatory problem. Unfortunately, before the circulation problem improved, Koufax developed an infection in this index finger. One needs good blood circulation to deliver oxygenated blood and infection-fighting white blood cells to an infected finger to clear an infection. With decreased circulation, even IV antibiotics can't get to the site where they are needed. Things were so bad at one stage there was concern that if the circulation didn't improve and the infection continued to spread, an amputation of the index finger might be necessary.[39]

This didn't happen. The circulation finally improved, and with this improvement the infection abated.

Koufax was on the DL for a long time, starting on July 17. When the index finger improved and after a brief period of rehabilitation, he came off the DL to pitch in game number 154 of the season, on September 21. Between that date and the end of the season he started two more games and pitched another in relief.

He started the first game of a three-game playoff series between the San Francisco Giants and the Dodgers. He lasted less than two innings and gave up three runs before being removed from the game. He was the losing pitcher as the Dodgers lost, 8–0. That was the end of Koufax's season as the Giants won the playoff series.

Koufax rested over the post-season and had no further problems. He came to spring training in 1963 and had no more difficulty with this index finger either that season or the rest of his career. He won 25 games in 1963 was named winner of both the Cy Young Award and National League Most Valuable Player Award.

Koufax had continued success from 1963 to 1966, experiencing no further problems with this index finger. This success, in addition to arteriogram findings, would tend to rule out the possibility of an aneurysm in Koufax's left shoulder. An aneurysm throwing clots distally to the left hand would be unlikely to go away on its own without any surgical intervention.

Thus, Koufax's traumatic event occurred when Koufax batted left-handed. This more than likely caused his circulation problem which almost resulted in the amputation of Koufax's index finger.[40]

Chapter 5

Ankle and Foot Injuries

Curt Schilling's Bloody Ankle

A torn tendon sheath at the wrist is similar to a torn sheath at the ankle. Curt Schilling had the latter injury in the playoffs and World Series in 2004.

Schilling pitched 20 years in the major leagues, retiring in 2007 with a fine record of 216 wins and 145 losses. In the post-season he has been outstanding with a record of 11–2 and an ERA of 2.23. He pitched for Baltimore, Houston, Philadelphia, Arizona, and Boston. His best years were for Arizona and Boston. With those two teams he won over 20 game three times and finished second in the Cy Young Award balloting in 2001, 2002, and 2004.

Schilling completely tore the tendon sheath around the peroneus brevis muscle tendon in his right ankle. The tendon is located on the outside of the ankle just below the fibula (ankle) bone. Like the tendon sheaths in the wrist, the tendon sheaths in the ankle help to hold tendons in their normal anatomic position. Schilling's right ankle was affected, the foot the right-hander uses to push off the rubber before throwing the baseball.

Schilling, playing for the Boston

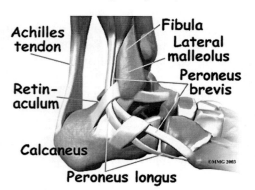

Inside view of structures of ankle. Medical records are not available, but possibly Curt Schilling tore the retinacular structure (part of tendon sheath), allowing the peroneus longus and brevis tendons to slide (sublux) from behind the ankle bone to the front of the ankle, impairing ankle function (used by permission of Medical Multimedia Group LLC).

Red Sox at the time, complained of some pain in the right ankle the last two weeks of the season. He was diagnosed as having tendonitis.[1] In the first game of the American League Division Series between the Anaheim Angels and Red Sox on October 5, Schilling aggravated the ankle injury, more than likely tearing the tendon sheath on a play in the seventh inning of a 9–3 victory for the Red Sox. While fielding a Garrett Anderson grounder, Schilling planted his foot to throw and threw wildly to first. Injured on the play, Schilling immediately grabbed his right ankle. He was removed from the game one batter later.

It would appear the full extent of the injury was not realized initially. Schilling was allowed to pitch in the first game of the League Championship Series against New York with no further treatment other than a local anesthetic at the site of his pain. In the game on October 12, Schilling fared poorly, allowing six runs in only three innings of work before being removed from the game. He had trouble with his balance and with pushing off the rubber, thus diminishing the velocity on his fastball.[2]

After the game, further tests were done which revealed the full extent of Schilling's problem. He had torn the tendon sheath of one of the peroneus tendons in his right ankle. Unless some novel treatment was found, he would not be able to pitch again in the playoffs.

A treatment was found. Red Sox medical director Bill Morgan came up with the novel idea of suturing the skin to the deep connective tissue on either side of the tendon in the ankle to prevent the tendon from subluxing in and out of place. The procedure, never done before, was tested on cadavers before being used on Schilling. Just before the sixth game of the playoffs between the Yankees and Red Sox, three sutures were inserted into the skin on either side of Schilling's peroneus brevis tendon, and local anesthetic was injected to relieve pain. The result was a success. Schilling pitched seven innings, giving up only one run, leading the Red Sox to a 4–2 victory on October 12. The three sutures Schilling had inserted in his ankle before Game 6 were removed immediately after the game.[3]

The Red Sox won the seventh game of the ALCS, 10–3. This marked a dramatic first-time rally from a three games to nothing deficit to win a seven-game ALCS.

It was apparent that Schilling would once again need to have the tendon sutured in place to be able to pitch in the World Series against the St. Louis Cardinals. After another quick fix before the second game of the World Series, Schilling was able to pitch six innings, giving up only two runs in the Red Sox's 6–2 victory. His sock became blood-stained in the process.

A side note: before the game against the Cardinals on October 24, four sutures were inserted instead of the three inserted during the American League Championship Series against the Yankees. But one suture was inadvertently inserted around a nerve, causing Schilling considerable pain. The extra suture was removed before Schilling started to pitch, and the rest is history.[4]

There were reservations expressed by Dr. Morgan as to whether a third procedure should be done if Schilling needed to pitch again. Permanent damage was the risk. As fate would have it, this was not the case as the Red Sox won the World Series in four games. The "Curse of the Bambino" was lifted; the Red Sox finally won a World Series, the first since the ill-fated sale of Babe Ruth from the Red Sox to the Yankees following the 1919 season.[5]

Schilling needed a more lasting fix to the torn tendon sheath after the World Series victory. He had a three-hour procedure to repair the injury, done by Drs. George Theodore and Bill Morgan at Caritas St. Elizabeth's Medical Center on November 9, 2004. At the same time as the tendon sheath repair, they did "debridement"—smoothing out of a small cartilage defect in the ankle joint.[6]

The famous bloody sock Schilling wore in Game 2 of the World Series was later enshrined in the Baseball Hall of Fame along with other Red Sox memorabilia to commemorate the end of the Red Sox's 86-year World Series title drought.[7]

David Freese

A similar injury, though not nearly as famous, is the injury to Cardinals third baseman David Freese. Freese started off 2010 as an early candidate for Rookie of the Year with a .296 average, four home runs and 36 RBI in 70 games. But he went on the DL on June 28 with a deep bone bruise in his right ankle.

Then a series of mishaps ended his season. First, he fractured his left big toe while working out with weights during rehab. Then, while at AA Springfield on a rehab assignment from the toe injury, he injured himself running the bases. He had doubled, and a single allowed him to try to score. While rounding third, Freese heard a "pop" and pulled up 30 feet shy of home plate.

He sustained a torn tendon sheath, according to Cardinals general manager John Mozeliak something "similar to the wrist injury Mark DeRosa" sustained. It was also similar to Curt Schilling's ankle injury. Freese required surgery to correct the torn tendon sheath.[8]

An article by Joe Strauss said the tendon "slipped from behind Freese's ankle (bone) to in front"[9] (something that would have happened to Curt Schilling had his tendon not been tacked down with sutures).

Reconstructive surgery on the problematic right ankle was done by Dr. Thomas Clanton at the Steadman Clinic in Vail, Colorado, on August 5, 2010. Later Freese required a minor cleanup on his left ankle, also done at the Steadman Clinic. Both ankle problems may have started with a car accident in January of 2009 when the floorboard of Freese's car slammed into his feet when he "plowed into a ditch."[10]

The 2011 season went better for Freese with a .297 batting average, ten home runs, and 55 RBI, helping to lead the Cardinals into the post-season. And, the post-season went even better as Freese ended up being chosen the NLCS MVP and World Series MVP. He will always be remembered for his key hits in game number six of World Series: a two run triple in the bottom of the ninth to tie the game and a home run to win the game in the eleventh. In the post-season Freese ended up batting .397 with 25 hits in 65 at bats with 5 home runs and 21 RBI.

Plantar Fasciitis

Heel pain manifesting as plantar fasciitis is a common problem in the general population. One would assume plantar fasciitis would be a common major league injury, but there isn't much news about it. There have been some isolated cases reported in the news in recent years: Shannon Stewart of the Oakland A's, Troy Glaus of the Toronto Blue Jays, and Albert Pujols of the St. Louis Cardinals. The conclusion: plantar fasciitis just doesn't make for big news unless the player might or does end up on the DL. Most players are able to play through the milder symptoms of plantar fasciitis, and newspapers rarely report these cases.

There are many activities in baseball that result in increased pressure on the heel and connective tissue (plantar fascia) of the arch of the foot. The primary cause of the pressure is running, often from sudden bursts of speed as well as sudden starting, stopping, and sudden changes in the direction. In addition, there are twisting and pivoting movements on the player's feet. These activities are experienced on the field by positional players, on the base paths by runners, and in the batter's box by the batter. These activities are repetitive in nature, done game after game. The wear and tear over the long season, and season after season, results in plantar fasciitis. With advancing age the normal healing process is slowed, hastening the development of the medical problem.

The technical name is plantar fasciitis, an inflammation indicated by the suffix "itis." Yet there is usually very little inflammation, but rather buildup of scar tissue from the degeneration of the plantar fascia tissue, the connective tissue that helps to form the arch of your foot, and the tissue that runs from the heel to the toes on the bottom of the foot. In addition to thickening of the plantar fascia, calcium deposits develop with this scarring and can lead to what is called a heel spur: a protrusion of bone coming off the heel bone, usually running parallel to the plantar fascia and deep beneath the skin. It cannot be felt by your hand. The spur is most often only seen on an X-ray of the heel and foot.[11]

The presence of a heel spur on an X-ray does not necessarily indicate a diagnosis of plantar fasciitis. Ten to 20 percent of the general adult population have a spur in one heel or the other. When you look selectively at the population with plantar fasciitis, the portion with a heel spur goes up dramatically, to 50 to 70 percent. In other words, having a heel spur does not make the diagnosis of plantar fasciitis, but if you do have plantar fasciitis, you are much more likely to have a heel spur.[12]

Baseball players, like the general population, have anatomic problems that can contribute to the development of plantar fasciitis. Flat feet, high arches, and the tendency to turn your foot in excessively (called pronation) are all factors. George Sheehan, the running doctor, cited a problem called "Morton's foot" as a possible contributing factor.[13] This is a condition where the second toe is longer than the first, unfortunately something you are just born with. In the older population, hammer toes and bunions can contribute to the problem. Other than recent information on Jim Edmonds of the Cardinals, research did not reveal any other major league players having hammer toes. There is no mention of Edmonds having plantar fasciitis.[14]

The treatment of the vast majority of cases of plantar fasciitis is conservative, not surgical (maybe one reason there are not a ton of major league players in the news as having this problem). Stretching of the arch and shoe orthotics that take some pressure off the arch are first-line treatments. As anatomically there is little or no inflammation noted, anti-inflammatory drugs such as aspirin, ibuprofen, and naprosyn, though helping the pain, do very little to lead to resolution of the underlying cause. Cortisone shots often help the pain in the short term, but in the long term do very little to clear up the cause — the damage and the degenerating tissue. Cortisone also has the rare but undesirable complication of rupture of the planter fascia secondary to soft tissue weakening. In one study, the rupture rate was 2.4 percent, with 2.67 injections the average.[15] Cortisone can also cause a reduction in the fat pad on the bottom of the foot (fat cell lysis). Less padding on the bottom of your foot is something to avoid as it leads to increased pressure on the plantar fascia.[16]

There are newer methods to relieve plantar fasciitis. ESWT, extracorporal shock wave treatment, one of these newer methods, was developed as a spin-off of another procedure used to break up kidney stones without surgery, called lithotripsy. The shock waves are directed to the tissues in the heel. The treatments lead to inflammation in the damaged tissues and growth of new, very small blood vessels, thus stimulating the healing process. At the same time it often breaks up some of the calcification damage present. One to three treatments are often used. Three systems for the delivery of the sound waves are pulses are currently available: OssaTron, Epos Ultra, and Orbasone machines.[17]

Another treatment, though not well known, is prolotherapy. Here a concentrated dextrose solution is injected into the site of the pain. The results or goals are similar to those with ESWT, increased inflammation leading to healing. Unfortunately, presently there isn't FDA approval for the use of prolotherapy for plantar fasciitis; it is considered investigational.[18] Injection of platelet-rich plasma is also investigational.

In the past (50 to 60 years ago) in the United States, x-rays were used to treat plantar fasciitis. X-rays cause inflammation leading to healing, the desired effect. One has to limit the dosage of the x-rays. In the U.S., x-ray treatments have not been used for some time because of the concern over the development of cancer post-treatment. In Europe, x-rays are still used to treat plantar fasciitis though with low dosages of radiation, probably much lower than the rads (radiation dosage) used by American physicians many years ago.[19]

The last resort, as it should be, is surgery. It can involve one of three things: debridement of the scar tissue, removal of the bone spur if present, and/or excision (separation) of the attachment of the plantar fascia at the heel bone. Most often the excision of the plantar fascia is partial, not complete (see Mark McGwire later in this text). Surgical excision is the most drastic treatment. All three possible surgical procedures can be done at once, or just one or two. At the major league level, any type of surgery usually makes the news. From the information researched, surgery for plantar fasciitis, at least on the major league level, is rare.

JOE DIMAGGIO

The Yankee Clipper, Joe DiMaggio, had probably the best-known case of plantar fasciitis and heel spurs of any major leaguer. He developed the heel problem in both feet in his early to middle 30s.

Joe DiMaggio played 13 seasons for the Yankees from 1936 to 1951, excluding the war years of 1943–1945. For the vast majority of his career, he manned center field for the Yankees. He is probably best known for his 56-game hitting streak in 1941, which still stands. He was a three-time MVP. His best season was 1937 when he hit .346 with 46 home runs, 167 RBI, and 215 hits. He had a better average from 1939 to 1941 (.381, .352, and .357) but he never had as many hits, homers or RBI as in 1937. He finished with a career .325 average and was subsequently inducted into the Baseball Hall of Fame in 1955.

DiMaggio's first trouble with his heels started on the left side. His obituary in the *Washington Post* in 1999 indicates this case of plantar fasciitis and heel spur had much to do with his limited playing time in 1946, only 132 games played.[20]

Richard Ben Cramer, in *Joe DiMaggio: The Hero's Life*, indicates that DiMaggio began having trouble with his left heel very early in the 1946 season, around May.[21] In June, he caught his spikes while sliding into second base and tore up his knee (Cramer doesn't say which one) and sprained his ankle. Afterward this injury, he favored the knee and in doing so aggravated the heel. Diagnostic x-rays were taken and revealed a three-inch heel spur.

DiMaggio played through the heel pain the remainder of the 1946 season. There was hope that with decreased physical activity in the off-season, the heel problems would improve. When his symptoms didn't improve despite plenty of rest, the decision was made to proceed with surgery. The surgery was performed on January 7, 1947, at Johns Hopkins University. A five and one-half inch incision was used to remove the three-inch bone spur (a possible plantar fascia release is not mentioned).[22]

Complications developed post-surgery, an infection along the incision.[23] He was treated initially with the relatively new drug Penicillin. When he failed to respond to the antibiotic, maggots were used to eat away at the dead tissue (yes, maggots). When the infection did finally clear up, he had developed a significant area on bottom of the foot devoid of any skin. A skin graft was done to cover the exposed area, using skin from his thigh. The graft worked. All healed well except for a persistent small hole on the bottom of his foot.[24]

Despite good progress, doctors still didn't expect DiMaggio to start playing center field until June or July. He wouldn't hear anything of it. He got a special padded shoe and played, only missing a few days at the beginning of the 1947 season.[25]

His other heel, the right one, began to bother him just a week and a half into the 1948 season[26] and bothered him all year. He stated that it felt "like an ice pick was stabbing me."[27] With the onset of the right heel problems, he had special shoes with high arches ordered.[28] He continued to have other health issues: he came down with a bad charley horse in his thigh, and in compensating for this injury made his heel worse.

When the off-season didn't improve his right heel symptoms, he again went under the knife, having surgery on the right heel on November 11, 1948, to remove yet another bone spur.[29] He did not develop complications of an infection this time, but the surgery did not cure his heel pain either. When testing the heel during an exhibition game against the Class B Greenville Majors, he had to come out of the game on April 10, limping. When he didn't improve the next two days, he was admitted April 13 to Johns Hopkins for observation and initiation of treatments. His treatments were "injections and X-rays,"[30] which were continued after his discharge on April 14. Other medical details, as so often happens, are lacking in the lay press information available.

DiMaggio's heel continued to bother him through April and May. He started participating in practice exercises — running, shagging flies, and batting — in early to mid–June. He didn't return to the starting lineup until June 28, more than two months into the season.[31]

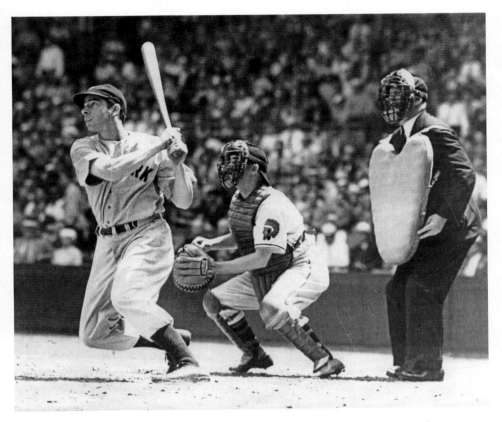

Joe DiMaggio batting in 1936 or 1937. Names of catcher and umpire are unknown (National Baseball Hall of Fame Library, Cooperstown, New York).

How did Joe DiMaggio's heel finally get better? Jack B. Moore in his book *Joe DiMaggio: Baseball's Yankee Clipper*, cites two different accounts told by the "Clipper" himself.[32] He cites an autobiography by DiMaggio called *Lucky to Be a Yankee* in which DiMaggio states that his symptoms gradually got better. Moore also cites an article on DiMaggio in *Life* magazine (August 1, 1949), quoting him as saying the heel pain just suddenly got better: "one morning I stepped out of bed, expecting the pain to shoot through the heel as usual. Nothing happened."[33] The heel, which had felt hot before, now was not: "Now it was cool."[34] Along the lines of sudden improvement is an off-hand reference to his mother, Rosalie DiMaggio, praying for Joe's improvement and then suddenly having her prayers answered.

Ultimately, DiMaggio's heel problems didn't cause his retirement. A variety of other ailments (shoulder, neck, muscle pulls, elbow, etc), led to DiMaggio's retirement. It is thought by many that he could have played on and still been productive. Despite what was then a large salary ($100,000), he decided to retire after the 1951 season at the age of 37, not willing to face continued injuries and further declining ability.[35] He passed the center field torch on to the next New York Yankees center fielder, Mickey Mantle.

MARK MCGWIRE

Mark McGwire played in the major leagues for 16 seasons (11½ with Oakland and 4½ with St Louis). He was the American League Rookie of the Year in 1987 and he broke Roger Maris's one-season record of home runs in 1998 when he hit 70 (a record later broken by Barry Bonds). It is a surprise that despite his great power numbers he never won an MVP award, finishing a close second to Sammy Sosa in 1998. He ended up hitting 583 home runs during his career, but because of questions of steroid use, he received only a 25 percent vote on his first year of Hall of Fame balloting.[36]

During the 1993 and 1994 seasons his future was in question because of left heel problems. He played only 74 games in those two seasons.

McGwire first developed a stress fracture in the left heel in early 1993, putting him on the DL for 43 days. Later he developed plantar fasciitis and a few other ailments that limited him to 27 games played in 1993. When conservative measures failed to alleviate his heel problems, he had surgery on September 24 performed by Dr. Donald Baxter, a foot specialist at Baylor University. Dr. Baxter's procedure was to release (surgical excision of attachment) 30 percent of the lateral plantar fascia and remove a small bone spur. This failed to resolve McGwire's heel pain, and he again suffered pain much of 1994 despite continued conservative measures.[37]

On August 30, 1994, McGwire had a complete release of the plantar fascia from its attachment at the heel bone. One would think that a complete excision of the attachment of the plantar fascia would lead to the loss of the arch of the foot, since the plantar fascia forms a fibrous band from the heel to the toes, but this is not the case. McGwire went on to play eight more seasons. When his career ended after the 2001 season, it was not plantar fasciitis that ended it, but a variety of ailments including a bad knee.[38]

Why had ESWT (extracorporal shock wave therapy) not been tried on McGwire's heel before any surgical intervention was considered? It was because the ESWT procedure as done by OssaTron was not approved by the FDA for the treatment of plantar fasciitis until October of 2000.[39]

ALBERT PUJOLS

Most baseball fans are well acquainted with Albert Pujols. He is the first major league player to start his career with ten consecutive seasons of 30 home runs, 100 RBI, and a batting average above .300. He was the unanimous National League Rookie of the Year in 2001, and he won the National League MVP award in 2005, 2008 and 2009. He has finished a close second place in the MVP balloting four other times.

In addition, Albert Pujols has suffered with plantar fasciitis. He began having trouble with his heels the last four months of the 2004 season, only his fourth season in the major leagues. Age 24 is very young to have this particular medical problem.

He had pain in both heels, but much worse in the left heel than in the right. The pain was described as a chronic soreness with an occasional sharp pain. Often during the 2004 season, he had to spend 30 to 40 seconds girding up to get out of bed in the morning.[40]

Cardinals trainer Barry Weinberg stated that every type of conservative treatment possible was used short of giving Pujols a cortisone shot. He was fitted with special cushion inserts to go into the heels of his cleats. Still, with all the difficulty Pujols had, he managed to play 154 regular-season games and 15 post-season games in 2004. When rest in the off-season didn't improve his symptoms to a significant degree, surgery for the problematic left heel was seriously considered in early November. Instead, on November 10 he received his first OssaTron treatment (ESWT) using shock sound waves (pulses). His response was excellent and he had very little discomfort for over a month and a half, but his pain gradually came back around the middle of January 2005. Because of his favorable response with his first treatment, a second OssaTron treatment was given.[41]

Once the 2005 season began, he again had some pain in the left heel, but not bad enough to warrant the one or two days off needed for a third ESWT treatment. He missed very little time in 2005 playing in 161 games plus nine post-season games.

Two weeks after the post-season ended, there was Pujols getting another OssaTron treatment. The subsequent off-season was uneventful. Upon returning to spring training in 2006, he again had some discomfort and he said he would probably undergo yet another ultrasound treatment for plantar fasciitis before the team's home opener on April 3.[42]

Since his four treatments by OssaTron over two years (late 2004–early 2006), Pujols has had no significant problems with his heel other than occasional flare-ups.[43]

Chapter 6

Stress Fractures

Stress fractures involve injuries to many different bones in the body — lower extremity, spine, and upper extremity. It seems appropriate for discussion to group them together, as the mechanism of the injury to the bones is similar.

Stress fractures are not caused by a single traumatic event (e.g., collision). With stress fractures, there are multiple small insults to the bone over time. The bone simply is not able to tolerate these repetitive stresses that are applied to it. It becomes damaged, thus the term stress fracture.

Quite often, and in many sports, stress fractures are due to training error — doing too much too soon, before the body is ready to perform at a peak level. In baseball such injuries, unless they occur during spring training after the long off-season, are more likely due to stresses applied over the long season, activities that tax the body to the limit over an extended period of time.

Most often a stress fracture is not visible on a plain x-ray film (no fracture line). This is not usually the case when trauma is involved; most often the plain film is abnormal when there is a trauma-induced fracture.

A proper understanding of stress fractures must include a proper understanding about the nature of bones. Bones are a dynamic organ system. Often when people consider the nature of the human skeleton, they think of the static set of bones one would note in a science or anatomy class, or maybe in a museum. These skeletons are static, unchanging. But human bones are dynamic, constantly changing and adapting to a changing environment.

Bone is both organic (has carbon in it) and inorganic (no carbon atoms). The organic consists of nerves, blood vessels, connective tissue, and cells of many types, including cells that make bone matrix and cells that break down bone matrix. The inorganic part, mainly consisting of calcium salts, is interwoven together within the bone matrix. The inorganic is also dynamic as there is an equilibrium state between the calcium in the bone and the calcium in the blood stream, as well as the calcium intake in one's diet.[1]

The bone consists of spongy bone and compact bone. The more porous spongy bone is more dynamic. It is said that the entire spongy bone in your body, the type that is more vascular, is completely replaced every three years. The compact bone, the harder of the two, is replaced completely in the body every ten years.[2]

Bone responds like muscles to stresses put on them. In addition to experiencing considerable muscle soreness from running the first time, this can put considerable stress on the bones, especially if one is unprepared adequately to start a running program. We will note the muscle soreness the next day after running if unprepared, but we will not notice bone soreness initially.

Training error is the most common cause of stress fractures.[3] One needs time to condition one's bones, just as one needs time to condition one's skeletal muscles, heart, and lungs. To put too much stress on our bones before they are able to adapt and strengthen in response to exercise over time can result in damage to them. This damage may not be noticeable right away. This slight damage builds over time if it is not allowed to heal, resulting in a stress fracture. It could begin in spring training, a period of intense training, and symptoms might not manifest fully until the regular season is well under way.

In baseball, it is not just training error. The baseball season lasts a long time, 162 regular season games in addition to all those spring training games, another contributing factor to development of stress fractures. There are repetitive activities such as throwing and batting that stress the bones to the limit; these lead to the bones becoming injured.

The stress fracture presents initially with pain both perceived and felt. The skin and tissue over the stress fracture site is tender. There might be some swelling at the fracture site, but usually not. Usually there isn't a fracture line seen on plain x-ray. An MRI or bone scan, though, will show the fracture in a very high percentage of the cases.[4] Often at onset, the player has pain with activity only, but if untreated the stress fracture symptoms progress, giving pain both with activity and with rest.

Most stress fractures heal with rest. Some do not. Not treated, a fracture line may eventually become visible on a plain X-ray. Depending on location and the severity of the fracture, surgery may be needed to insert a rod in the shaft of the bone or brace it with metal pins or screws. Even bone grafts to aid healing are needed for certain fractures.

Some locations are worse than others. Fractures of the neck of the femur (just adjacent to the hip) are much more serious than other stress fractures and much more likely to result in the bone breaking completely if not recognized and treated. These are more likely to need a rod put into the shaft of the bone to stabilize the fracture, preventing possible breakage (see example of Ryan Ludwick). Frank Thomas' navicular fracture in his foot is a type seen more often in basketball players and is notorious for not healing well. Surgical intervention is often needed to get the fracture to heal. A pin or screw is needed, and sometimes a graft of bone tissue to the fracture is required.

The exact incidence of stress fractures compared to all possible injuries is not clear. "A great deal of variation exists among studies reporting stress fractures as a portion of total athletic injuries."[5] No studies that specifically looked at the incidence of stress fractures in baseball were found, compared to all other injuries.

Generally speaking, stress fractures are more likely to be in the lower extremities (pelvis, legs, and feet). One study in the *American Journal of Sports Medicine* looked at a broad spectrum of athletes and indicated that bone scan-positive lower extremity stress fractures make up more than 90 percent of the total stress fractures seen at a sports medicine clinic over a 3.5-year period.[6]

This makes sense as the lower extremity bones do most of the work in supporting our body against gravity. Any sport that requires running (e.g., baseball) would result in more frequent lower extremity stress fractures.

Stress fractures are common, especially in runners. Studies have shown this injury to be 4.7 percent to 15.6 percent of all running injuries. Track and field runners, jumpers, and distance runners have a higher incidence of lower extremity stress fractures than baseball players, though no studies were found of baseball players that directly make this comparison.[7]

Upper extremity stress fractures do occur in baseball players (mostly because of throwing the baseball and swinging the bat). A review study in *Clinics in Sports Medicine* in 2006 specifically looked at the occurrence of upper extremity stress fractures and simply noted that certain types occur more so in baseball players compared to other sports. These fractures noted are ribs, clavicle (collar bone), humerus (upper arm), elbow, and forearm (ulna). Stress fractures of the hands or wrist in baseball players were not mentioned even though gripping and swinging the bat might cause this type of fracture.[8]

Previously discussed was Jose Canseco's hamate (wrist bone) fracture. Even though the bone broke completely in a rather sudden manner, there was a stress fracture preceding the complete break. Rest had been prescribed prior to the development of the fracture line, but a period of rest in Canseco's case was not successful in preventing further injury. At the time of the acute fracture, Canseco was swinging the bat.

Lower Extremity Stress Fracture

PAUL O'NEILL

Outfielder Paul O'Neill played 17 years in the majors, eight with Cincinnati and nine with the New York Yankees. It is with the Yankees that he is best remembered. He was involved in the post-season seven straight years with the Yankees, including four World Series titles with the Yankees (plus one with the Reds). He had a career .288 average with 281 homers and 2,105 hits in 7,318 career at-bats. He even stole 141 bases in his career. His best years were with the Yankees, with at least 100 RBI in four straight seasons, 1997–2000.

In his last season he sustained a stress fracture.[9] On Friday, September 7, he was running from first base to third base when he felt pain in his left foot. After this he had trouble even walking. An MRI on September 10 revealed a stress fracture of his fourth metatarsal. The appearance of the fracture on an MRI would tell the difference between an acute fracture and a stress fracture. It was thought O'Neill would be out only two to three weeks, during which time he was to wear a protective boot.

As it turned out, he returned in four weeks, in time to play in the Yankees' 2001 post-season which went well until they lost the World Series to the Arizona Diamondbacks in seven games. O'Neil had 11 hits in 38 post-season at bats in 2001, including two home runs.

MARK MULDER

Mark Mulder, then of the Oakland Athletics, suffered a stress fracture near the top of the right femur bone in August of 2003.[10]

Mulder was originally diagnosed with tendonitis in the right hip. A precautionary MRI revealed he had a stress fracture. The location of the fracture should not be a surprise, as Mulder, a left-hander planted his right leg when he threw across his body, putting stress on his right femur. From the discussion in newspaper articles, the location of the stress fracture was near the greater trochanter.

Nothing is mentioned of the femur needing to be pinned, as in the next case, Ryan Ludwick. Treatment for Mulder involved placing him on crutches, which he apparently did for almost a month.

RYAN LUDWICK

Ryan Ludwick played for the San Diego Padres and

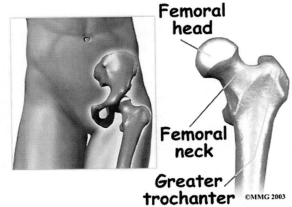

Location of greater trochanter relative to other structures of hip is indicated (used by permission of Medical Multimedia Group LLC).

Pittsburgh Pirates in 2011. In 2008, while playing for the Cardinals, he posted several career highs; he played in 152 games with a .299 average, 161 hits, 37 home runs, and 113 RBI in 538 at-bats. This, though, was his first *full* season in the majors, as his six-year major league career had been marked by numerous trips to the DL for various injuries. Along with these injuries, Ludwick had been up and down between the major leagues and the minor leagues.

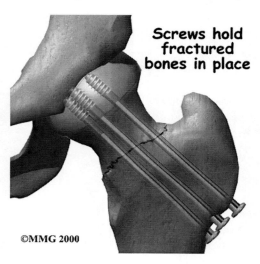

Screws hold fractured bones in place

©MMG 2000

Possible site of Ryan Ludwick's hip pinning if stress fracture involved neck of femur bone (used by permission of Medical Multimedia Group LLC).

His most serious injury, a stress fracture, occurred in 2002 while playing for the Oklahoma RedHawks minor league team. He had been up with the Texas Rangers in June and played 21 games in center field, but after hitting only .235, he was sent down to the Rangers' Triple-A affiliate.[11]

Ludwick began having pain in his left hip in August of 2002. It initially thought to be a hip flexor strain. The pain became so severe that Ludwick even experienced trouble just walking after each game.[12]

He had tests, most likely an MRI, and was diagnosed with a stress fracture of the femoral neck of the hip, a very serious injury. Bo Jackson's baseball career was basically ended when he fractured the femur at the femur neck while playing football (see later discussion). Ludwick also feared his baseball career might be at an end. Fortunately for Ludwick, the fracture line extended only halfway though the neck of the femur. Still, without surgery the injury could have gotten worse. To stabilize the fracture, a metal rod was inserted into the femur. Ludwick had the surgery on August 22, 2002.[13] It is uncertain where Ludwick's hip was pinned.

Ludwick faced a long rehabilitation, but despite this he was ready for spring training in late February 2003, with the Rangers. He did not make the major league roster out of spring training and was sent back to Oklahoma City. He did well enough there to make the Pacific Coast League All-Star team before being recalled to the Rangers. He made a brief appearance for the Rangers before being traded to the Cleveland Indians.

Unfortunately, while playing for the Indians that September, Ludwick suffered yet another in his long list of injuries, a dislocated knee-cap while sliding into third base. The injury was so severe that it required surgery to correct a tear in the patella (knee cap) tendon, another season-ending injury. To add insult to injury, he had to have a second surgery on the same right knee in early 2004 because of the build-up of scar tissue.[14]

After an entire year (2006) at Detroit's Triple-A affiliate, he was signed by the Cardinals. For them Ludwick was able to stay at the major league level for much of 2007 and all of 2008, avoiding any significant injury. In 2008, as previously stated, he had a career year with the St. Louis Cardinals, and was even named to the National League All-Star team. He again had another good year for the Cardinals in 2009 before being traded to San Diego in the middle of the 2010 season.

Ryan Ludwick, as of this date, has had no further problems with the stress fracture of the femur bone in his left hip. He still has a metal rod or pin in his left hip which will remain there unless he has problems with it.

FRANK THOMAS

For Frank Thomas, then of the Chicago White Sox, the years 2004 and 2005 were very difficult. He began having problems with his ankle/foot in June 2004. He first felt pain in the ankle while fielding a grounder on June 17. When symptoms didn't get better with time, he went on the DL on July 10. Tests were run, an MRI and a bone scan and he was found to have a stress fracture of the navicular bone near his ankle.[15]

At the time of diagnosis, the team podiatrist, Dr. Lowell Weil, recommended that Thomas have foot immobilization and bear no weight on the foot.

Thomas' symptoms didn't get better as the year passed. He missed the rest of the 2004 season. Finally, on October 6, he had surgery to correct the problem. During the procedure Thomas had a bone graft (bone removed from another location and placed where the fracture is to aid in healing). He also had two screws inserted to reinforce the fracture site.[16]

Thomas at this point in his career was mainly serving as a DH. The reason for right-handed-hit-

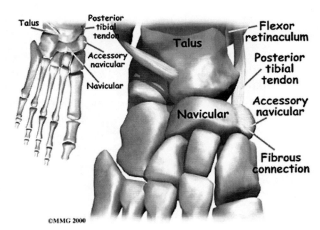

Top view of bones of foot and ankle showing possible location of Frank Thomas's navicular bone stress fracture (used by permission of Medical Multimedia Group LLC).

ting Thomas' continued problems with his ankle was described by White Sox trainer Herm Schneider. He said, "Thomas has had foot and ankle problems, and the combination of his size (270+ pounds) and his style of hitting — which puts maximum pressure on his left leg — makes him vulnerable."[17]

In 2005 Thomas came off the DL on May 30. He only played 34 games before he went back on the DL on July 21. He had another stress fracture in the navicular bone of his right foot/ankle, but this fracture was not exactly at the same location where Thomas had had his previous surgery. He missed the rest of 2005 and played only 34 games while batting .219 with 12 home runs in 105 at-bats.[18]

Thus, the two-time MVP (1993, 1994) played in only 74 games in 2004 and 34 games in 2005, with significant playing time lost to navicular stress fractures in his left foot. Even though an exam on November 3 showed good healing, it is not surprising that the Chicago White Sox decided to buy out Thomas' option year on his contract for $3.5 million instead of paying his last year's option salary. They just did not want to take a chance on him staying healthy at age 38. This made Frank Thomas a free agent.[19]

The Oakland A's decided to take a chance on Thomas. They signed him for a base salary of $500,000 with as much as $2.6 million in possible incentives. They did not sign Thomas until after their team orthopedist, Dr. Jerrald Goldman, administered a series of stress tests on the foot/ankle. Goldman was satisfied with the results.[20]

Thomas rewarded the A's for taking a chance on him in 2006. There are no indications Thomas has had further problems with his left foot. He was able to play in 137 games in 2006, batting .270 with 39 home runs and 114 RBI. In 2007, Thomas played 155 games for the Toronto Blue Jays and finished with 30 doubles, 26 home runs, and 95 RBI.

Thomas's 2008 season was limited because he had a quadriceps strain and quadriceps tendonitis. This limited him to only 71 games played, sandwiched around two trips to the DL, not related to his previous left foot stress fracture.[21] Thomas did not play in the major leagues after 2008. We will have to see if his lifetime average of .301 with 521 home runs, 1,494 runs, 1,704 RBI and 1,667 walks are good enough to get him elected to the Hall of Fame. Will a player with great stats and two MVPs get into the Hall of Fame if he has spent a large chunk of his career as a designated hitter?

Upper Extremity Stress Fracture

As mentioned several times before, baseball requires repetitive movements. With the upper extremity this is mainly throwing or catching the ball and swinging the bat. Stress fractures of the upper torso usually occur where muscles, ligaments, and tendons attach to bone. Stress is applied, pushing the bone to the limit of its tolerance.

The main difference between upper and lower extremity stress fractures is that gravity is not a common factor in injuries in the upper extremity, except maybe in the spine. Since weight-bearing structures are not an important factor in upper extremity stress fractures, they should occur less frequently than lower extremity fractures. In the baseball research done here, this was not found to be the case, as there was little difficulty finding a plethora of upper extremity stress fractures.

As opposed to many sections in this book, this section starts with a list of upper extremity stress fractures found. This is by no means a complete list. It should be no surprise that the majority of those injured by upper extremity stress fractures (16 out of 19) are pitchers.

ELBOW   Jack Morris (Detroit Tigers) July 1989 — pitcher[22]
        Adam Loewen (Baltimore Orioles) 2007, 2008 (ended career as pitcher)[23]
        Randy Wells (Chicago Cubs) end of 2008 — pitcher[24]
        Derrick Turnbow (California Angels) — pitcher[25]
        Antonio Alfonseca (Florida Marlins), 2005 — pitcher[26]
        Cesar Jimenez (Seattle Mariners) 2007 — pitcher[27]
        Taylor Tankersley (Florida Marlins) 2009 — pitcher — had surgery[28]
        Joel Zumaya (Detroit Tigers) 2010 — pitcher — had surgery[29]
        Doug Brocail (Texas Rangers) 2002 — pitcher[30]
SHOULDER BLADE   Brandon McCarthy (Texas Rangers) 2007 — pitcher[31]
GLENOID (shoulder socket)   Brad Radke (Minnesota Twins) 2006 — pitcher[32]
CORACOID (shoulder blade)   Joel Zumaya (Detroit Tigers) 2008 — pitcher[33]
RIBS   Phil Hughes (New York Yankees) 2008 — pitcher[34]
      Bobby Crosby (Oakland A's) 2005 — shortstop[35]
      Matt Morris (San Francisco Giants) 2006 — pitcher[36]
      Tim Wakefield (Boston Red Sox) 2006 — pitcher[37]
HAND (Hamate Bone)   Jose Canseco (Oakland A's) 1989 — outfielder[38]
HAND (Third Metacarpal)   Nick Johnson (NY Yankees) 2003 — first basemen-DH[39]
SPINE (lower back [twice])   Francisco Cordero (Texas Rangers) 2001 — pitcher[40]

The elbow is a pivotal point for things going bad for a pitcher. He can tear a ligament or a flexor muscle tendon or suffer from ulnar nerve neuropathy, loose bone fragments in the elbow, bone spurs, and ultimately career-threatening arthritis.

Considerable stress is put on the elbow in the pitching motion. Another problem that can occur: the bone itself can be pushed beyond its ability to adapt, causing a stress fracture. Rest usually heals this, but not always. Surgery sometimes helps to reinforce the bone with metal, but not always.

ADAM LOEWEN — ELBOW STRESS FRACTURE

Adam Loewen is not a household name. Sure, he was the fourth overall pick in the 2002 amateur draft by the Baltimore Orioles, a highly regarded high school pitcher from Surrey, British Columbia (DOB 4/9/84), but now he is not pitching anymore nor is he with the Baltimore Orioles.

Loewen missed virtually all the 2007 season with a stress fracture diagnosed early in the season. He had had a promising rookie season in 2006, starting 19 games for the Orioles. His ERA was not very good (5.37), but at 22 years old his prospects for improvement were very good.

The 2007 season started off well enough. Loewen made the team out of spring training and was projected to be the Orioles' fourth starter for the season. But from spring training on, Loewen experienced progressively intensifying pain in his left pitching elbow. Despite this pain he was still able to manage six starts in 2007 before finally being placed on the DL. His record at that time was two wins and no losses with a respectable 3.56 ERA. But there was an early sign of trouble as he averaged only five innings per start. In his last start before going on the DL, he again lasted only five innings, this time taken out because his elbow pain simply got so severe he could not continue to pitch.

Dr. Andrew Cosgarea, the Baltimore team physician, did the initial evaluation on Loewen. A plain X-ray revealed nothing, as it often does with a stress fracture. A bone scan done on May 4 revealed a stress fracture of Loewen's elbow (the exact bone is not mentioned). Following consultation with Dr. James Andrews, Loewen was placed on the DL. Initially it was thought he would only be sidelined for eight weeks.[41]

Sometimes things don't go as expected. When the healing of the stress fracture didn't progress as expected, surgery was considered. On June 14, 2007, Dr. Andrews inserted a titanium screw (4½ inches) into the elbow to aid the healing process (bone not mentioned, though the olecranon process of the ulna bone in the elbow is the most likely site). With the surgical procedure, Loewen, already on the extended 60-day DL, missed the rest of the season. There was still optimism for the 2008 season. Loewen was young and should heal just fine; he would only be 24 in 2008.

But the 2008 season brought more of the same, and his stats were much worse. Loewen made the team again out of spring season. In his first four starts he had no wins and one loss with an ERA of 7.85. Loewen thought his poor performance in early 2008 was due to his prolonged period of inactivity in 2007. But after his fourth start on April 24, when he lasted only two and two-thirds innings, he finally admitted he had been bothered by the return of pain in his left elbow. In the latest start he had a dull pain at the start of the game, which gradually became sharper and sharper as the game progressed. The pain "affected the way he threw the baseball and hindered him from controlling his fastball." He was immediately placed on the DL. He would need further evaluation.[42]

Once again Loewen made the trek to Birmingham, Alabama, to see Dr. Andrews. Andrews gave encouraging news, noting no structural damage to the elbow. Loewen was placed on a throwing program to last three weeks before being activated off the DL.[43]

Loewen came back off the DL only to go back on it on July 8, 2008. Evaluation at that point: Loewen would need another surgery on his problematic elbow, and this time would need to be away from pitching at the major league level for another year and a half. There was no guarantee that he wouldn't have more problems if he continued to pitch.

Loewen had been a good hitter in high school and had also hit .353 with one home run and 38 RBI while at Chipola Junior College in Florida. In light of this hitting ability, he decided to forgo another surgery and try to make a comeback as a position player instead of trying to continue to pitch. Batting for decent average might be a difficult proposition initially as he had not had an at-bat in his six years as a professional. The plan: he would rest his elbow until the pain abated completely. Then he would try some batting practice and hopefully catch on in the 2008 fall instructional league, where he would continue batting and also play a position, first base or the outfield.[44]

Loewen was put on waivers by the Baltimore Orioles (he was out of options). It was thought to be a routine matter. The Orioles had every intention of signing him to a minor league contract after he cleared waivers. To Baltimore's surprise, the Surrey, British Columbia, native decided in October to sign with the Toronto Blue Jays instead.[45]

In 2009 Loewen played for the Blue Jays' Advanced-A team in Dunedin, Florida. He played 103 games with 391 plate appearances. He batted .236 and hit 22 doubles, though with only 31 RBI. On the downside, he had 114 strikeouts, almost once every three times to the plate. But one would have to call this minor league experience a success when you consider Loewen had not hit live pitching in over six years.

In 2010, at the Double-A level, Loewen did even better with a .246 average, 13 home runs and 70 RBI, though once again he had a high strikeout rate with 143 strikeouts in 537 plate appearances. In 2011, for Triple-A affiliate Las Vegas, Loewen had a .306 average with 46 doubles, 17 home runs, and 85 RBI in 585 plate appearances.

Loewen finally made it back to the major leagues as an outfielder and DH for the Toronto Blue Jays in 2011, playing 14 games, though batting only .188 with 6 hits in 32 at bats. He signed as a free agent with the New York Mets in 2012.

Adam Loewen is not a household name but exhibits a bad outcome for a stress fracture of the elbow. He had to quit pitching and become a position player. At least he was able to make the switch in positions.

A better outcome is the stress fracture Jack Morris sustained in 1989. He also has a better-known name.

JACK MORRIS — ELBOW STRESS FRACTURE

Jack Morris amassed 254 career wins and 186 losses in 18 years pitched, the vast majority of his career for the Detroit Tigers (14 years), only pitching for Minnesota, Toronto, and Cleveland late in his career. He is best known for the 1991 post-season with the Twins. He won four total games, including two in the World Series against Atlanta. His ten-inning, 1–0 win in the clinching seventh game against Atlanta is truly a memorable moment in baseball history. Morris was named MVP of that Series. Morris also had the most wins in all of baseball during the 1980s with 162.

Once again, the elbow is a battleground for injuries, and a stress fracture is just one possible injury. In 1989 Jack Morris suffered this particular injury during his worst season. He finished with 24 starts, a 6–14 record and a high 4.86 ERA. His season started off poorly as he lost his first six starts. He won two games before suffering his seventh loss of the season on May 22. About this time, Morris admitted to his manager, Sparky Anderson, that he had been pitching hurt.

Dr. David Collon, the Detroit Tigers' team physician, evaluated Morris. It is unknown if any specialized tests other than just a plain X-ray were obtained. Certainly in 1989 CT scans and bone scans were available. Collon commented that Morris had a small fracture involving "the support structures of the inner side of the elbow." The fracture appeared to be "a number of weeks old." Morris headed to the disabled list, the first time he had been on the DL since coming up to the Tigers as a rookie in 1977.[46]

Jack Morris ended up on the disabled list for nine weeks, returning on July 24 against Milwaukee. He had mixed results, giving up seven runs in five and one-third innings. Prior to that start, he had made two starts at the minor league level, but only pitching eight innings in rehab. That he was rusty in his first major league start back from the DL is not surprising.[47]

Morris suffered no further ill effects from his stress fracture. The following year, 1990, he had a league-high 36 starts and 11 complete games. He won 18 games for Minnesota in 1991 and 21 games in 1992 for Toronto before his career tapered off in 1993 and 1994.

BRAD RADKE — GLENOID SCAPULA STRESS FRACTURE

There is no law that says you can't have more than one medical problem at a time causing similar symptoms. For instance, a pitcher can rip up his elbow. He can have a torn UCL, torn flexor muscles, bone spurs, and ulnar nerve compression all at the same time, all with similar symptoms. Brad Radke is an example of a stress fracture occurring at the same time as a shoulder labral tear.

Rare today, Brad Radke pitched his whole career for one team, the Minnesota Twins (1995 to 2006). His career record was 148–139 with a 4.22 ERA. His record might be better if he had not pitched on some bad Twins teams, including eight straight losing seasons from 1993 through 2000. Radke was a workhorse for the Twins averaging 204 innings per season.

The last two years (2005 and 2006), Radke pitched in pain. Radke's MRI in 2005 had shown a torn labrum and he knew it (a SLAP lesion — superior lateral anterior posterior tear). But rather than get it fixed and go through extensive rehab, he decided to retire after the 2006 season. He said, "Now I'm like, well, you could've (had surgery), and then I slap my face and tell myself to wake up. That was the end. I was just so mentally burned out and physically, too. There was no way I could have gotten myself better.... The last couple of years were pretty tough. It really took a lot out of me. It was time. It really was."[48]

Radke knew mentally he was not up to doing the extensive rehab necessary to come back from a torn labrum repair. The last year he had another problem, a stress fracture of his shoulder. It involved the glenoid bone, the part of the scapula that cradles the fibrocartilagenous labrum. The head of the humerus bone articulates with the labrum.

There is pain; then there is worse pain. The pain Radke suffered in early to mid–2006 became much worse towards the end of the season. An MRI in mid–August showed nothing new. In order to cope with pain, Radke received two cortisone shots in his shoulder at intervals over the next three and one-half weeks. This didn't help. When the pain became so severe that Radke had considerable trouble simply playing catch, the MRI was repeated. That one showed a stress fracture of the glenoid.[49]

Twins team orthopedist Dr. Dan Buss called the injury "an extremely rare problem." Radke rested completely for two weeks. He then attempted a come-back. Why? The Twins were close to participating in the post-season. Wouldn't they want one of their best pitchers pitching? In such a situation, some degree of pain can be tolerated as long as it is not unbearable. Radke did come back, pitching again on September 28. He went five innings, throwing 57 pitches, allowing three hits and an unearned run.[50]

Maybe there was at least one more effort left in his arm. The Twins called on him to pitch the third game of the AL Championship Series against the Oakland A's. A feel-good ending just wasn't to be. The Twins, already down two games to none, lost the third game, with Radke the losing pitcher. He lasted only four innings and 83 pitches, giving up four runs and two home runs in the 8–3 loss to the A's. It would be the last major league game Radke would ever pitch. He announced his retirement on December 19, 2006.[51]

Radke suffered the last two seasons of his career with a shoulder labrum tear which he chose not to have fixed. At the end of 2006, he suffered a rare glenoid shoulder stress fracture.

Rib Stress Fractures

There have been several pitchers (Matt Morris in 2006, Tim Wakefield in 2006, and Phil Hughes in 2008) who have had rib stress fractures. Pitching requires a twisting motion to pull the arm through the pitching motion. More often than not this motion is going to damage muscle, tendons, or ligaments. Rarely, the muscle and tendon stress applied to bones (ribs) can result in a stress reaction in the bone instead (stress fracture).

MATT MORRIS

Matt Morris pitched most of his 11-season career with the St. Louis Cardinals. He won 121 games against 92 losses. He also pitched for the San Francisco Giants in 2006–2007 and finally for the Pittsburgh Pirates in 2007–2008. It was while pitching for the Giants in 2006 that Morris suffered a rib stress fracture.

When a pitcher's stats suddenly deviate from his usual performance, one must suspect that the pitcher is injured. Matt Morris fits that description. He pitched much less effectively the last month of the 2006 season and pitched in pain on the right side of his back, just under the scapula.

An initial MRI test in late August showed nothing. But an MRI with special views on October 2 revealed a stress fracture of a rib as well as a stress reaction (precursor to fracture) of two other ribs. There was no time on the DL as it was the end of the season. There is no indication he ever had further problems with the rib stress fracture.[52]

TIM WAKEFIELD

Tim Wakefield chugged along through 19 seasons in the major leagues. He pitched the last 17 years for the Boston Red Sox and recorded 200 career wins against 180 losses. Most of his longevity has to be attributed to the pitch he threw, the knuckleball. It requires less effort than most pitches and is less taxing on the body. Tim Wakefield's stress fracture of his right ribs in 2006 may therefore come as a surprise to many.

He started having pain in his back around June 3, 2006. An MRI of his spine on July 7 was negative. When the pain persisted, a bone scan and CT scan were obtained around the middle of July which revealed the stress fracture. Wakefield was placed on the DL.[53]

Wakefield did not pitch for the Boston Red Sox from July 17 until September 13. Boston missed him as their record without him was 22–31, and they dropped out of first place, ending up third in the American League East division and out of the playoffs. There had been several other Boston pitchers injured in the same season.[54]

Wakefield recovered to pitch 31 games in 2007. Over the next four seasons he went 10–11, 11–5, 4–10 and 7–8 before retiring prior to the start of the 2012 season.

PHIL HUGHES

Phil Hughes of the New York Yankees was in the infancy of his career in 2008, just his second season for the Yankees at the age of 22. He was a first-round pick (23rd overall pick) of the Yankees in the 2004 free-agent draft.

He started off 2008 poorly and was 0–4 in six starts with an ERA of 9.00 (bad stats, think injury!) when placed on the DL on May 1 with a stress fracture of the ninth rib on the right side. He did not pitch a major league game from April 29 until September 17.[55]

Hughes recovered nicely in 2009. He went 8–3 with a 3.03 ERA in 51 games, of which seven were starts. He pitched in nine games in the 2009 post-season for the World Series Champion Yankees with no wins and one loss.

In 2010, once again a starter, Hughes thrived, going 18–8 for the Yankees.

Chapter 7

Neck, Back, Spine
and Disk Injuries

The most common back and neck injuries are simple muscle and tendon strains (called mechanical back problems). When back and neck pain last longer than a couple of weeks, then one has to consider possible disc-related problems.

Lower Back

DISC AND SPINE PROBLEMS

Spine (low back and neck) problems can occur for various reasons: damage to muscles, tendons, and ligaments around the vertebrae, or to discs between the vertebrae. Often, the herniated disc as an aggravating factor is easier to understand than other spine problems.

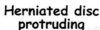
Herniated disc protruding

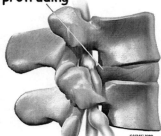

Between each pair of vertebrae in the spine is a fibro-cartilagenous disc. In proper position, it is just fine. As one ages, the disc loses flexibility and can become damaged. Normally it is held in place by ligaments, but pressure can push part of the disc outside of its normal space. The disc can have various types of damage. There are nerves that protrude out each side of the vertebra. If the

One possible cause of back pain, lumbar disc herniation. Disc is pressing on nerve root next to bony vertebrae in back (used by permission of Medical Multimedia Group LLC).

disc is damaged, it can become herniated, impinging on the nerve going to the neck, arms, back, or legs. Or the disc can simply be worn out with the space between vertebrae narrowed, as in degenerative discs.

Certain vertebrae discs are more likely to get damaged than others. These are the lower cervical (neck) vertebrae just above the shoulders and the lower back vertebrae just above the pelvis.

Discs can be damaged suddenly as with a fall, or they can get damaged over time by overuse. Why some people get disc problems and others don't is uncertain. It is like any disease process. Why do only some get it?

Some disc problems will be discussed under trauma, such as with sliding injuries. Only overuse injuries are discussed here.

Ralph Kiner

Did Ralph Kiner have disc problems or not? Disc problems were one of the most common reasons to do back surgery even before modern methods to make a more accurate preoperative diagnosis with an MRI or a CT scan. The surgery would be based largely on clinical symptoms and in 1955 would be exploratory, requiring a larger incision to track down the problem and treat it properly. A larger incision than the ones used today would have greater long-term morbidity and require a longer rehab.

Hall of Famer Ralph Kiner played mainly for the Pittsburgh Pirates during his ten-year major league career (1946–1955). He had seven straight years hitting at least 35 home runs, five with at least 40 home runs, and two over 50 home runs. He had five straight years with over 100 RBI. For all his effort, he never finished better than fourth in the MVP voting, as the Pirates were not very good, finishing only once above the .500 mark. They were never close to being in the World Series.

In the book *Baseball Forever: Reflections on 60 years of Baseball,* by Ralph Kiner and Danny Peary, Kiner's back problems are discussed.[1]

At the relatively young age of 32, while playing for the Cleveland Indians, Kiner began having problems with his back (strained ligaments and a tender nerve near the spinal column, he was told). The back pain was especially bad when he swung the bat. It became apparent after consulting several medical doctors that to continue to play baseball, Kiner would have to have surgery, but he was also told that even with surgery he had only a 50–50 chance to play again. With salaries not very substantial in 1955, Kiner didn't like his odds and decided to retire instead of having the surgery.

Did Ralph Kiner have disc problems or not? Did he have a herniated disc? His case illustrates the difficulty in tracking down an exact diagnosis in older references. In an age before CT scans and MRIs and without surgery, the exact etiology of Kiner's back problems is not known. Like Don Drysdale's case noted earlier, without the surgery Kiner's diagnosis is speculative.

Randy Johnson

Randy Johnson (the Big Unit) did have a diagnosed overuse disc problem. Johnson ended his career in 2009 with 303 wins and 166 losses. He pitched for 22 seasons for Montreal, Seattle, Houston, Arizona, the New York Yankees, and San Francisco. He won five Cy Young Awards and seems a shoo-in for the Hall of Fame the first year he is eligible.

Johnson also had three surgeries for bulging discs in his lower back: September 12, 1996, October 26, 2006, and August 3, 2007.[2] He was limited to eight games started in 1996 and ten in 2007. Nothing is mentioned in the articles researched about exactly which discs at which vertebra level were herniated. References simply state it was Johnson's lower back and that the disc herniated in the second surgery was the same one that resulted in the third surgery.[3]

Symptoms leading up to the surgeries are mentioned. An article on July 16, 1996, mentioned that Johnson's right calf didn't feel quite right though he didn't have much back pain.[4] In 2007 he had a sharp pain in his hamstring (which one not mentioned).[5] Both times symptoms were mentioned as affecting his delivery of the ball to the plate.

One would imagine that Johnson's height (6 foot 10 inches) and that he threw very hard might make him prone to have disc problems in his lower back. At least one person, Mark McGwire, who also had disc problems, expressed this opinion in an interview in 1996.[6]

Prior to Johnson's third surgery, he was having a sharp pain in his hamstring that was also affecting his delivery. Conservative measures were tried to avoid this third surgery. As often tried, two cortisone injections were given in his back via the epidural method to reduce swelling around the compressed nerve. The first injection helped some but the second did not. One can assume physical therapy was used in conjunction with the injections. When those fail, surgery is a common choice for a herniated lumbar disc causing sciatic (radicular) pain.[7]

Johnson, according to his stats, recovered from his first and third surgeries in good shape, especially after the 1996 surgery as he won four Cy Young Awards from 1999 to 2002. The recovery after the 2006 surgery did not go as well, possibly because he simply tried to come back too soon after this surgery.[8] That he was in his 40s at the time did not help his prospects.

The third surgery allowed Johnson to pitch two more years, though in a limited fashion in 2009. Johnson was able to pass the magical 300-win milestone in 2009 at age 45.

Joe Crede

The treatment of herniated or prolapsed disc problems by surgery has improved since disc surgery has been introduced. In addition to being able to make a more accurate diagnosis, the tendency has been to make smaller and smaller holes to insert instruments to take out damaged and herniated discs, and to remove less and less disc.[9] More recently, removing disc fluid from the disc causing the bulging or herniated disc part has been tried. Joe Crede is an example of these trends. With any disc surgery, conservative measures, including physical therapy, are used prior to and after any surgical procedure.

Joe Crede was selected by the Chicago White Sox in the fifth round of the 1996 amateur draft. His best seasons were 2003 to 2006, when he averaged 500 at bats per season, 27 doubles and 23 home runs. His best season was 2006, when he hit 30 home runs with 94 RBI.

He had had some problems with his back since 2004, but the situation became much worse in 2007. In 2004 he was noted to have two herniated discs. Between 2004 and 2007 he received four epidural injections (of cortisone probably).

Symptoms in 2007 were much worse. When he went on the DL (he only played 47 games), his pain was so severe he was having trouble sleeping at night, standing up straight, or sitting for extended periods of time. Another epidural injection was considered but after consultation with Dt. Frank Phillips at Rush Memorial Hospital in Chicago, Dr. Andrew Dossett at the W. B. Memorial Clinic in Dallas, Texas, and Dr. Robert Watkins at the Marina Spine Clinic in Marina del Rey, California, he decided to have minimally invasive surgery. Dr. Watkins made a small incision and sucked out some fluid near the nerve.[10]

In 97 games in 2008, Crede had 335 at bats with 17 home runs and 55 RBI. Then, on September 2, he landed awkwardly while making a diving stop. He appeared to be back at square one. He again went the route of multiple consultations, and then had a procedure done in September, this time by Dr. Andrew Dossett in Dallas, Texas. Details here were less clear. Crede was to become a free agent after the season. In November, his agent, Scott Boras, told the press that Crede had a minor procedure during the fall.[11]

An article posted at ESPN.com in September of 2009 noted that Crede struggled in 2009 after signing a contract with Minnesota. He ended up batting only .225 with 15 home runs and 48 RBI in 90 games. In addition to an assortment of minor injuries, he ended up on the DL from August 22 to September 8 for back problems. After coming off the DL, he only played one more game the rest of the season.[12]

Dr. Dossett was scheduled to do a minor procedure on Crede at the end of September to suck out fluid from the disc to try to relieve some of the pressure on the nerves in Crede's lower back. Crede was expected to be fine by spring of 2010. As it turns out, though, Crede, a free agent, was not signed in 2010 and did not play in the major leagues that year.[13]

In 2011 Crede signed a minor league deal in 2011 with the Colorado Rockies with an invitation to spring training.[14]

Don Mattingly

Not all back problems related to lower back disc problems are surgically correctible. A degenerative disc problem is usually not surgically correctible.

Don Mattingly did not have a herniated disc, but a degenerative disc problem. Back problems contributed significantly to the decline in his career stats and eventually to his decision to retire in February of 1997 at the age of 35.[15]

Prior to his problems with his back, in 1987 Mattingly looked like a shoo-in to go into the Hall of Fame. From 1984 to 1987 he averaged over .330 and averaged 211 hits, 30 home runs, and 121 RBI per season with a .550+ slugging percentage. He still holds the Yankees record for hits in one season, 238 in 1986. But after 1987 he hit over 20 home runs with 100+ RBI only once (1989), and his slugging percentage was never above .500.

Mattingly had had a back injury while playing football in high school, but had done well with few back problems up until his injury on June 4, 1987. Sadly, this injury occurred just after he had tied the major league record for consecutive games with a home run, eight. The back injury happened in a very simple manner while Mattingly was fielding ground balls prior to a game against Milwaukee. His pain was severe enough that he had to be admitted to the hospital and ended up in traction for three days at NYU Medical Center. An MRI showed two damaged discs. His wife, Kim, said he had protruding discs. The newspaper report appearing on June 9 in the *Detroit Free Press* noted, from a source close to the Yankees, that Mattingly "had no nerve damage, no pain in his leg and no muscle or reflex loss, which would indicate a more serious problem."[16]

In 1987 Mattingly played 141 games but missed getting 200 hits for the first time since 1983. Mattingly rebounded to have a good year in 1989 (158 games played, 23 home runs, and 113 RBI) before his back became much worse in 1990. "It is not surprising the Yankees finished last in the American League East in 1990. After all, Don Mattingly was reduced to mere mortality by a chronic back ailment...."[17] Mattingly missed 60 games last year because of persistent back troubles linked to a degenerative disc condition."[18]

Surgery for Mattingly's back was discussed, but not recommended. Mattingly saw Yankees team physician Dr. Stuart Hershon and noted back specialist Dr. Robert Watkins in California. Other means of dealing with Mattingly's back pain had to be found besides surgery.

Mattingly was forced to alter his stance because of his back problems. In the past, when he was hitting line drives all over the field, he hit in a "crouched pigeon-toed stance." In an article in *The Sporting News* in August of 1990, Mattingly reported, "It's a position I just can't get into any more. I'm going to have to find another comfortable way to hit."[19] He was constantly trying to find an effective hitting position that did not tax his back much. He wasn't succeeding.

Mattingly's work ethic suffered because of the back. Before the back prob-

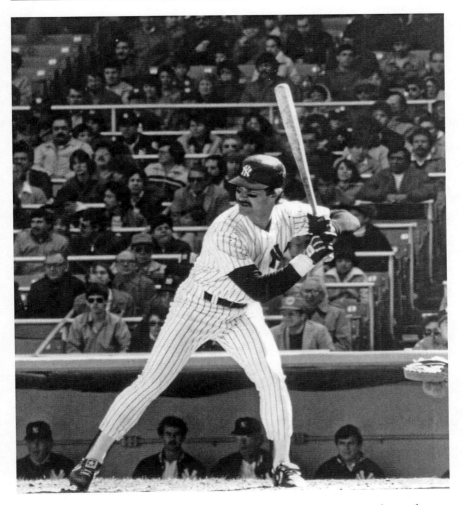

Don Mattingly of the New York Yankees in his typical batting stance, date unknown (National Baseball Hall of Fame Library, Cooperstown, New York).

lems, he would take 300 swings every day in batting practice. Now he could not take more than 50 to 75 swings per day. He also had to shorten his swing and hit more balls the opposite way.[20]

In 1992, he played in 157 games with 184 hits, a .288 average, 17 home runs and 86 RBI. These are good stats, but not great, especially not for Don Mattingly, who was in the fourth year of a five-year, $19.3 million contract. It is difficult to assess the 1994 and 1995 seasons, both strike-shortened, but the power numbers were definitely down — only six home runs in 1994 and seven in 1995.

Finally, in Mattingly's 14th year with the Yankees, they made the playoffs for the first time during his career. He did his part in the playoffs, hitting .417 with ten hits in 24 at-bats, yet the Yankees still lost to Seattle in the first round of the Division Series. During the regular season, Mattingly had hit only .288 with seven home runs and 49 RBI in 128 games.

When he continued to have trouble with his back, he sat out the entire 1996 season, unfortunately missing the Yankees' first World Series title since 1978. He never participated in a single World Series game during his entire 14-year Yankees career.

He attempted to prepare for the 1997 season and had some interest from the Kansas City Royals, but ultimately he decided against playing another season. He stated, "I wasn't willing to pay the price it was going to take to succeed."[21]

David Wells

David Wells pitched through an assortment of injuries during his career in the majors. Previously mentioned was his Tommy John surgery. He also had significant back problems during his 21-year career.

In his book *Perfect I'm Not*, Wells first mentioned back problems while pitching for the Cincinnati Reds in 1995.[22] He had just been traded by the Detroit Tigers to the Reds on July 31 as the Reds were trying to make a stretch run to make the playoffs. The Reds had already lost Jose Rijo to elbow problems. Rijo had gone on the DL on July 18 and would have Tommy John surgery on August 22.

Wells started off just fine for the Reds, winning four of his first five starts. Then, he had two bad starts in a row, against Pittsburgh and Colorado, not making it past the fifth inning in either. An article in *The Columbus Dispatch* on September 15, 1995, noted a remarkable turnaround in his next game. He pitched a complete game in an 8–1 victory over San Diego.

In the article, his success was attributed to two things. First, he liked to stay in the game. After two shaky games in a row and then a shaky first inning against San Diego, Wells got mad and became more determined. Second, his turnaround was attributed to correcting bad mechanics. He said, "My mechanics were screwed up my previous two outings, so I got with Gullie (pitching coach Don Gullett)."[23]

In his book he paints a very different picture.

> I wince through four innings against the Pirates, getting lit up for eight hits and four runs. I then spend the next five days stretching, twisting, and getting messaged [for his back]. Feeling much better, I go back to the mound against the Colorado Rockies, where I stiffen up again, almost immediately. I've got the needle inside me twenty-four hours later — and after the sting, my back works great. My next start rolls in as a complete-game four hitter against the Padres,

and I won't throw another flat-out bad outing all season. Cortisone becomes my new best friend.[24]

The two stories are probably not too different from each other. It is quite possible Wells' back problems led to bad mechanics. But just working on his mechanics was not going to correct his back problems.

Wells continued to experience back problems over the next several seasons, getting one cortisone shot after another in his back. In 2000, while pitching for the Toronto Blue Jays, his life took a turn for the worse. Wells finished with a 20–8 record, finishing third in the Cy Young Award voting for the American League. He also had a league-leading nine complete games. But these results do not tell the complete picture, as Wells said every one of his complete games came after a cortisone shot.[25] No form of therapy helped, only the cortisone. Nine shots of cortisone in a season are way too many.

It would appear from his book that Wells was rather adamant that he needed the shots, and someone complied in giving them to him.[26] Not good! By 2000 the doctors should have known better. There are potential complications in the form of deterioration of tissues over the long haul.

In July 2001, while pitching for the Chicago White Sox, Wells' back problems really went south. The cortisone shots were not working anymore. Therapy was not working anymore. Wells' season was over after making only 16 starts.

He again describes his situation well in his book.

July. I'm done. With two weeks of shots and stretching, and rest, and chiropractors, and every therapy known to man all failing me miserably, I can no longer stand up straight. I can no longer sit in a normal chair. I can't put my socks on. I can't walk comfortably. And there's no way in hell I could ever, *ever* survive ten minutes with my kids. That's what puts me over the top. That's what makes me finally pull the trigger on surgery. Put into that context, the decision is simple.[27]

It would seem logical Wells probably had an MRI in 1995. Nothing is said in Wells' book nor in any newspaper articles, but for cortisone to work it needs a specific target. Wells probably had some disc problems with his back as far back as 1995.

An MRI was repeated in July of 2001. It confirmed a severely herniated disc at the L4 and L5 area. Surgery confirmed the herniated disc and revealed, as Wells said, "a little piece of chipped bone lodged under the nerve in my spinal column. To get that sucker out of there the doctors had to pull the nerve away from the spine, then scrape around and yank the bone out. The procedure ended up being a bigger deal than expected, which I realized the second I woke from surgery."[28]

Wells had severe pain immediately after surgery. Wells said, "I now had a nasty, burning pain shooting down through my ass and into my right leg"[29] (in his book, Wells was never short on colorful descriptions).

Rehab initially consisted of doing nothing other than some walking for a period of six weeks. Then the rehab switched to everything he tried before surgery, including watching his weight. He did not pitch again in 2001.

He convinced George Steinbrenner during the 2001 off-season that he was recovered from his 2001 back surgery. The Yankees, Wells' favorite team, signed him for 2002. He pitched with few back problems in 2002 and finished with 19 wins against 7 losses and an ERA of 3.75. His book indicates no further problems with his back in 2003 either, and he finished the season with 15 wins against 7 losses.

In review, it could be said that in addition to his herniated disc, Wells could have suffered a stress fracture in his lower back along the way. It can be speculated that all the cortisone shots he received in his back may have been a factor in the development of a stress fracture, and this fracture may have resulted in the loose bone fragment found at his surgery.

Jose Canseco, Kevin Brown, Todd Helton, Ben Sheets, etc.

Also having lumbar disc surgery were Jose Canseco in 1999,[30] Carlos Hernandez (twice) in 2001,[31] Kevin Brown in 2002,[32] Ben Sheets in 2004,[33] Todd Helton in 2008,[34] and Mark Kotsay in 2009.[35] There have been many more.

UPPER BACK DISC

Chris Duncan

Disc disease is usually in the lower lumbar discs just above the pelvis. Neck (cervical) problems are usually in the vertebrae just above the shoulders (upper back). These areas sustain the most stress.

In the past, if a person had a herniated disc in the neck causing pain and radiation of pain down the neck and arm, the disc space involved (adjacent vertebrae) would be fused using a bone graft. This is the standard of care for cervical herniated disc problems *not* helped by conservative measures including physical therapy, epidural cortisone injections, and traction.[36] The problem with disc fusion is the limitation of range of motion for the neck that results from such care (10 percent or more). For most of us such treatment is just fine. But in a baseball player, any limitation in movement is not good, especially for a major leaguer to perform at the high level necessary.

Just recently, disc replacement surgery has been approved. A metal insert replaces the damaged disc, maintaining the disc space necessary to prevent pressure on the nerve. As with any relatively new procedure, long-term results are not well known. What will be the problems ten to 20 years after the surgical implant? As would be expected, the device should last a long time with a low level of use. But what of a job or activity that puts lots of demands on the device? What of the long-term demands on the device when it is put into a relatively young person?

Though not the same, Bo Jackson's artificial hip serves as a cautionary parallel example.[37] Bo Jackson suffered a fracture-dislocation of the hip. The blood supply to the femur head was impaired and the femur head died, necessitating an artificial replacement (metal/plastic) of the joint because of debilitating arthritis that developed. It was nice that Bo Jackson came back to play baseball briefly, but this was not very wise. The femur/hip is a weight-bearing joint subject to extra stress just in normal activity. To try to perform at the major league level with an artificial hip is not a good idea. First, the hip replacement is not made — either in the short term or long term — to sustain the stress of playing a major league sport. Just to jog on the artificial hip is not advisable. The wear on the joint is excessive. That Jackson needed a second hip replacement (revision) in 1995 after playing baseball for two years on his first artificial hip should not be a surprise.

The disc in the neck does not get as much stress as the hip does. But certainly the demands on the neck from playing in the major leagues, especially when swinging the bat or twisting to catch or throw a ball, may be too much for an artificial disc replacement to tolerate. Telling this to a young, competitive major leaguer, who possibly could make millions of dollars playing baseball, may be a difficult task.

With all that said, Chris Duncan of the St. Louis Cardinals had cervical disc (C5-C6) replacement surgery on August 4, 2008, with a metal-and-plastic prosthesis. The disc was removed in three pieces. The surgery was performed by the Chief of Cervical Spine surgery at Washington University Medical Center in St. Louis, Dr. K. Daniel Riew. This is thought to be the first time the procedure was performed on a professional athlete. The exact prosthesis brand used is not mentioned.[38]

Duncan began experiencing some neck discomfort in 2007, but attributed it to an awkward sleeping position. During spring training 2008 the pain got worse, and Duncan missed one week of practice. The pain progressed to right shoulder pain especially aggravated by throwing (he threw right-handed, though he hit left-handed). When he began to experience weakness, he underwent an MRI on June 30 which showed a bulging disc.

After a hard slide on July 10, where Duncan slid into Philadelphia shortstop Jimmy Rollins, his condition deteriorated more. He began to experience a burning pain down the arm that was bad enough to impair his sleep. He had numbness in his shoulder, numbness in his hand, and "no feeling whatsoever in his right index finger and thumb."[39]

A re-exam on July 22, which probably entailed another MRI, showed a herniated, or ruptured, disc. In the last two weeks leading up to Duncan's August 4, 2008, surgery, he could not even drive his car, the pain was so severe.

A disc fusion was considered, but when Duncan was told the fusion could restrict neck movement by 10 percent he chose to have the disk replacement surgery.

Duncan's recovery went well after his surgery. Almost immediately he began to experience less pain. In spring training Duncan hit .306 with four home runs and 19 RBI.[40]

Duncan started off the 2009 regular season well, but had a bad slump at the end of June. Between June 29 and July 21 he had only 1 hit in 31 at bats and had no RBI, dropping his batting average to .227. The exact reason for Duncan's slump is not clear. The Cardinal organization was apparently not happy with falling production from their starting left fielder. After the July 21 game against Houston, an 11–6 loss, Duncan was first optioned to the Cardinals' Triple A affiliate Memphis and then traded to Boston for infielder Julio Lugo. Duncan went straight to Boston's Triple A affiliate, Pawtucket, where he remained the rest of the 2009 season, not even hitting .200 for the remainder of the season in 27 games and 94 at bats. The Cardinals replaced Duncan with Matt Holliday who they obtained from the Oakland A's.

In 2010 Duncan signed a minor league contact with the Washington Nationals. He did just fair with their Triple-A affiliate, batting only .191 in 82 games with seven home runs and 27 RBI, but his season ended with left hip problems. With arthritis forming in the hip, he had a hip arthroscopic micro-fracture procedure in August of 2010.[41] (This is a procedure to attempt to get the hip joint to grow some new cartilage and is more commonly done on the knee.)

With continued hip problems, Duncan had a second hip arthroscopy to repair the hip labrum[42] (see section on hip labrum problems to follow). It would appear that hip problems on top of the neck disc problem mean Duncan's baseball career is over.

Larry Walker

Larry Walker has a better-known name than Chris Duncan. He did not get disc replacement surgery or a disc fusion surgery while he was playing. It is unknown whether he had such a surgery after he quit playing. But Walker's neck problems were a big reason why he retired after the 2005 season.

Larry Walker's major league career spanned 17 years during which he mainly played for the Montreal Expos and Colorado Rockies. It was with Colorado that his best years came. In 1997 he won the MVP Award and had one of the best years in modern baseball. He hit 49 home runs, drove in 130 runs, and hit .366. He ended up with a career .313 average and a high career slugging average of .565, won three batting titles, and was a seven-time Gold Glove winner. He garnered a 20.3 percent vote on his first year, 2011, on the Hall of Fame ballot.

He was traded to the Cardinals in 2004 and played on their National League champion team in 2004. It was during 2005 that he started having cervical disc problems from a herniated disc in his neck.

Problems started right out of spring training and got worse as the season went on.[43] An article in the *Denver Post* in October of 2005 describes his injury well. "He tried to fight through it, but the injury soon turned his life upside down, making for fitful nights trying to find the right position to sleep. Before every game, he comes for an hour-and-a-half of treatment. Massage, hot packs, cold packs, electric stimulation; you name it. At times, the pain has been excruciating."[44]

According to one source, Walker also received four cortisone shots in his neck, the last one given the last week of the 2005 season.[45] It didn't help his batting in the post-season for the Cardinals as he ended up with only three hits in 28 at-bats. The Cardinals were eliminated by the Houston Astros in the National League Championship Series that year.

Walker retired at the end of the 2005 season instead of having surgery on his herniated disc and trying to play on. As stated, it is unknown if he eventually had the neck surgery after his retirement.

Chapter 8

Arthritis and
Labral Tears in Hip

Every year there appears to be one particular injury that makes more news than others. In 2009 that appeared to be injuries to the cartilage and surrounding tissue (labrum) of the hip.

It is confusing. We have two joints that have cartilage and connective tissue called the labrum. Injury to the shoulder labrum is very common and has been known about for some time. Injury to the labrum of the hip is less well known and not as common. It makes sense that one injury would be more common than the other. The shoulder is a shallow joint which allows considerable movement and flexibility, making it more prone to injury. That baseball taxes that movement to the limit, especially when throwing the baseball, make injuries to the shoulder labrum even more common.

The hip has limited movement mainly because there is a rim of bone surrounding the head of the femur. This is a deep socket joint. The strong muscles surrounding a joint also add to stability. The muscles in the hip are much stronger than the muscles of the shoulder, which adds extra support to the hip.

A classic example of the differing stability of the two joints is the process of dislocation of the joint (the head of the humerus-shoulder or head of the femur-hip). Dislocations of the shoulder are common, usually due to a fall on an outstretched arm. Dislocations of the hip are very rare, the most common mechanism being a car wreck.

The best-known case of a hip dislocation is Bo Jackson (see previous discussion). It did not occur while playing baseball but while playing football. Bo Jackson was tackled from behind by a 200+ pound defensive player while running full speed down the sideline. His femur completely came out of socket and then back into the socket with a fracture of the hip bone at the same time.

Jackson's femur's blood supply was cut off, the cartilage in the head of the femur died due to aseptic necrosis, and he needed a hip replacement because of traumatic arthritis.[1]

Research revealed no history of hip dislocations noted at the major league level. Often injured Nick Johnson, at the time playing for the Washington Nationals, had a fracture of his femur from a collision with Austin Kearns on September 23, 2006.[2] Johnson had to have a rod placed and screws inserted that were removed 16 months later; he did not dislocate his femur.[3]

Dislocations of the shoulder are common. Most collisions occur between two fielders, a fielder and runner, or a fielder and a wall or ground around the ball park (a traumatic injury). A classic example is Oakland A's second baseman Mark Ellis's injury when he collided with shortstop Bobby Crosby in 2004.[4]

It is really not that hard to find histories of shoulder dislocations in major league baseball. The shoulder, more unstable and vulnerable to traumatic injury, is also more prone to overuse injuries because of its increased range of movement. The extra movement puts extra strain on the joint.

There are other injuries to the hip. An injury to the hip labrum of the hip (cartilage and fibrous tissue in the hip bone) is being diagnosed with increasing frequency.

Until recently, the treatment of such an injury was often worse than the injury. Arthroscopic techniques for the hip joint have improved. The injury is diagnosed more often on suspicious symptoms that in the past would have been considered chronic muscle or tendon injury. In addition diagnostic tools, including MRI with dye injected into the joint (MRI arthrography), have made diagnosis of labrum injury easier.

One would suspect that a hip labral injury in the past, if untreated, would simply result in an arthritic hip. No arthroscopic treatment had been perfected for the early hip labral tear injury. If available, the history for a couple of major league players who were forced to retire because of hip problems might have been altered, one more so than the other.

Pitchers put alternate stress on one hip or the other. A right-hander winding

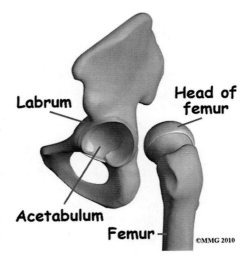

Location of fibrous cartilaginous labrum in hip joint attached to acetabulum of pelvic bone but also against the head of the femur bone when the joint is functioning (used by permission of Medical Multimedia Group LLC).

up first rocks back on his right hip, and when he throws puts weight on his left hip. Over an extended period of time this can wear on the cartilage in both hips.

Charlie Hough

Charlie Hough (216 career wins against 216 losses), who pitched for 25 years in the major leagues, was not a particularly hard thrower. He threw a knuckleball. But for whatever reason — bad genetics, bad mechanics, or bad luck — he wore out his right hip. He had hip replacement surgery for an arthritic hip in 1995, the year after he retired.[5]

It is not known if Hough had a labrum injury that could have been repaired, slowing down the arthritis process. He was 47 years old when he had his hip replacement. It is known that he had significant problems the season prior to his hip replacement, but not if he had problems in 1993, the season prior to his final year, or earlier during his long career with the Los Angeles Dodgers, Texas Rangers, Chicago White Sox, and Florida Marlins.

Albert Belle

Albert Belle's career ended at a much younger age than Charlie Hough. He was forced to retire because of a degenerative hip in 2001 at the age of 34. He had nine straight years of 100 RBI or more, yet failed to garner even the minimum vote in his second year of eligibility for the Hall of Fame despite his great statistics. His stats are very comparable to Hall of Famer Kirby Puckett, who was forced to end his career prematurely because of glaucoma and resulting visual problems, but Puckett was a popular player with the media and Belle was not. Belle is the only major leaguer to hit 50 doubles and 50 home runs in the same year — 1995.

Belle began having hip problems in the summer of his last year, 2000. He was diagnosed with hip bursitis in September. He missed the last week of the season. He did extensive rehab that off-season, but it was very obvious early in spring training of 2001 that he had a significant disabling hip problem, and he was forced to go on the 60-day disabled list and never came off it. Because of this, the Baltimore Orioles collected from the insurance company a significant portion of the $39 million ($13 million per year) left on the original five-year contract for $65 million that Belle had signed in 1998.[6]

Research did not reveal whether Albert Belle had an arthroscopy of his hip in 2001, though there is a good chance he did even though it was not as common a procedure as it is today. If Belle did not have the arthroscopy in 2001, then he probably had one later on.

After his retirement, Belle had a treatment of his hip that is becoming more common in younger patients (under age 60). It is called hip resurfacing. Belle had this procedure done in March of 2007.[7]

The total hip replacement chops off the top of the femur (head and neck) and puts in a metal ball. The newer procedure puts a metal cap over the head of the femur, preserving more bone, and puts a metal cup into the acetabulum (part of the pelvis).[8] Short-term results of the resurfacing procedure are encouraging, but long-term results are not known yet.[9]

Mike Lowell

Mike Lowell of the Boston Red Sox had a hip arthroscope and labrum repair in November of 2008. He is quoted jokingly as saying the procedure should be called the "Mike Lowell" procedure.[10] But Jason Isringhausen, while pitching for the St. Louis Cardinals, had the procedure done for significant labrum damage earlier than Lowell, his first procedure following the 2004 World Series and again two years later in September 2006.[11] Many, many others had the hip procedure before Mike Lowell did. Sorry!

Jason Isringhausen

Jason Isringhausen has pitched 15 years for the New York Mets, Oakland A's, St. Louis Cardinals, and Tampa Bay Rays. He first became a full-time closer for Oakland in 2000 and holds the Cardinals' career record for saves with 217.

He first began having trouble with his hip in 2004, the year he set the Cardinals' single season record for saves with 47. His first procedure showed a significant tear of the hip labrum.[12] Isringhausen then saved 39 games in 2005 and 33 in 2006 though in 2006 had a significant number of blown saves.

Dr. George Paletta, the Cardinals' team physician, performed the first procedure on Isringhausen in November 2004. Dr. J. Thomas Byrd, the team physician of the Tennessee Titans, performed the second hip procedure because there was some arthritis forming and some rubbing caused by a bone formation in the anterior part of the neck of the femur which needed trimming (re-contouring). Some debridement of damaged cartilage was also necessary. It is thought that because of the continued deterioration in the hip joint, Isringhausen may eventually need "some manner" of hip replacement after he retires.[13]

Isringhausen's gradual deterioration in his hip condition, as noted on successive surgeries, may not bode well for the many players having hip arthroscopies in 2008 and beyond. Eventually all these players might be at risk of a bad outcome. One could speculate that the more severe the labrum damage requiring repair, the more significant the eventual hip problems may be later in life, including arthritis.[14]

General Hip Arthroscopies — Several Other Players

Who has had hip arthroscopies for hip labrum damage? One article cites third basemen Mike Lowell of the Boston Red Sox, third basemen Alex Rodriguez of the Yankees, second basemen Chase Utley of the Phillies, first basemen Carlos Delgado of the Mets, third basemen Alex Gordon of the Royals, and pitcher Brett Myers of the Phillies. These players are also mentioned in an article posted at usatoday.com on July 1, 2009.[15] Of all the players having the hip surgery, other than Jason Isringhausen, only Carlos Delgado has needed a second hip arthroscopy on his troubled hip. He had this done in mid–February of 2010, and then needed a third arthroscopy done that September.[16]

Why the sudden increase in hip arthroscopies? In the article "Hip injuries are on the rise," New York orthopedic surgeon and hip specialist Dr. Bryan T. Kelly is quoted as saying. "I think the main reason is improved recognition of pathology. Now we are beginning to recognize that a lot of problems that seem to be muscle strains and muscle pulls (in the groin area) are ending up these (hip) problems."[17]

In the same article, Phillies team physician Dr. Michael Ciccotti asks, "Are these injuries occurring more frequently or are we just more aware of them and more precise at diagnosing them and treating them?"[18] This is very significant question, one relevant in the discussion of any type of baseball injury.

Chapter 9

Acute Muscle, Connective Tissue and Tendon Tears

Acute muscle, connective tissue (sports hernia), and tendon tears, wherever the location, are some of the most common injuries in baseball. In the news more often lately is the oblique muscle injury.

Side Splitters — Oblique Injuries

Baseball involves a twisting motion at the waist. Both throwing and hitting a baseball involve twisting at the waist with rotation of the arms in relation to the spine. Thus, a common injury in baseball is to the muscles involved in twisting, most commonly a muscle in the abdomen called the internal oblique muscle. It moves from the ribs and midline fascia of the upper abdomen to attach with a long insertion to the upper pelvis (iliac crest) and the thoraco-lumbar fascia of the lower back.

In the past, the injury was simply called a rib muscle strain or abdominal muscle strain, but more recently has been called an oblique muscle strain. Once thought to be an uncommon injury, it certainly has been getting much attention recently. One source says the increased frequency of this injury is secondary to the strengthening of bigger muscles in the chest and arms and a lack of flexibility of smaller muscles, such as the oblique. The source also speculates that one reason for the more common occurrence of this injury is that baseball players are bigger and stronger than in the past, as they often engage in year-round strengthening exercises. The past use of steroids could also have played a role in bigger muscles and an increase in the frequency of this injury.[1]

A system has been proposed to grade the injury from one to three, with one being the mildest injury to three being the worst injury (more detail on muscle injuries later). Grade one usually doesn't limit activity much, but still must be treated with care (only small muscle fibers have been torn). A grade two injury doesn't impair normal activities but definitely limits twisting movements. A grade three injury would show a significant muscle tear on an MRI exam, can be due to the muscle actually tearing off its attachment at the lower three ribs, and significantly limits even normal activities.[2] A grade one injury can heal within a week or two. A significant grade three tear of this muscle may necessitate the player shutting down completely for six weeks. One author suggested time off from baseball (on the DL) equal to two weeks times the grade of injury.[3]

How many major league players get oblique strains per year? Two sources quote Stan Conte, director of medical services for the Los Angeles Dodgers, who estimates that between 2002 and 2007 there was an annual average of 20 professional baseball players with oblique strains on the DL. Of these, half were pitchers and half were position players.[4]

For a batter, an injury to this oblique muscle significantly hampers batting until the injury is healed. For position players, fielding and throwing can also be a problem. In 2006 the most notable oblique muscle injury was Albert Pujols.[5] Pujols' injury may have cost him the 2006 MVP award. He had to be completely shut down for two weeks in June after a great start. Also suffering this injury in 2006 were Chipper Jones, David Eckstein,[6] Nomar Garciaparra, Jeff Kent,[7] Johnny Damon, and Casey Blake.[8] In early 2007 Bobby Abreu of the Yankees suffered this injury.[9] In 2008 there were Gary Sheffield, Brandon Inge, Magglio Ordonez, and Paul Konerko, to name just a few.[10] This muscle twists the abdomen in swinging a bat and if not allowed to completely heal, the muscle can tear again, slowing down the recovery time.

With pitchers, this oblique muscle tear is just as serious an injury. It can shut a pitcher down for up to two months. The twisting motion required for pitchers in throwing the baseball is significantly impaired by this injury. Especially impaired is the follow-through motion, the period of rapid acceleration when the pitcher goes from the cocked position to the release of the ball. Pitchers with this injury in 2006 included C. C. Sabathia,[11] Mark Prior,[12] and Brett Tomko.[13] Mike Hampton had this injury in early 2007 before being shut down completely by an even worse elbow injury.[14] Jon Lieber of the Phillies had significant problems with this injury early in 2007.[15] Chris Young of the San Diego Padres was on the disabled list for two weeks in 2007 with this injury.[16]

Aaron Cook, the Colorado Rockies' opening day starter, ended up missing 79 days on the disabled list from August 10, 2007, to the fourth game of the World Series, showing how long a more severe injury can take to recover.[17]

In 2008 there were just as many of these injuries in the majors as in 2007.

The 2009 season was in its infancy when Chris Carpenter, the Cardinals' often injured pitcher, was injured this way. Carpenter missed five weeks, the injury occurring while he was swinging a bat, not pitching.[18] Carpenter's oblique injury may have cost him the 2009 Cy Young Award.

A position player suffering an oblique tear in early 2009 was Chipper Jones of the Braves, who had had a similar injury in 2006.[19]

The 2010 season brought its share of oblique injuries, including the Phillies' Joe Blanton,[20] Joel Pineiro of the Angels,[21] Yovani Gallardo of the Brewers,[22] and the Rangers' Tommy Hunter,[23] all pitchers. Matt Tolbert of the Twins, a utility player, also experienced this injury.[24] There were many more.

Billy Wagner strained his oblique muscle just three pitches into his first appearance in the 2010 playoffs between the Giants and the Braves at AT&T Park. First, Wagner tweaked the muscle in the 10th inning of the Braves' Game 2 victory while attempting to field an Edgar Renteria bunt down the third base line, just barely avoiding a collision with Atlanta third baseman Troy Glaus.[25]

Wagner aggravated the oblique injury while fielding yet another bunt, this time by Andres Torres. He turned briefly to look at the Giants' Renteria sliding at second base and then threw to first. Immediately after the play he gripped his side in pain and had to be helped off the field on what was ultimately the last play of his career, a career in which he recorded 422 total saves, 37 in his last season with the Braves.[26] (Wagner had previously announced his retirement before the playoffs.)

And the list goes on. With an estimated 20 of these injuries every year, there are sure to be many that have not been mentioned. In the future there will be many more.

Sports (or Sportsman) Hernia

A hernia is a protrusion of an organ or other bodily structure through a weak area in the muscles or tissues that surround it. The most common types of hernias are abdominal, inguinal, hiatal, femoral, umbilical, etc. One kind of abdominal hernia is the sportsman or sports hernia, a condition that can cause chronic groin pain, most often in the athlete. This is "an occult hernia caused by weakness or a tear of the posterior inguinal wall without a clinically recognizable hernia."[27]

This is a lot of technical language. Most people, especially males, know what an inguinal hernia is. On an annual physical exam, males are checked for an inguinal hernia. The doctor sticks his finger up the patient's scrotum and asks him to cough. If a bulge is felt where a bulge should not be noted, the patient has a hernia. If a bulge is not felt, but the patient has pain and is a high performance athlete, he could have what is called a sports hernia. This is

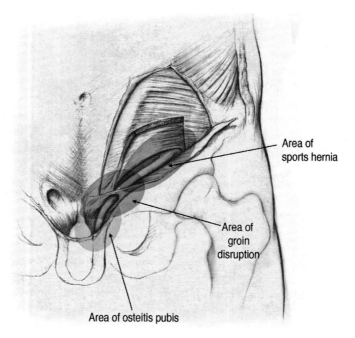

Location of difficult to diagnose sportsman, or sports, hernia relative to other possible causes of groin pain in a male baseball player. Surgical repair to alleviate symptoms is most often necessary (© 2002 Christy Krames).

often caused by an athletic activity that tears lower abdominal muscles, leading to a lower abdominal wall weakness that allows a hernia to develop.

All that said, the sports hernia is difficult to diagnose. If the athlete has pain that limits his performance, a diagnosis is needed. The most common cause of pain in the groin is a simple muscle strain. Often with rest the pain will resolve. Then no further pain is noted. With a sportsman hernia, after a period of rest, the pain recurs once the athlete returns to physical activity.[28]

Often the diagnosis is made by excluding other possible problems. A wide variety of tests can be done in evaluating a sports hernia, including urinalysis, rectal exam, plain X-Rays, ultrasound, CT scan, MRI, or bone scan. These simply rule out other possible causes of the groin pain. One possible diagnostic test indicated in the *British Journal of Surgery* in 2000 is called a herniography. Dye is injected into the abdomen and the patient is asked to strain. X-ray pictures are then taken. If the test shows the hernia, it makes the diagnosis easy. If the test is negative, this does not rule out the existence of a sports hernia.[29]

Most often surgery is required to correct the defect and relieve the pain. There are several surgical techniques used to correct the hernia (some using the minimally invasive laparoscope). "In the motivated patient, after surgical repair, 95 percent are free of pain and able to return to competitive sports."[30]

CHRIS DUNCAN

Other than his cervical disc problems, Chris Duncan of the Cardinals had yet another unique injury, a sports hernia. In an article on September 10, 2007, in the *St. Louis Post-Dispatch*, Tony LaRussa, the manager of the Cardinals, noted that Duncan had had a lower half injury or abdominal strain that had bothered him since the end of July. It apparently had been affecting his batting, as Duncan had been in a slump, batting only .175 since July 22. Apparently, on September 8, Duncan, while running from first to third on a ground ball single by Aaron Miles, aggravated his problem to the point that something more had to be done.[31]

As with many newspaper articles, much medical information is left out. For instance, what medical tests had been done on Chris Duncan? What might have caused the sports hernia to occur in the first place?

An article in the *Washington Post* on September 23 stated that Duncan thought his vigorous off-season weight lifting might have caused the hernia, though the article did not explain the gap in time between the weight lifting and the onset of pain in late July.[32]

Chris Duncan had surgery on his sports hernia on September 20, 2007.[33]

In a *Washington Post* article, there was a mention that Duncan's brother Shelley might also have a sports hernia.[34] An article in the *New York Post* in November of 2007 indicated that Shelley had surgery for the sports hernia ten days after the 2007 season ended for the Yankees.[35] Was the cause of the hernias the lifting of weights the Duncans did during the 2006–2007 off-season, or was the cause bad genetics?

IAN KINSLER

Even more recent than Chris Duncan's sports hernia, Texas Rangers second baseman Ian Kinsler and Cleveland Indians outfielder Grady Sizemore were diagnosed with sports hernias. Kinsler, who went on the disabled list on August 18, 2008, opted to have surgery in early September, effectively ending his 2008 season.[36]

GRADY SIZEMORE

In September of 2009, outfielder Grady Sizemore had surgery in Philadelphia done by Dr. Bill Meyers. Sizemore had suffered the injury in spring training of 2009 and had played the rest of the season with the injury. Sizemore's

20-minute lower abdominal procedure was his second surgery in a week. He had season-ending arthroscopic surgery on his elbow prior to the hernia repair.[37]

RAUL IBANEZ

Raul Ibanez of the National League champion Philadelphia Phillies had surgery to repair a sports hernia in November 2009, after the World Series was over. Dr. Bill Meyers repaired Ibanez's hernia.[38]

JOSE BAUTISTA

In 2010 Toronto Blue Jay Jose Bautista had surgery for a sports hernia. The hernia did not affect his stats in 2010. Bautista played in 161 games hit a career-high 54 home runs with 124 RBI, 109 runs, and 100 walks. He stated the injury occurred in May and he simply played through it. It apparently affected him most when he ran.[39]

It is not uncommon with some injuries that if the pain is tolerable and the player's performance is not much affected during the season, then surgery is put off until the season is over.

NICK PUNTO

The 2011 season had barely begun when Cardinals reserve infielder Nick Punto had to have surgery for a sports hernia. Punto's history is typical. He had been limited in his spring training because of a "nagging" discomfort in his groin area.[40]

Noteworthy is that Punto had been on the DL for the Minnesota Twins in 2010 for what was thought to be a groin strain. No mention was made as to whether the injuries in 2010 and 2011 were related.[41]

General Muscle and Tendon Tear — not shoulder, wrist, or hand

The following section is devoted to more muscle/tendon strains and pulls. Stephanie Bell, in an article at ESPN.com, expresses noteworthy feelings about all these muscle/tendon injuries (other than oblique injuries and sportsman hernia) writing, "Muscle injuries: Also referred to as a "pull," twinge" or "tear," the oft-reported muscle strain is the ultimate definition of boring when it comes to baseball injuries, but it is so commonplace that we would be remiss if we did not address it."[42]

These injuries can be found in almost any sports medicine book[43] (e.g., *Sports Injuries: Mechanisms, Prevention, Treatment* by Fu and Stone). The tendency is to grade the muscle injury depending on the severity. In the past, some of the classification depended simply on observing whether the patient recovered quickly or possibly needed surgery to correct the problem. With the advent of MRIs, used almost routinely at the major league level, it is possible to grade injury to muscles more accurately.

As noted in the discussion of oblique tears, muscle tears can be classified. Grades one, two, and three is the simplest classification of muscle tears, which are mild, moderate, and severe respectively. Within each group there is some variation. Mild grade one changes may result in only a sore muscle for several days and little or no missed time on the DL. The player simply plays through the injury. An MRI might show no damage, as changes may be on a microscopic level.

Grade two often involves some "tearing or disruption of a moderate number of muscle and tendon fibers, which result in moderate pain, swelling, and disability in association with an abnormal (weak or painful) contraction of the involved muscle."[44]

It would appear there is great latitude as to what a grade two tear is. If a trip to the DL is involved, the duration depends on the severity of the injury and the player's ability to heal.

A grade three strain involves a complete disruption of the muscle/tendon unit. Surgery to repair muscle/tendon function is sometimes necessary.

Hamstring

Ken Griffey Jr.

Hamstring strains or tears are one of the most common of all baseball injuries. This group of muscles in the back of the thigh, just below the buttocks, is very important in running. In baseball, running usually involves short, quick bursts of energy. This quick stop-to-start movement is especially taxing on the hamstring muscles. The hamstrings are also important in throwing and pitching, but less so than in running. Acute tears can also occur due to bracing against an immovable object (the mechanism of Ken Griffey's worst hamstring tear). Acute tears are included under the category of overuse injury.

Hamstring injuries can be due to trauma. Trauma, a muscle contusion, would be caused by a direct blow to the muscle. In baseball this can happen with any type of collision, though the hamstring muscles, located in the back of the thigh, are not usually injured in this manner. Quadriceps muscles, in the front of the thigh, are much more subject to trauma injuries. As one would expect, this injury is more common in football, in which frequent collisions are caused by blocking or tackling.

Ken Griffey Jr. has had some nasty hamstring injuries. He went through his first eight years with few injuries, mainly a bad wrist fracture. After 2000 he was injured almost as much as he enjoyed good health.

Ken Griffey Jr. needs little introduction. He retired in 2010 with 630 home runs, 1,836 RBI, 2,781 hits, and a .284 batting average. He started his career as the first overall pick of the 1987 free-agent draft by the Seattle Mariners. He spent very little time in the minors, making his debut in 1989 at the young age of 19. He hit at least 40 home runs every year from 1996 to 2000. He won ten consecutive Gold Gloves from 1990 to 1999 while playing center field for the Mariners.

Griffey did so well that he became known by the simple nickname "Junior." Consider Joe DiMaggio's nickname, "The Yankee Clipper," or Ted Williams' nickname, "The Splendid Splinter." More recently, one would note Albert Pujols' nickname "Prince Albert." These are the types of nicknames often reserved for greatness.

On February 10, 2000, Junior Griffey was acquired by the Cincinnati Reds for pitcher Brett Tomko, outfielder Mike Cameron, pitcher Jake Meyer, and infielder Antonio Perez. Griffey's dad, Ken Griffey Sr., had played for

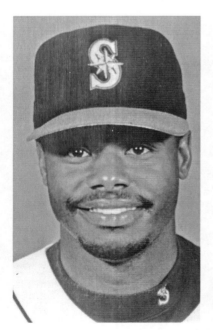

Cincinnati for many years. Subsequently, Junior signed a contract with the Reds for nine years for $112.5 million, with a club option for a tenth year. Unfortunately, this was also the start of a series of yearly injuries; Griffey's stats never again would approach what he achieved during his tenure with Seattle.[45] Where has this scenario been heard before?

In 2000 and 2001, Griffey had chronic problems with his left hamstring. It was sore much of the season in 2000. Contemporary articles did not indicate any specific cause for the chronic injury pattern in early to mid–2000. That changed on September 11, as he aggravated previous problems, partially tearing the hamstring and missing the rest of the season simply by running fast. In the seventh inning against the Chicago Cubs, Griffey tried to score from first on a double by Dmitri Young. He appeared to have injured it as he pulled up slightly between second and third. He subsequently slid into home plate, but indicated the slide was not what caused the injury.[46]

Seattle Mariner Ken Griffey Jr. in 1996 (National Baseball Hall of Fame Library, Cooperstown, New York).

During spring training in 2001, Griffey

injured his left hamstring again, this time simply rounding third base. He missed a few games, but did not end up on the DL until April 28, when he tweaked his partially torn left hamstring while running to first base after a checked swing.[47]

Problems with his right hamstring started in 2002. He suffered a mild strain in June. He previously had been on the DL (April 8 to May 23) for a partially torn patella tendon suffered during a rundown between third base and home on April 7. Then he injured the right hamstring again during an all-out effort to run to first base to avoid grounding into a double play on June 7. He succeeded in avoiding the double play, but ended up on the DL from June 25 to July 21.[48]

Tony Jackson, in *The Cincinnati Post* on June 8, wrote, "The fact that the injury occurred in Griffey's healthy right hamstring, as opposed to his chronically gimpy left hamstring, was an encouraging sign."[49] No injury is really encouraging, and Griffey eventually ended up on the DL when the injury didn't respond to conservative therapy.

Griffey again injured a hamstring muscle when he suffered a partially torn right hamstring on July 10, 2004, (on DL from July 11 till August 3). But this injury pales in comparison to the injury to the same hamstring he suffered on August 4, 2004. This time he completely ripped the tendon of the right hamstring right off the bone.[50] This injury falls more under the category of traumatic injury, as it occurred when Griffey slid into the outfield wall to prevent a nasty collision with the wall. It is listed here because it is just one of a string of hamstring injuries Griffey suffered during his career.

The play: Griffey started in right field for the first time in his 16-year career at SBC Park in San Francisco (maybe a bad sign to begin with). He raced to cut off a ball hit in the gap before the ball hit the wall. He slid, bracing himself against the wall with his right leg; the right leg hyperextended in the process. Griffey "walked" off the field with what was later diagnosed as a completely ruptured right hamstring.[51]

It soon became very apparent that this injury was potentially career-ending. For Griffey to continue playing baseball, surgery was required to reattach his hamstring with tendon to the pelvis bone. Griffey had surgery of a unique nature on August 16, 2004. Dr. Tim Kremchek, well-known orthopedic surgeon and the Cincinnati Reds' team physician, used three titanium screws to reattach the hamstring muscle to the bone.

Post-op care was difficult. In order for the hamstring to heal properly in the right position, Griffey had to wear a sling to keep the right leg bent behind him all the time for six weeks. If he got around at all, he had to support himself with a scooter. Inactivity of this type had to be difficult for any professional athlete. Griffey described the experience as "miserable."[52] He counts this as the worst of his surgeries and rehabs.

Griffey had surgery on August 16. He was finally cleared to walk on October 1. He did that until he was given the okay to play golf and swing a bat in December. He started running the bases and making quick movements on the baseball field in spring training. He was just fine on Opening Day.[53]

In 2005 Ken Griffey did well; he was able to play 128 games, ending up with a .301 average, 35 home runs and 92 RBI. He won the Comeback Player of the Year award in the National league.[54]

However, 2005 was not an injury-free year. Griffey had problems with his left knee, requiring surgery. Ending his season on September 4, he had arthroscopic surgery to remove loose bodies from the knee. At the same time some scar tissue from his 2004 right hamstring operation was removed.

In his remaining career with Cincinnati (until July 31, 2008), there were no further trips to the DL for hamstring injuries. Griffey did go on the DL in April of 2006, but this trip was for an inflamed tendon behind his right knee. He did have another muscle injury shortening his season in 2007, but it was a high left groin strain sustained simply as he braced to make a throw from the outfield on September 19. The 2007 season had been one of Griffey's more durable since 2000, as he played in 144 games while hitting .277 with 30 home runs with 93 RBI.[55]

In 2008 Griffey had left knee problems requiring off-season arthroscopy by Dr. Kremchek. It was not anything out of the ordinary for a 39-year-old male who had played 20 years of major league baseball. Torn cartilage and some knee degenerative changes were noted, but no further hamstring problems landed the All-Star on the DL. Griffey played the vast majority of his games in 2009 with the Mariners as the DH, decreasing the likelihood of significant injuries with less running into walls in the outfield.[56]

After being utilized little in 2010 with the Mariners, Griffey decided to retire.[57]

Jose Reyes

Ken Griffey Jr.'s hamstring problems didn't begin until he was over 30 years old. Jose Reyes' hamstring problems started at a much younger age.

Both Jose Reyes and Ken Griffey Jr. made it to the major leagues at a young age, 19. Reyes was thought to be a can't-miss athlete even at age 19, one of *the* best prospects in all the minor leagues.

During his nine seasons with the Mets, he justified this early assessment. From 2005 till 2008 he has had four seasons of 190-plus hits, 12-plus triples, 99-plus runs, and 56-plus stolen bases. His best year was 2008 he had 204 hits, 37 doubles, 17 triples, 113 runs scored, 16 home runs, and 56 stolen bases. From 2005 to 2007 he lead the league in stolen bases with 60, 64, and 78 respectively.

Early on, when he had problems with his hamstrings there was some concern about his durability. At age 19 he missed three weeks at Triple-A Norfolk and five more days after joining the Mets, with a strained right hamstring. He suffered another strain of the right hamstring in spring training in 2004, on a headfirst slide into second base. He had an MRI on March 15. This hamstring injury, combined with a stress fracture of his left fibula Reyes sustained later in the year, caused him to miss considerable time (most of August and September with the stress fracture).[58]

Questions about Reyes' durability were somewhat erased during seasons 2005 to 2008. Reyes played 161 games in 2005, 153 in 2006, 160 in 2007 and 159 in 2008.

The hamstring bug bit him again in 2008. In April he again injured a hamstring, this time his left. An MRI fortunately revealed only a mild strain. In contrast to previous hamstring injuries, this strain was closer to Reyes' knee, while the injuries in 2003 and 2004 were located higher up, more proximal. He aggravated the April injury on June 17, while he was running to first base (a typical mechanism of injury).[59] These injuries to his left hamstring did not result in a trip to the DL. Reyes played through these injuries, and ended up playing 159 games in 2008.

The right hamstring bug again bit him in 2009, and he spent considerable time on the DL in 2009.

Research revealed no article in 2009 that specifically stated how and when Reyes initially injured his right hamstring muscle. One article in *Newsday* (Long Island, New York) by David Lennon in October noted no specific initial injury but did state Reyes aggravated the injury when he snapped the frayed tendon on June 3 during a rehab game.[60]

One article at newyorkmag.com in October of 2009 gave a timeline for Reyes' 2009 problems, though it did not specifically mention the June 3 incident.[61] On May 15, Reyes missed three games because of tightness in his right calf. He aggravated the injury on May 20 when running to first base after hitting a ground ball. He went on the disabled list May 21 and never came off of it in 2009. An MRI obtained in June, probably after aggravating the injury further on June 3, revealed a slight tear of the tendon behind his knee — a hamstring muscle.

The rest of 2009 season consisted of adding orthotics to Reyes' shoes, rehab therapy, slight running, and gradual working back into playing shape after periods of rest. Reyes even received experimental injections of Platelet Rich Plasma in an attempt to heal the tendon. This is a new method of healing chronic tendon and muscle tears using the patient's own blood (platelets) injected into the site of injury. This new therapy is supposed to stimulate the release growth factors and in doing so stimulate the body's own healing processes.[62] In Reyes' case the treatment didn't work.

During rehabilitation, Reyes, while running the bases with some extra intensity on September 29, injured the right hamstring in a different place. This was only thought to be a mild strain. The assessment was that this less severe injury would heal on its own. But the original hamstring injury was not going to respond to conservative treatment. Surgery was necessary.

There actually are three muscles that make up the hamstring in each leg. On the medial (inner) thigh are the semimembranosus muscle and semitendinosus muscle. In the lateral (outer) posterior thigh is the biceps femoris. Generally, it is difficult to interpret from newspaper articles exactly where the problem lies, as most articles don't specify where the injury is. An injury to the hamstring muscle could be anywhere from the buttocks to knee, involving any one of the three muscles, though most tears are where the muscle joins the tendon.

Jose Reyes' more severe, chronic injury was noted to be behind the knee. In fact some articles early in 2009 indicated the strain was actually a high calf muscle strain, not a hamstring tear at all, an easy mistake to make considering that those muscles are in close proximity. A later article says the injury was to an accessory hamstring muscle. One article finally identified the specific tendon injured as part of the semitendinosis muscle. The tendon that was torn did not heal, and Reyes did not play a single major league game after May 20.[63]

Who better to repair this damaged hamstring tendon than someone who is an expert in treating this type of injury? The Mets' team physician, Dr. David Altchek, deferred treatment to Dr. Daniel E. Cooper, the Dallas Cowboys' team physician. Successful surgery to clean up the scar tissue was performed on October 15, 2009.[64]

In 2010, Reyes hit .282 in 133 games with 29 doubles, 10 triples and 11 home runs. He even stole 30 bases. The 2011 season started off very well. On July 2, 2011, Reyes was leading the National League with a .354 average with 124 hits, 65 runs scored, and 15 triples. He then injured his left hamstring running to first base in the first inning of a July 2 game against the New York Yankees. Reyes was removed from the game the very next inning.[65]

When Reyes didn't improve an MRI was done which revealed a grade 1 strain and Reyes was put on the DL. He missed almost three weeks, including the All-Star break, and then went on the DL with a left hamstring strain again for most of August. He had again injured himself running out a ground ball, this time in the first inning of an August 7 game against the Atlanta Braves at Citi Field. This time an MRI showed a strain in a different part of the left hamstring.

Despite Reyes' two trips to the DL for hamstring problems in 2011 he still ended up winning a batting title with a .337 average, though stolen bases and triples were scarce after Reyes' first hamstring injury of the year. He did finish the year with the required number of plate appearances, though he only had 586 PAs in 126 games played.

Despite the knowledge that Reyes had not played more than 133 games in a season since 2008, the Miami Marlins signed him to a $106 million, six-year contract with an option for 2018 that might make the contract worth $120 million. The Mets, Reyes' former team, never made a formal offer.

GROIN STRAIN

Nomar Garciaparra

Nomar Garciaparra's injury in 2005 gives an example of the classical muscle injury initiated by a quick burst of speed. It is not always the hamstring muscle and tendon that is injured in such manner.

Occasionally when muscles tear, they tear in the middle of the muscle, but the vast majority of muscle tears are near the attachment of the muscle to the tendon or the tendon to the bone. Nomar Garciaparra's injury is no different.

Nomar was a six-time All-Star and Rookie of the Year in 1997, three years after he was taken in the first round (12th pick overall) in the 1994 draft by the Boston Red Sox. He spent the greater part of his career (nine seasons) with the Boston Red Sox as a shortstop. He twice led the league in hitting, hitting .357 in 1999 and .372 in 2000. He seemed a certain future Hall of Fame member till a series of injuries hit.

He had several wrist injuries — in 1999, 2001, and 2004. He had an Achilles heel injury in 2004,[66] and this left groin muscle injury in 2005.

After playing for the Red Sox, Nomar played for the Cubs, Dodgers, and A's. It was while playing for the Chicago Cubs in 2005 that he sustained the severe groin injury that forced him to miss three months of that year.

On April 20, in a game in St. Louis, he injured his left groin muscle. He hit a ground ball and, when attempting to run to first base to avoid a double play, he collapsed when leaving the batter's box. It was one of those injuries that could be seen over and over from replays from the Cubs' telecast on WGN. It was obvious the injury was severe, as Garciaparra was in considerable pain and could barely move. He had to be carried off the field.[67]

The injury was a complete tear of the tendon of a left groin muscle off the bone, what is called a grade III tear. It was not said exactly which groin muscle, as there are six on each thigh that form a complex that attach to the pubic bone. In fact, where they attach is in very close proximity to the attachment of the more proximal abdominal muscles (from above the pubic bone).

The tear, though complete, probably did not encompass a great deal of muscle separation from the pubic bone, as the treatment chosen was not to reattach the muscle's tendon to the bone but rather to clean up torn tissue around the tear and then reinforce both connective tissue around the tear and the abdominal muscle tendons from above. The muscle and tendon attachment would heal with rest and without being re-attached.

This method of treatment was chosen after consultation with several specialists familiar with this type of injury, an injury actually much more common in hockey and soccer than in baseball.[68] Surgery took only 30 minutes. It was performed by Dr. Bill Meyers at Hahnemann Hospital in Philadelphia.[69] Because the surgery was less extensive in nature, the recovery would be quicker.[70] Even with the less invasive surgery, Garciaparra was still on the DL from April 20 until August 5, 2005, just over three months.[71]

CALF INJURY

Pedro Martinez

Pedro Martinez made his major league début at age 20. His career record was 219 wins and 100 losses with an ERA of 2.93 and 3,154 strikeouts in 2,827⅓ innings. He won three Cy Young awards.

Martinez missed considerable playing time from 2006 to 2009 while recovering from surgery to correct a rotator cuff tear, the surgery done in early October 2006. In 2006, while Martinez was having trouble with his shoulder, he was also having problems with calf muscle strains, suffering this injury in each of his legs over the last month and one-half. One injury sometimes leads to another injury in another location.

His right calf strain was sustained on August 14. The strain was first noticed when he was warming up to pitch against the Phillies in Philadelphia. It obviously hampered his delivery as he hit two batters and balked in another run, all in the first inning, giving up six runs. He ended up pitching only that one inning.[72]

An MRI on August 15 revealed a mild right calf strain, though severe enough to place him on the 15 day DL, Martinez's second trip to the DL since June, when he was on the DL for an inflamed hip (June 29 to July 28). Caution was needed for the calf strain as this was the leg he pushed off when he made his delivery to the plate.

Martinez came off the DL on September 15. On September 27 he noticed some tightness again after pitching, but the tightness was worse in the left calf, not the right. An MRI on September 28 revealed a torn tendon in the left calf, essentially ending his season and negating any chance that he might pitch in the playoffs for the Mets that year. (Possibly favoring his right calf caused the injury to the left calf.) It was revealed shortly thereafter that he had been struggling with his right shoulder, too, and he had rotator cuff surgery the first week of October. Surgery for his calf injuries was not deemed necessary.[73]

To compound the Mets' dilemma El Duque, Orlando Hernandez, who had been pitching very well the last month and was the projected first-game starter in the playoffs in the Division Series against the Dodgers, injured his right calf on October 3. He was simply jogging in the outfield when the injury occurred.

An MRI exam confirmed that Hernandez had sustained a strain.[74] The 40-year-old Hernandez ended up missing the playoffs completely, hurting the Mets' chances, and the Mets, having beaten the Dodgers in the Division Series, eventually lost to the Cardinals in the National League Championship Series.

BICEPS INJURY

Mo Vaughn

Mo Vaughn had a productive career although he had a tendency to strike out a lot. He was signed as the 23rd overall pick out of Seton Hall University in the 1989 amateur draft by the Boston Red Sox and had his most productive years with the Red Sox and Anaheim Angels. He was named MVP of the American League for the Red Sox in 1995 when he hit 39 home runs and led the league with 126 RBI. Actually, 1996 was even better for Vaughn as he had 44 home runs, 143 RBI and a .326 batting average, but he finished fifth in the MVP voting.

Vaughn signed a $60 million six-year free agent contract with the Anaheim Angels after the 1998 season.[75]

Vaughn suffered a torn distal biceps muscle and tendon just above his elbow (proximal to elbow — pitcher's elbow muscle tears are just below the elbow). The injury started as a "little knot or cramp in his left biceps" occurring in the sixth inning of a game on August 2, 2000.[76] He apparently felt a pop while playing but only reported it later — most likely the injury occurring during a swing of the bat. After a massage, he was back on August 4 and played the rest of the season despite the injury, though he noted that after the injury he just didn't feel right. He simply thought the problem was mild tendonitis and treated it thusly. For instance, Vaughn was seen applying ice on his left biceps on August 12.[77]

Vaughn ended up 2000 playing in 161 games, with a .272 average, 36 home runs and 117 RBI, but he led the league with 181 strikeouts. He started his off-season workouts including weights as usual, but by December he noticed considerable weakness in his left biceps. An MRI revealed a complete tear of Vaughn's left biceps, necessitating surgery. A complex, two and one-half hour surgery was done February 6 by a Dr. Bernard Morrey at the Mayo Clinic. The surgery was complex, not only because the muscle was reconstructed, but because a tendon graft from the back of Vaughn's leg was needed to reconstruct the distal biceps tendon.[78]

Vaughn missed the entire 2001 season and then was traded to the Mets on December 22 in exchange for pitcher Kevin Appier.[79] Vaughn's career with the Mets was short-lived. He had a decent year in 2002 with 26 home runs and 72 RBI, but his 2003 season was cut short by an arthritic left knee which ultimately led to his retirement at age 36 in 2004.[80]

TORN ACHILLES TENDON

Ryan Howard

Ryan Howard, the 31-year-old slugging first baseman of the Philadelphia Phillies, tore his left Achilles tendon on the very last play of the fifth game of the 2011 NLDS against the Cardinals.[81] Howard injured the Achilles in a manner similar to Nomar Garciaparra. He hit a grounder to the first base side of the infield. On running out of the batter's box, he stumbled and fell. When he got up he was barely able to walk and had to be helped off the field as the Cardinals celebrated their victory.

The injury was initially thought to be severe, and an MRI later confirmed that the left Achilles tendon was ruptured. Surgery was done on October 12, 2011.[82] Howard was still recovering at the start of the 2012 season and was activated on July 6. This season would also end early, when he broke his right big toe on September 29.

Conclusion

It would be impossible to list all the muscle/tendon injuries in baseball. These injuries are almost as common as pebbles of sand on the beach. They are some of the most common injuries in baseball, though most are not unique to the sport.

PART II. TRAUMATIC INJURIES

Chapter 10

Sliding Injuries

Baseball trauma, which is not as common as overuse injuries, can be divided into several categories: sliding injuries, either to the person sliding or the one being slid into; collisions between players on the field; collisions between players and parts of the baseball field (turf, bases, walls around the playing field, parts of dugouts, or equipment, etc.); and impact injuries caused by a baseball either thrown or hit. In this discussion, trauma is broken down into each category with the mechanisms of injury. Following general discussion of trauma, there is a special discussion on head trauma and concussions, which are caused by many different mechanisms.

At all levels of baseball, professional and recreational, sliding is one of the most common mechanisms of injuries. In recreational softball, for instance, one study estimated sliding injuries account for 71 percent of all traumatic injuries.[1] This author could not find a similar study for professional baseball, but a general scan of the literature would indicate the percentage is probably significant.

Sliding injuries can occur to the runner sliding into a base or to the fielder standing on or near the base. This book will look at injuries to the runner first, noting whether the slide is head-first or feet-first, as this obviously results in different types of injuries.

Injury to Runner

UNKNOWN MANNER OF SLIDING

Bob Horner

On August 15, 1983, Bob Horner, third baseman of the Atlanta Braves, broke his right wrist (navicular bone) on a slide into second base. References don't mention whether this was a head-first slide, but do indicate Horner was trying to break up a double play. He fractured his wrist and missed the last 43 games of the 1983 season.[2]

Bob Horner was unfortunate to fracture the same wrist the following year (May 1984) in the very same place (the scaphoid bone). This later injury was not during sliding but while diving for a ball hit near his position at third base.

Not only did Horner miss the rest of the season from the second injury, the navicular fracture did not heal completely, and on December 18, 1984, he needed a bone graft as well as a screw inserted to get the fracture to finally heal (a bone graft is done from small pieces of bone from someplace else in the body put in the area of the fracture to aid healing). Dr. Peter Carter, an orthopedic doctor in Dallas, Texas, performed the surgery. The procedure was innovative. The bone graft had been done before, but the use of the reinforcing screw was a relatively new idea.[3]

It is quite possible that Horner's first fracture never healed completely and made him more prone to get a second fracture of the same bone by a non-sliding mechanism.

HEAD-FIRST SLIDES

The head-first slide became more common in the 1960s to 1970s, around the time Pete Rose was doing it frequently.[4] Before that, feet-first slides were the norm.

Why do it? Dr. David A. Peters, an engineer with Washington University, said that based on engineering principles, the head-first slide is faster, except in the case of first base, where the player typically runs through the base rather than slides.[5] Two studies done and published in journals in 2002 and 2003, however, show no significant statistical difference.[6] The study published in the *Clinical Journal of Sports Medicine* notes a .02 second difference in individuals studied between head-first and feet-first slides, the former 3.65 seconds and the latter 3.67 seconds.[7] This difference is made a big deal of by some, but the study indicates the difference is not statistically significant.[8] Neither study was done on professional baseball players.

The major concern with head-first slides is hand injuries, as that body part is exposed. In order to avoid this injury, some advocate that when running on the bases the player should hold a glove in each hand to avoid hitting the bag with an open hand, decreasing possible injuries to the exposed fingers and thumb.[9]

Shawon Dunston

A classical head-first sliding injury, though not well known, occurred to Shawon Dunston on June 15, 1987. The manner in which it occurred is what makes it classical. Dunston executed a head-first slide in the bottom of the ninth in a 3–2 loss to the Philadelphia Phillies. Initially it was thought to be just a sprain, but x-rays revealed an oblique fracture of the fourth metacarpal (the bone in the palm of the hand just proximal to the ring finger). The injury was severe enough to require surgery, probably with a pin being put in to stabilize the fracture.[10]

Dunston returned to the lineup on July 12. The Cubs were very happy to get Dunston back as they had also lost their starting second baseman, Ryne Sandberg (sprained ankle), while Dunston was on the DL.

Alex Gordon

One doesn't need to go back in time very far to find another hand fracture from a head-first slide. In spring training of 2010 (March 7), Kansas City Royals third baseman Alex Gordon fractured his thumb when sliding head-first into second base on an attempted steal. He slammed his thumb into the left foot of Texas second baseman Joaquin Arias.[11] The fracture fortunately was minimally displaced, though Gordon ended up on the DL from March 8 until April 18.[12]

After the injury Gordon was quoted as saying that he'll "probably stop [head-first sliding] from now on."[13]

Rafael Furcal

Even more recently, Rafael Furcal broke his left thumb while sliding into third base on April 11, 2011.[14] He was on the DL for six weeks. It wasn't a good year for Furcal as 12 days after he returned, he went back on the DL for a left oblique strain, an injury suffered during a rundown play.[15]

Kenny Lofton

Another head-first sliding injury was a bit unusual. It was one of those uncommon slides into first base. It is often said that one should not slide into first base unless one is trying to avoid being tagged out on an errant throw. The reasons are that one does not get to the base any faster than by running through the base,[16] and one might get injured.

Kenny Lofton, in an ill-advised attempt to beat the throw from first baseman Mike Stanley to pitcher Pedro Martinez, injured himself as he slid into first base head-first. Lofton was running down the baseline full-speed when he made his slide, a last-second, all-out extra effort to try to beat Martinez to the bag just as Martinez was receiving the throw. It was on October 11, 1999, during the fifth and deciding Divisional Series battle between the Cleveland Indians and the Boston Red Sox.[17]

The result: Lofton dislocated his left shoulder and tore his rotator cuff. To add insult to injury, Lofton was called out on the play and Cleveland lost the game. It was speculated soon after the injury that Lofton might be out an extended period of time, and even miss the start of the next season, especially considering he had to have surgery done by Dr. James Andrews in December of 1999.[18]

In a very pleasant surprise, Lofton was able to return to play in the 2000 opening day game for the Cleveland Indians at Camden Yards in Baltimore.

Lenny Dykstra

Lenny Dykstra, then the center fielder for the Philadelphia Phillies, was well known for his frequent slides into first base. After grounding to an infielder, he just had to do everything he could possibly do to beat that throw to the bag. That included sliding. Dykstra is quoted as saying, "I've dived into first that way a million times and never got hurt."[19]

So, on August 16, 1992, in an attempt to beat the throw to first, he once again dived head-first at first base — and this time he broke the second metacarpal (beneath the index finger in the palm) in his left hand. Dykstra ended up on the DL, his third trip to the DL in 1992.[20]

Rick Manning

Terry Pluto, in his book *The Curse of Rocky Colavito*, mentions two head-first sliding injuries that occurred to Cleveland Indians players (other than Kenny Lofton who is not discussed in Terry Pluto's book).[21] These injuries did not affect a hand, arm, or shoulder as one might expect. Both injuries entailed significant back injuries which affected the players' careers in a very adverse manner.

Rick Manning was the center fielder for the Indians for eight and a half years of his total 13 years in the majors (he played for Milwaukee the other years). His career stats are not great (.257 career average). But they might have been greater if not for his injury that occurred June 4, 1977, a head-first slide into second base. At the time it appeared the injury was not severe, as Manning was able to finish the game. In fact he even played three more games before his back pain became much worse. It got so bad he could barely run.[22]

He needed a back brace for six weeks because of his pain. Apparently the severity of the injury was not apparent on initial x-rays. One month after the injury, repeat x-rays revealed a fractured vertebra. Manning played only 68 games that year, sidelined from early June till September.

In Manning's first two seasons (1975 and 1976) for the Indians he batted .285 and .292. After the injury he only batted a best of .270 in 1982. It is thought that the injury affected his swing. According to Terry Pluto, he was never the same hitter.

Joe Charboneau

A more career-damaging sliding injury occurred to Joe Charboneau. Charboneau burst on the scene for the Cleveland Indians in 1980. His stats were good despite missing some games with a pelvis injury. He batted .289 in 131 games with 23 home runs and 87 RBI. This was good enough for him to win the American League Rookie of the Year award.

During spring training of 1981, while playing an exhibition game in Tucson, he injured his back during a head-first slide into second base. Pluto relates that Charboneau felt a pop in his back during the slide.[23] The day after the injury, he could hardly move. He was examined by a doctor who came to the clinical diagnosis of a ruptured disc. Another doctor who saw him said he just had a strain, but the first opinion was probably correct (today he would have had a better diagnosis with an MRI of the spine, but not in 1981).

Because of the second opinion, a strain, Joe Charboneau was allowed to continue to play. By as he played it became more and more obvious that something more serious than a strain was affecting his back. He stood stiffly and swung weakly.

In the first half of 1981 he was only able to bat at a .208 clip. The 1981 season was interrupted in June of 1981 by the players' strike. The break in the season did give him time to rest, but when the season resumed after the strike, he didn't do any better. In early August he was sent down to the Class AAA Charleston minor league team, later returned to the Indians, and finished with a .210 average.[24]

Charboneau had surgery to repair the ruptured disc after the 1981 season. The following spring of 1982 he hit well, but this didn't last. He ended up hitting .214 in only 56 at-bats in 22 major league games. He had only hit six home runs in the majors after his back injury in 1981. He basically became a singles hitter and lost any running speed he had before the injury. He was released in early 1983 and never played in the major leagues again.[25]

FEET-FIRST SLIDES

After mentioning these cases, it is easy to see that sliding into a base can cause serious injury to a player. Cases previously mentioned, except possibly Bob Horner, resulted from head-first slides. Feet-first slides can also result in significant injuries to the knee, ankle, and leg.

Sliding is an activity that is practiced like any repetitive activity to insure proper technique and avoid injuries. When it comes down to actually sliding, decisions to slide need to be made instantaneously. For the runner to try to change his mind (slide vs. not slide, slide left vs. slide right, head-first vs. feet-first) in mid-slide can have bad consequences — Tommy Davis, for instance.

Research revealed numerous injuries from feet-first slides. It is one of the most common traumatic injuries found. Only a few examples follow.

Pete Reiser

Pete Reiser's baseball career gives examples of numerous types of traumatic injuries a player can possibly experience while playing the game of baseball.

In the book *Pete Reiser: The Rough-and-Tumble Career of the Perfect Ballplayer*, by Sidney Jacobson, Reiser was noted to have two significant sliding injuries which occurred in the more traditional manner of sliding feet-first.[26]

In 1946, he had a head concussion. When he returned, he sustained a calf injury. Despite this, manager Leo Durocher continued to play him. The Dodgers were running nip-and-tuck with the Cardinals, and Durocher needed his star out there. Finally, Reiser injured himself sliding in the third-to-the-last game of the season against Philadelphia.

Reiser walked in the first inning of that game. In Rudy Marzano's book *The Brooklyn Dodgers in the 1940s*, he reports that despite Reiser's calf injury, Durocher gave him the steal sign. Reiser took a lead to get ready to steal. A quick pickoff throw darted to first base behind the runner. To avoid the tag, Reiser slid back into the bag feet-first and caught his left foot on the bag.[27]

As had happened before, Reiser had to be carried off the field on a stretcher. X-rays revealed a fractured fibula (the outer bone in the upper part of the ankle). Reiser was lost for the last two games of the Dodgers' season and

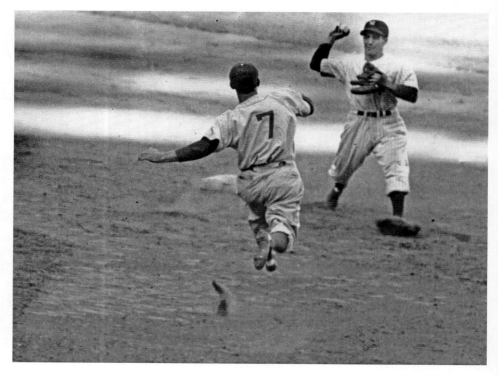

Pete Reiser going into a feet-first slide during a game in the 1947 World Series between the Dodgers and the New York Yankees (National Baseball Hall of Fame Library, Cooperstown, New York).

the two-game playoff against the St. Louis Cardinals. The Dodgers had finished tied with the Cardinals on the last day of the season. The Dodgers lost both games of the playoff though it is uncertain whether Reiser's presence would have made any difference.

In 1947 Reiser again injured an ankle sliding, this time during the third game of the Dodgers/Yankees World Series. Reiser had walked in the first inning and attempted to steal second base. On his feet-first slide he was called out, and he collided with the Yankees' Phil Rizzuto, injuring his right ankle. Reiser was taken out of the game the next inning.

X-rays after the game revealed that Reiser had a slight fracture; the exact bone broken is not mentioned. Reiser, upset about the x-ray findings, pleaded with the doctor not to tell anyone about the results of the tests. "Just put a tight bandage on it," he told the doctor, "say it's a bad sprain, and that I'm through for the series."[28]

Apparently, though, Reiser was not through for the series, as he ended up playing the next day, though not as a starter. Despite Reiser's limp, Dodgers manager Burt Shotton put Reiser in to pinch-hit in the ninth inning of Game 4 of the Series. The Dodgers were behind 2 to 1 with two outs and a runner

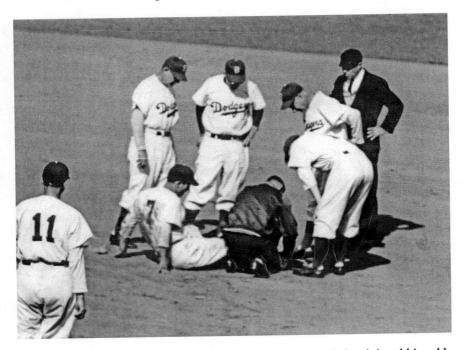

In the first inning of the third game of the 1947 World Series Reiser injured his ankle on a similar play. He was attempting to steal second base after reaching first on a walk (National Baseball Hall of Fame Library, Cooperstown, New York).

on second. The pitcher for the Yankees, Bill Bevens, who was working on a no-hitter, ran a count to 3 and 1 to Reiser, and then he was ordered to intentionally walk him — a bad decision, as it turned out. Reiser limped down to first base and was replaced by a pinch-runner, Eddie Miksis. Ironically, Miksis would come around to score the winning run on Cookie Lavagetto's double, the only hit of the game off Bevens.

Reiser would only end up getting eight at-bats in the 1947 World Series, with two hits. Ultimately, the Dodgers would lose to the Yankees in seven games.[29] As in many of these situations, it is uncertain if Reiser's injured right ankle had anything to do with the final outcome.

Reiser apparently continued to have trouble with this bad right ankle into the 1948 season, and because of the ankle and other injuries including chronic dizziness, Reiser was reduced to playing part-time. He appeared in only 64 games, and half of those appearances were as a pinch-hitter.[30]

Nothing is mentioned about Reiser's ankle after 1948, but by then his problems related to his repeated head concussions led to his eventual retirement from the game (see later discussion).

Tommy Davis

Another Dodger with a significant ankle fracture from a feet-first slide was Tommy Davis. He was coming off two National League batting championships, having batted .346 in 1962 and .326 in 1963. He had an off year in 1964, batting only .275, but there was hope he could bounce back in 1965.

According to Davis's autobiography, *Tales from the Dodger Dugout*, he suffered a significant ankle fracture on May 1, 1965.[31] His description of the events is helpful.

> We were playing the Giants in front of a crowd of 50,000 at Dodger Stadium (Chavez Ravine in Los Angeles). I was on first and Ron Fairly hit a ground ball to Orlando Cepeda at first base. I ran to second, thinking I'd break up a double play and slide under Jose Pagan (shortstop). But the closer I got to Pagan, who was on the inside of the base, the more I realized he wasn't going to get the ball. Cepeda had just gone to first base. I didn't have to do what I did.[32]

Thus he changed his mind in mid-slide as he was going to the bag. Sometimes altering your planned slide at the last moment can have dire consequences. It did for Tommy Davis. The spikes on his right foot caught in the clay before reaching second base, twisting his right ankle and foot backward. He suffered a spiral fracture where the bone was twisted. He had to be carried off the field. The bone was damaged badly enough that it had to be manipulated back into place.

Often surgery with pinning is necessary with such fractures to avoid significant deformity, especially if the fracture is near a joint. Not to achieve proper anatomic positioning can result in premature arthritis later in life.

Sometimes, though, even with good positioning arthritis can result (see following example of Robin Ventura).

Tommy Davis missed the rest of the 1965 season. Davis reports that Hall of Famer Monte Irvin had a similar injury in April 1952, after a breakout season in 1951 for the New York Giants. Irvin's career was cut short because of this injury. Davis was concerned that the same thing might happen to him, though it did not.[33] Davis went on to play 11 more years for various teams, though he never matched the great stats and two batting titles he had in 1962 and 1963.

Robin Ventura

Robin Ventura played in the major leagues from 1989 to 2004 (16 years), mainly playing third base. From 1989 to 1998 he played for the Chicago White Sox. Then he played three years with the New York Mets, and subsequently one and one-half seasons each with the New York Yankees and the Los Angeles Dodgers. He has a lifetime batting average of .267 with 1,885 hits and 294 home runs in 7,064 at bats.

Robin Ventura had one of the worst possible feet-first sliding injuries that can occur and is an example of late complications that can develop from such a severe injury. On March 21, 1997, during a spring training game against the Boston Red Sox, Ventura was attempting to score from second on a Ray Durham single. Left-fielder Juan Williams threw the ball to catcher Bill Haselman, who easily applied the tag to Ventura. There was very little contact between the catcher and the sliding Ventura.[34]

Ventura was out, in more ways than just because the successful tag had been applied. He had caught his spikes on the dirt as he slid home, bending his right ankle severely, almost to a right angle. The unnatural bend in the ankle persisted after the play was over. Ventura had sustained both a dislocated ankle (out of socket) and compound fractures of the fibula and tibia, the bones just above the ankle (a compound fracture is so severe the bone sticks out of the skin). He also sustained torn ligaments. He was carried of the field on a stretcher and taken to the hospital.[35]

That same day Drs. James Bascarden and Donald Slevin at Sarasota Memorial Hospital did surgery on Ventura's ankle. Ventura required metal screws put in his ankle to put it back together.[36] That Ventura came back at all that season was amazing. He was out four months but was able to play 54 games for the White Sox after his return from the DL.

His recovery seemed complete in 1998 as he played in 161 games, batting .263 with 21 home runs and 91 RBI in 590 at bats.

During the next three seasons with the New York Mets (1999 to 2001), he began to have some problems once again with his right ankle. Though his problems weren't severe, functioning well while playing baseball necessitated him receiving one or two cortisone shots in the ankle during each year.

He still managed to play over 141 games in each year, with a high of 161 in 1999.[37]

In 2002 his ankle began to get worse and he required cortisone shots every month just to continue to play. He still managed to play 138 games in 2003, split between the New York Yankees and Los Angeles Dodgers. In 2004 he became severely limited by pain in his right ankle. He did manage to play 102 games, but he was forced to retire because of his ankle.[38]

By 2005, even though he wasn't playing baseball anymore, the ankle became even worse. He began to have trouble getting up in the morning because of the pain. He required a cane to walk five days out of seven. His wife had to do most of the driving for him, dropping him off as close to destinations as she could. Ventura was now disabled because of his right ankle.[39]

Without medical records to examine, it is difficult to state exactly what was happening at this point. It would appear Ventura was having trouble with the ankle joint, possibly due to premature arthritis from the 1997 injury. He could also have had a condition called avascular (also called aseptic) necrosis, a condition where the bone in the joint actually dies. If the bone dies, the cartilage next to the bone (that cushions the joint) also dies. Arthritis is the result.

The deterioration in the joint was apparently bad enough, and the long-term prognosis for the joint grim enough, that Ventura consulted Dr. William Bugbee, a San Diego specialist. The options: fuse the joint (causing quite limited motion) or have a bone graft from a cadaver to replace the deteriorating bone and joint. Dr. Bugbee had done the bone transplant procedure over 250 times before.[40]

Ventura had the ankle bone transplant surgery on November 18, 2005, with bone from a cadaver inserted and the deteriorating bone removed. Obviously, the bone from the donor had to approximate the size of the bone to be replaced; the cadaver had to have a joint approximately the size of Ventura's. The article at MLB.com indicates that part of the shin bone down to the ankle, including some cartilage, was used. The shin bone is part of the distal tibia (one of the two bones in the lower leg that forms the top part of the ankle). Although the article at MLB.com doesn't say so, the use of the shin bone would indicate that the distal tibia was replaced.[41]

Rehabilitation after surgery required six months of therapy and at present Ventura is walking fairly well. He attended 2008 spring training, but not as a player attempting a comeback. Activity was limited; he didn't do any batting, fielding ground balls, or running.

Ventura suffered a severe injury to his ankle while sliding feet-first. He later developed complications in the ankle (probably arthritis) resulting from the original injury. Thanks to modern medicine he was able to replace the damaged bone and at least walk reasonably well. In 2012 Ventura became manager of the Chicago White Sox, and reported being able to walk and play golf without any pain.

INJURY TO FIELDER BY SLIDING RUNNER

With sliding there can be an injury to the runner sliding into the base, or to the fielding player who is standing at or near that base. Second base is a common site for these injuries. Quite often there is a collision between the runner coming from first to second base and the fielder on the base, usually either the shortstop or second baseman. In certain circumstances the runner deliberately tries to "take out" the fielder in order to break up a potential double play.

Home plate can be a dangerous place for collisions: a runner runs or slides into home plate, and the catcher tries to block the plate to prevent a run from scoring. Often the collision is a deliberate attempt by the runner to knock the ball out of the catcher's hand. If the catcher drops the ball, the runner is safe.

Also, that catcher is standing in the runner's way, blocking his path to home plate. The runner can use whatever means necessary to get past the catcher. He can slide to the side of the catcher to avoid the tag, he can jump over the catcher, he can run right through the catcher, or he can slide under the catcher, while attempting to touch that plate with his foot or hand. Fortunately for the catcher, he is wearing a protective vest and leg guards, though even these things cannot prevent a significant injury. The fact that the catcher has to pay attention both to the throw and the runner coming down the line at the same time increases his chance of getting injured.

Collisions can also happen at first or third base. At first the runner is most often going full-speed down the line to run right through the base to beat the throw. Poor first baseman, second baseman, or pitcher for that matter, if were to get in the way.

Albert Pujols' Slide into Josh Bard

Fielders at various positions can be injured by the sliding player, and home plate is often the site of the collision. One doesn't need to go back in history very far to find such an injury. An article at sportsillustrated.com on May 22, 2008, highlights this problem. Josh Bard, the Padres' catcher, was injured by a slide at home plate by Albert Pujols on the May 21 game between the Cardinals and Padres at Petco Park in San Diego. Pujols was trying to score from second base on a hit to right field by Troy Glaus. The throw from Brian Giles arrived at home plate at the very same time as Pujols. Bard, who was attempting to block the plate with his leg, was hit on the leg by Pujols' slide. Bard's left leg was twisted and he suffered a high ankle sprain. He was placed on the DL the next day and was predicted to be out four to six weeks. The slide by Pujols was a good, hard slide. The fans in San Diego didn't think so. Pujols was booed several times after this.[42] Fortunately they didn't throw any debris on the field.

Bard ended up on the DL much longer than six weeks, from May 21 till July 24, 2008.[43]

Brian McCann Slides into Orlando Hudson

Second base, as previously stated, is a most frequent place for sliding injuries, and most injuries there are not due to controversial slides.

On Saturday, August 9, 2008, Gold Glove second baseman Orlando Hudson was injured on a wild play during the sixth inning of a game between the Atlanta Braves and the Arizona Diamondbacks at Chase Field in Phoenix.

Atlanta came into the sixth inning trailing Arizona, 3 to 2. Atlanta rallied to score seven runs in the inning, eventually winning, 11 to 4. During this sixth-inning rally, a throw came in to pitcher Juan Cruz after a single by Atlanta catcher Brian McCann (Cruz was probably the cut-off man on the throw from the outfield). Cruz tried to cut down McCann at second as he tried to advance from first to second on the play. Right-hander Orlando Hudson was covering second, facing toward the infield. Cruz's throw was errant to the right of the bag, and Hudson had to reach to his left with his glove to get the ball. At the same instant Hudson reached, McCann was sliding into second. McCann slid into Hudson's glove hand, bending Hudson's left wrist back in an awkward fashion, stripping the glove off Hudson's hand. Hudson's wrist was injured.[44]

The severity of the injury was quickly apparent: Hudson had dislocated a bone in his wrist. He had surgery Saturday night after the game to reduce (put back into place) the dislocated bone. Ligament damage in the wrist was noted and this was fixed in a separate procedure on Monday, August 11, by hand specialist Dr. Don Sheridan.[45]

Sammy Sosa's Bad Slide

There have been many controversial slides noted in the literature, some better known than others. The most controversial is one where the runner slides into a base with his spikes up. It is bush league. If it were basketball, the runner could be called for a flagrant foul and tossed from the game. In baseball the runner could get also get tossed from the game or later be fined by the commissioner's office, though that rarely happens. Or there could be a third result.

On July 29, 2005, as noted on the website for the *International Herald Tribune*, Sammy Sosa slid into home plate with his feet up, attempting to score in the tenth inning of the game between the Orioles and Texas Rangers, exposing his spikes. The third result happened: the benches for both sides cleared. There wasn't any indication a brawl resulted, as fortunately order was quickly restored.[46]

On the slide, Rod Barajas of the Baltimore Orioles — the catcher — sustained a very nasty bruise on his arm, and the spikes-up maneuver didn't help Sosa as the umpire declared him out at the plate on the throw from Gary Matthews.[47]

Ty Cobb Slides into Carl Mays

It is well-known that Ty Cobb often deliberately slid into a base or fielder with his spikes up. He was even rumored to have sharpened his spikes to inflict more injury into the fielder he slid into. Many opposing players hated Ty Cobb for pulling just such stunts.

One particular instance of Cobb using his spikes-up slide to bring about injury occurred in a game between the Boston Red Sox and the Detroit Tigers. Mike Sowell, in his book *The Pitch That Killed: The Story of Carl Mays, Ray Chapman, and the Pennant Race of 1920*, notes the instance, though does not give an exact date.[48] Carl Mays, the submarine-style pitcher of the Red Sox, liked to throw the ball near Cobb's head. In late 1915, Cobb swore revenge. In a game in which Mays threw several pitches near Cobb's head, Cobb got his revenge. He deliberately pushed a bunt between the pitcher and the first baseman in such a way that the first baseman had to field the ball and then toss the ball to the pitcher, Mays, covering the bag. As Mays arrived at first base, Cobb leaped at him feet-first, putting a nasty gash in Mays' leg, and in the process sent Mays stumbling to the ground. Cobb is quoted as telling him, "The next time you cover the bag, I'll take the skin off your other leg."[49] Obviously, the inflicted injury was intentional and in retaliation for Mays throwing pitches very close to Cobb's head.

Joe Medwick's Slide into Marv Owen

Another particularly nasty slide occurred during the seventh game of the 1934 World Series between the Detroit Tigers and the St. Louis Cardinals. In the sixth inning of the game at Detroit, with the Cardinals leading, 7 to 0, Joe Medwick hit an RBI triple to right field. He slid very hard into third base, spiking Marv Owen. Owen allegedly spiked Medwick in retaliation. The two players nearly came to blows. Medwick later scored to make it St. Louis 9, Detroit 0.[50]

When Medwick went back to his place in left field in the bottom of the sixth inning, the fans in Detroit became irate. They thought Medwick had deliberately tried to injure Owen. The Tigers fans began pelting Medwick with soda bottles, fruit, and all manner of trash. Medwick left the field three times, but every time he returned he was once again pelted with the debris. Baseball Commissioner Kenesaw Landis, in attendance at this game, in order to protect Medwick and to resume play, ordered St. Louis to replace Medwick with another player.[51]

Fortunately, neither Marv Owen nor Joe Medwick was seriously injured. Results could have been much worse. The Cardinals, despite being without Medwick in their lineup, continued their rout of Detroit to win the final game of the World Series, 11 to 0, defeating Detroit four games to three.[52] The "Gas House Gang," as they were called, won the Cardinals' third world championship.

Tommie Agee Slides into Joe Morgan

The fielder at second base can be injured by a slide made deliberately to prevent a double play (throw from second base to first base by shortstop or second baseman). Prior to 1978 (see discussion later of Hal McRae rule) the runner coming into second base could basically give the fielder a body block and even go outside the baseline to do so. Joe Morgan's knee injury is an example of this.

Joe Morgan was a Hall of Famer who played 22 years in the major leagues. He played his first nine with the Houston Astros and then gained most of his recognition in the eight years he played for the Cincinnati Reds, where he won two MVP awards (1975, 1976). He also won five Gold Gloves for his play at second base.

Morgan, in his book *Joe Morgan: A Life in Baseball*, notes that he was injured in early April of 1968 on a play at second base.[53]

On the play, Tommie Agee of the Mets came hard into second base, basically throwing a body-block on Morgan in an attempt to break up a potential double play. As Morgan's body was fully extended with his leg and knee rigid, the body block injured his left knee. Morgan reports he injured his "mediate" cruciate ligament (most likely a tear of the anterior cruciate ligament, which crisscrosses inside the knee to lend extra stability to the knee). This injury required surgery, and Morgan was out for the rest of the year. Morgan called this the only significant injury he had in his league career. In 1968 Morgan played in only ten games the whole year, his longest stint on the DL of his career.[54]

Morgan doesn't express hard feelings about the incident in his book. He calls the body block an example of hard-nosed play. He also looks at the positive aspects of the injury. With the missed days, he had time from the dugout to study the game of baseball intensely (especially stealing technique). It was helpful in his maturity as a major league player. He found benefit from his misfortune. Fortunately, his knee injury did not significantly impair his play after the 1968 season.

Larry Dierker, in *This Ain't Brain Surgery: How to Win the Pennant Without Losing Your Mind*, presents a different side to the discussion of this injury. He says the players thought Agee's slide was way out of line — out of the baseline — and overtly violent in nature, making this slide both controversial and with significant resultant morbidity.[55]

Alex Rodriguez's Slide into Dustin Pedroia

On May 22, 2007, there was a controversial slide by Alex Rodriguez into Dustin Pedroia that didn't involve spikes. The slide was featured on sports.aol.com fanhouse with a video of the slide. Rodriguez was trying to take out Pedroia, the Red Sox second baseman, to prevent a double play on a ball originally hit to third baseman Mike Lowell by Jorge Posada. Rodriguez slid past the bag on the infield side and appeared to put his elbow into Pedroia's side. The double play was not completed, though just barely. It is uncertain whether this was due to Rodriguez's slide or not. Pedroia remained in the game, as apparently no significant injury was sustained, a fortunate thing. The consequences could have been much worse: a broken rib or injury to the face, for instance.[56]

Hal McRae Rule

Controversial slides occur often when a runner tries to take out the fielder at second base. One such controversial slide led to a rules change. It occurred during the 1977 ALCS between the New York Yankees and the Kansas City Royals. In the second game, Hal McRae took out second baseman Willie Randolph, breaking up a double play and allowing an important run to score. McRae barreled into Randolph with a body-block while sliding out of the baseline.[57] This led to a rule change in 1978. In this new rule, the batter running to first and the runner coming into second are both out if the umpire judges the runner going into second has intentionally interfered with the fielder's attempt to catch a thrown ball or to throw the ball to complete any play.

An article by Rich Marazzi in the September 2004, *Baseball Digest* outlines several instances where interference might be called: (1) A runner executes a roll block; (2) A runner throws his body at the fielder's body by using a sideways motion; (3) A runner hooks or trips the pivot man's legs; (4) A runner slides in a manner where his body is three feet outside or inside the direct line between first and second base; (5) and — added in 2004 — a runner deliberately makes contact that begins after passing the bag, on the shortstop side of second base.[58]

These rules were added to protect the fielders from injury. Unfortunately, the rule changes were too late for some, such as Joe Morgan in 1968.

Chapter 11

Collisions Between
Players, Non-Sliding

Runner Collides with Fielder

SCOTT ROLEN

Scott Rolen is an example of two injuries that occurred because of collisions of the non-sliding nature (his labrum injury has been previously discussed). The first injury occurred while Rolen was fielding his position during the 2002 National League Divisional Series between the Cardinals and the Arizona Diamondbacks. Arizona had runners on at first and second. The runner at second was Alex Cintron. Junior Spivey hit a ground ball to Rolen. As he went to field the ball, Cintron ran into him, injuring his shoulder. Cintron was called out due to runner interference. The injury sustained by Rolen was severe enough that he had to be removed from the game. Rolen had a CT scan and was diagnosed with a shoulder sprain of his non-throwing left arm (not a dislocation). He missed the rest of the playoffs.[1] On the positive side, it was the end of the year and Rolen was able to rest during the off-season, and did not miss any more days the next season.

Scott Rolen's other shoulder injury occurred at first base on May 10, 2005. He did not slide into first base. He was running to first base to beat a throw to the first baseman, Hee Seop Choi. He collided with Choi, a rather large individual.

Rolen is 6 foot 4 inches and 240 pounds, but Choi is even bigger at 6 foot 4 inches and 250 pounds. As it sometimes happens, the throw to Choi turned him inward, facing towards Rolen's path. Rolen sustained an injury to his non-throwing left shoulder. He had the left arm extended when he ran into Choi.[2]

It seems as though major league baseball, and other sports for that matter, order MRIs on almost any injury at the drop of a hat. The MRI is a very expensive test. But when you are paying players millions of dollars to play baseball, it makes one want to know exactly what is going on. The information is very useful. It makes the future more predictable. Scott Rolen had two MRIs. The first one didn't show any significant problem. The second, using special views, a special MRI (maybe with dye injected into the shoulder), revealed the tear of the labrum.

Whether due to trauma or overuse, a labral tear can be a very significant injury, as the head or round part of the upper humerus bone sits in the socket of the scapula (shoulder bone) and is supported there by the cupped labrum. Sure, muscles, ligaments, capsule, and tendons also hold the shoulder in place, but the shoulder just doesn't move correctly without the labrum holding the head of the humerus in place as it glides in motion.

Rolen had arthroscopic surgery to repair the tear on May 13. He was placed on the disabled list from May 12 to June 17. He attempted to come back after that, but he just wasn't the same player. His throwing wasn't affected by the shoulder injury, but his batting definitely was. He batted only .207 (18 for 87) with only eight RBI in 25 games and was put on the DL again on July 22, 2005, with left shoulder cuff inflammation.[3]

Because of continued problems after the first arthroscopy, the shoulder was arthroscoped again. Scott Rolen's shoulder second surgery was by performed Dr. Tim Kremchek (Cincinnati Reds team physician), a shoulder specialist, on July 25, 2005. Rolen missed the rest of the season. During the second arthroscopy, more extensive repair was done. Kremchek thought in addition to the labrum problem, Rolen had suffered a shoulder dislocation that caused loosening of the shoulder capsule. He put screws into the capsule to the labrum in the back (four) and front (one) of the joint.[4]

Rolen was able to resume playing baseball the next season with only minor problems with the shoulder, having little difficulty with the shoulder until the end of the 2006 season. He received a cortisone shot at the end of 2006 leading into the playoffs and World Series.

The story wasn't over. In 2007 Rolen again had trouble with his left shoulder. His decreased power statistics showed it. He had impaired movement in the shoulder, a frozen shoulder. He was having problems with his swing at the plate as his left hand was lower than it usually was.

Rolen had a third arthroscopy on September 11, 2007. This time the labrum was fine. During the third arthroscope, Dr. Kremchek removed scar tissue, cleaned out a thickened bursa sac, and did manipulation of the shoulder under general anesthetic to increase Rolen's range of motion, in the process increasing flexibility in the shoulder.[5]

Rolen's problems with the left shoulder continued, all as a result of the

2005 collision on the base paths. None of the problems were thought to be related to his 2002 collision.

Rolen was traded between 2007 and 2008 from the Cardinals to the Toronto Blue Jays for Troy Glaus. In 2008 Rolen played only 115 games for Toronto, batting .262 with 11 home runs and 50 RBI. His power numbers were down considerably when compared to the time period from 1998 to 2004 where he averaged close to 30 home runs a year. In 2009 Rolen spent time between Toronto and Cincinnati. His stats were modest compared to previous years, with 128 games played, 11 home runs and 67 RBI.

Things appeared to have turned around for Rolen in 2010, when he hit .285 with 20 home runs and 83 RBI in 133 games. But 2011 was another bad year for Rolen with his left shoulder. This time it wasn't the main joint in his shoulder, but the acromioclavicular (shoulder-clavicle) joint. It is uncertain if this joint was also injured in his 2005 collision and was only now giving him problems. Nothing was said, though that is a possibility. That injury limited Rolen to 65 games played in 2011, and he had to have surgery to remove bone fragments and bone spurs from the joint on August 3.[6] He missed the rest of the season.

DERREK LEE

Derrek Lee of the Chicago Cubs had an injury at first base, also on a collision between the runner and the first baseman. In this case, though, when the runner ran into the first baseman, it was the first baseman that was injured. It was a freakish play. On April 19, 2006, the Dodgers' Rafael Furcal led off with a bunt that went to the right of the pitching mound. Reliever Scott Eyre dove for the ball and then flipped the ball with his glove to Derrek Lee at first base. The ball sailed over Lee just as Furcal collided with him. Lee had his right arm (the arm without the glove) in front of him at the time of the collision and suffered a rather severe injury, broken distal ulna and distal radius bones (the two ends of forearm bones) in his wrist.[7]

He had a cast put on and was out from April 20 until August 29.[8] The Chicago media was quick to point out that the injury occurred less than two weeks after Lee signed a five-year, $65 million contract.[9]

The next season, Lee was able to play 150 games, though his home run totals (46 to 22) and slugging percentage (.662 to .513) were down from 2005 to 2007. Lee denied the wrist had anything to do with the drop-off in his stats.[10]

Lee's stats in 2008 were similar to 2007. In 2009 he improved and they were more similar to what he had in 2005 with a .306 average and 35 home runs and 111 RBI in 141 games played. He was less productive in 2010–2011.

HANK GREENBERG'S WRIST INJURY

The manner in which Hank Greenberg's wrist was injured was similar to the way Derrek Lee injured his wrist. Greenberg was playing first base and had his arm extended to receive a throw when his wrist was injured by the passing runner. Greenberg had fractured the same wrist the year before by a completely different mechanism. Like Lee, Greenberg had just signed a lucrative one-year contract for $25,000, making him one of the highest paid players in major league baseball in 1936, a time when anything other than a one-year contract was very unusual.

Greenberg played 13 years in the majors with a big interruption of nearly four seasons for World War II. He played all but one season for the Detroit Tigers, playing his last season in 1947 for the Pittsburgh Pirates. He had a career average of .313 with 331 home runs and 1,276 RBI. He was a two-time MVP (1935 and 1940) and was elected to the Hall of Fame in 1956.

In 1936 he was coming off one of his better years, an MVP year with an amazing 98 extra-base hits (46 doubles, 16 triples, and 36 home runs) and 170 RBI. But on April 29, 1936, he collided at his first base position with base runner Jake Powell, a Washington Senators outfielder.

Greenberg in his autobiography *Hank Greenberg: The Story of My Life*, describes the events of 1936 well.

> I got off to a flying start, hitting around .350 and leading the league in runs batted in. In Washington in early May, in the twelfth game of the season, Marvin Owen fielded a ground ball at third base. He flipped it over to me at first base and I stretched out to get the throw, which was fading into the baseline. The batter was Jake Powell, and he ran into me coming down the line. I always felt he could have avoided the collision, but I guess he felt he was entitled to the base path, and if he could knock the ball out of my hand, which he did, he would be safe.... Unfortunately, I cracked the same bone in my left wrist as I had in the 1935 World Series. As a result, I was out for the rest of the season.[11]

In the previous World Series, 1935, Greenberg was playing for the Tigers against the Chicago Cubs. In the seventh inning of the second game, Greenberg reached first base after being hit by a pitch. He tried to score on a base hit by Pete Fox. Gabby Hartnett, the catcher for the Cubs, had the plate blocked. In Greenberg's slide into home, Hartnett fell on Greenberg. Greenberg's wrist snapped back from an initial curled position.

The result: the wrist was injured. Initial x-rays were negative. The wrist appeared sprained, and because of pain and swelling Greenberg missed the rest of the World Series, which the Tigers won in six games. Only after the World Series did repeat x-rays show that the left wrist was fractured. This is the same wrist Greenberg fractured again in 1936.

RAY FOSSE'S COLLISION

Another famous collision between a runner and a fielder occurred in the 1970 All-Star Game. The collision was between the runner, Pete Rose, and Ray Fosse of the Cleveland Indians, the American League catcher. Technically speaking, a runner deliberately running into someone is not a sliding injury, especially when the runner makes no attempt to slide and runs right through the fielder in an attempt to score and knock the ball out of the fielder's hand at the same time.

In the 1970 All-Star Game, the score was tied 4 to 4 going into the bottom of the 12th inning. Pitching for the American League was Clyde Wright. There were two out when Pete Rose hit a single and moved to second on a base hit by Billy Grabarkewitz. Jim Hickman hit a single and there went Pete Rose, rounding third and determined to score.

Amos Otis fielded the ball and threw it home. Ray Fosse was blocking the plate. The ball arrived the same time as Rose. Rose, instead of trying to avoid the tag, ran right into Ray Fosse, like a running back plowing right over a tackler. The ball arrived just after the collision. Boom! Down went Fosse, and Rose scored the winning run. Rose had a bruised thigh muscle after the collision. Fosse's injury was much worse.

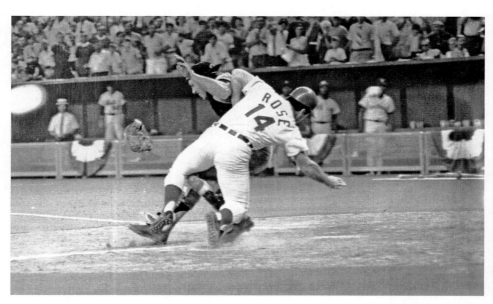

The National League's Pete Rose collides with American League catcher Ray Fosse as he scores the winning run in the All-Star Game in Cincinnati, Ohio, on July 14, 1970. Fosse suffered an injured shoulder on the play and was taken to a local hospital (AP Photo).

In *The Curse of Rocky Colavito*, Terry Pluto describes Ray Fosse the best. Fosse was a rising star.[12] He had made his first All-Star team. Before the All-Star break, Fosse was hitting .313 with 16 homers and 45 RBI. Herb Score, the broadcaster for the Indians, said, "Ray had everything. He was a tremendous defensive catcher and handler of pitchers. He was a leader. He threw pretty well, and not only could he hit, but he hit for power. I know this. He was the best catching prospect I've ever seen with the Indians."[13] This book came out in 1994. The collision at home plate changed the rest of Fosse's career.

After the collision, he was able to hit .297 after the All-Star break, but he hit only two home runs and he had only 16 RBI for the rest of the season. He played seven and a half more seasons and hit only 39 more home runs and retired with a lifetime .255 batting average.

Initial x-rays had revealed nothing unusual. Possibly the shoulder swelling present at the time of his initial x-rays interfered with the radiologist's ability to come to a proper diagnosis. If they had done a CT scan or MRI, it would have shown the full extent of the injury, but unfortunately in 1970 these tests were not available. Fosse's arm hurt the rest of the 1970 season. He altered his swing because of pain in his shoulder. He developed bad habits. He was never the same after the injury.

A final note: new x-rays were taken the next year, 1971, when Fosse was having another problem, back pain. Finally x-rays revealed that Fosse had indeed fractured his humerus and sustained a shoulder separation the previous year (the latter is an injury to the clavicle/scapula — shoulder blade — joint). Unfortunately, at this point it was damage done; nothing medically available in 1971 could help one year after the initial injury.

Buster Posey — Collision Between Runner and Position Player

Buster Posey, a 24-year-old catcher for the San Francisco Giants, was injured on May 25, 2011, in a collision at the plate very similar to the collision that occurred between Pete Rose and Ray Fosse.

Posey, Rookie of the Year in the National League in 2010, played in 108 games in 2010, hitting 18 home runs, and driving 67 runs and batting .305. He was an integral part of the Giants' post-season run to a World Championship title in 2010, hitting .288 with 17 hits in 59 at bats. At the time of Posey's injury he was hitting .284 with 4 home runs and 21 runs batted in.

The injury occurred at AT&T Park in San Francisco in top of the 12th inning. The Florida Marlins' Scott Cousins made a mad dash to home plate from third base on a sacrifice fly to Giant right fielder Nate Schierholtz.

The fly ball was shallow, but after tagging the base Cousins still beat the throw, which Posey was unable to corral. Cousins, thinking Posey might catch the ball, lowered his head and collided his shoulder into Posey knocking him backward.

Cousins told the press, "I felt like he [Posey] was blocking the dish. It's the go-ahead run to win the game, I got to do whatever I can to score."[14] It was the winning run for the Marlins, as they won the game 7 to 6 in the 12th inning.

Almost instantly after the collision it was obvious Posey had a significant injury as he was seen writhing in pain and was unable to get up on his own. MLB replays showed that Posey's left ankle and leg had been bent back awkwardly underneath him. He had to be helped off the field not putting any weight on the affected left leg.

An MRI revealed significant damage to ligaments and bone. Surgery was done on May 29 which addressed torn ligaments and a fractured fibula. Two screws were inserted to reposition and repair the ligaments and the ankle joint was smoothed. The fractured fibula was only minimally displaced and did not need any fixation, such as with a metal plate, to hold the fracture in place.

The surgery was done by Giants orthopedist Dr. Ken Akizuki with assistance from Podiatrist Dr. Larry Oloff and Dr. Mike Dillinger, a physician with extensive experience in traumatic injuries, such as what might occur in football.

Posey was to be on crutches for two months and then had the screws removed in a second surgical procedure on July 22, 2011. After this second surgery Posey's long rehabilitation process began.

Posey's injury prompted two debates. Should a runner be allowed to simply plow into the catcher blocking the plate in an attempt to bowl him over and knock the ball away? Several articles appeared on the subject. The second debate focused on whether a solid hitter like Posey should be playing behind the plate where the risk for injury is greater even with the catcher wearing extra protective gear.

Giants manager Bochy, a former catcher, thought Cousins play was unnecessary and Cousins ought to have a fine and a suspension. He thought the play should have been an automatic out for the runner. His contention was that Posey was not blocking the plate and there was an avenue for Cousins to slide avoiding a tag. But, Cousins chose to go after Posey and spear him. "Buster had no chance there. He's trying to catch the ball," Bochy said.[15]

No fine or suspension of Cousins followed.

Ray Fosse, the catcher who was injured by Pete Rose in 1970, was asked about a possible rule change. His response was that the rules should be left alone.

"The game has been around more than 100 years, and now they're going to start protecting catchers?" Fosse told the *San Francisco Chronicle*. "In high school, you can't run over the catcher. But that is high school. The idea is to score runs. If the catcher has the ball and he's standing there, the runner has to stop? Is that the protection?"[16]

Former All-Star catcher Bob Boone was asked by ABC news about Posey's injury. His reply questioned Posy's positioning at the plate to receive the throw at the time of the injury. He thought that contributed to the injury. When questioned about a rule changes he added, "We don't want guys to get hurt. Of course we don't. But, it's part of the action of the game."[17]

Giants General Manager Brian Sabean was asked about moving Posey to first base where he would not be subject to the abuse a catcher usually faces on a day to day basis. He rejected it saying that Posey was a fine catcher, one of the best in the business at his position, and a major asset to a team.[18]

Posey thought his greatest value to his team was as a catcher.

"I guess the way I look at it is this way: I feel my value as a baseball player is probably greatest as a catcher," he said.[19]

This author is unaware of any measures yet taken up by the commissioner's office to ban such collisions initiated by the runner, collisions done deliberately to knock the ball out of the catcher's hand with or without the catcher blocking the plate. And, in 2012 Buster Posey was back behind the plate catching for the San Francisco Giants.

Fielder Runs into Fielder

When players are running for a popup or a fly ball, one fielder can run into another fielder. One fielder needs to call off the other fielder by yelling, "I got it," but it does not always work. Maybe one fielder doesn't hear the other, or maybe in the heat of the moment, one fielder forgets to call "I got it" to the other. Or both fielders call for the ball and it is too late for either one to get out of the way. There have been some very nasty collisions caught on tape. These collisions can lead to many types of injuries, including head concussions.

Larry Brown Collision

Once again, Terry Pluto in *The Curse of Rocky Colavito* gives us another great example of a collision by the mechanism just mentioned, between two fielders going for the baseball. This collision occurred on May 4, 1966, between Indians shortstop Larry Brown and outfielder Leon Wagner.

Larry Brown was the starting shortstop for the Indians from 1963 to 1969. He is not famous, with only a .233 career batting average, but his injury gives a classic example of a severe fielder-to-fielder collision.

A fly ball was hit to left field at Yankee Stadium by Roger Maris. It looked like it might be a foul ball, but the wind blew it back onto the field, the ball falling between Brown and Wagner. Brown denied hearing Wagner call for the ball. Collision: the two cracked heads. Brown was the worse for it with "convulsions and bleeding from the ears, nose, and mouth."[20] "Brown was carried off the field with a fractured nose, fractured cheekbones, and a frontal and basal fracture of the skull. Wagner received a broken nose and slight concussion."[21]

Brown subsequently was in a coma in intensive care for three days and in the hospital for 18 days. The injuries looked severe enough to prevent Brown from playing the rest of the season, but in fact he missed only 43 days. He probably came back too soon from such a severe injury. Apparently he just couldn't stand seeing some other player, Chico Salmon, starting in his place at shortstop, according to Terry Pluto. Plus these were the years of one-year contracts and no job security, a good motivation for a player to come back too soon from an injury.

Terry Pluto notes that Brown's batting average fell from .253 to .229 in 1966, but in 1964 Brown's average was only .230. Brown was never a very good hitter, and it doesn't appear his severe head injury from this collision had any long-term effects as Brown continued to start at shortstop for the Indians up until 1969.

NICK JOHNSON

A more recent severe injury to a fielder in a collision with another fielder occurred on September 23, 2006. At Shea Stadium, in a game between the Washington Nationals and the New York Mets, Nats first baseman Nick Johnson was severely injured, suffering a fractured femur.[22]

The play happened in the eighth inning. David Wright was at bat against reliever Jason Bergmann. He lofted a ball to the outfield over Nick Johnson's head. Unfortunately, the ball fell exactly between the charging right fielder, Austin Kearns, and Johnson as second baseman Jose Vidro also approached the play. Neither Kearns nor Johnson pulled up, and neither called the other off. Kearns and Johnson ran into each other, both running at full speed.

Vidro heard a crack. Johnson was down and in great pain. It took 15 minutes to stabilize Johnson's right leg. Then he was put on a stretcher and taken to the hospital.

Bad news! Johnson had a fracture of the large bone in his upper right leg, the femur. Exactly where the femur was broken was not mentioned. The fracture was severe enough to require a titanium rod and three screws. Johnson missed the rest of the 2006 season, though he still posted career-best numbers in games (147), hits (145), doubles (46), homers (23), RBI (77), runs (100), walks (110), slugging percentage (.520), and on-base percentage (.428).

Then there was the long 16 months it took to get back to playing, Johnson missing the entire 2007 season.[23]

Initially Johnson was expected to be back from his September 2006 surgery in time for 2007 spring training. But by spring training he was having trouble with certain skills necessary to play. He could bat, but skills that required a quick first step such as running to first base, moving to get a ball on the ground to the left, or pivot and throw, he could not do.

Johnson was thought to have hip bursitis and had two cortisone shots with only mild improvement. Because of continued problems with pain in his hip and his knee, he saw a hip specialist at the Mayo Clinic who recommended removing the rod and screws in his hip in August 2007. Once he had this surgery, the whole rehab process started all over again.[24]

Johnson finally recovered from his femur fracture to play in 2008, but on May 13, facing the Mets, he injured his right wrist while swinging the bat. Unfortunately, an MRI revealed a tear in one of the ligaments in his wrist (which one is not mentioned). Conservative treatment was unsuccessful, and he required surgery on June 24, ending his season once again.[25]

One could write a book just on Nick Johnson's injuries. He has been on the disabled list every one of his nine seasons in the majors, playing 38 games in 2008, 133 in 2009, and only 24 games in 2010. Since coming up with the Yankees in 2001 and then moving on to the Expos, Nats, Marlins, and back to the Yankees in 2010, he was out with a bruised heel, a fractured cheekbone, a lower back strain, a fractured right hand (stress fracture), a bruised right wrist, and a sprained right wrist.[26] In 2010 he had two wrist surgeries, one for inflamed tissue and one for an unstable tendon.[27]

Johnson has had so many injuries the newspapers even have trouble keeping them all straight.

Mark Ellis

Mark Ellis, the Oakland A's starting second baseman for several years, missed all of 2004 after a fielder-to-fielder collision. Ellis dislocated his right shoulder diving for a ground ball hit up the middle by the Chicago Cubs' Sammy Sosa. He collided with shortstop Bobby Crosby resulting in a torn labrum.[28]

Since this was his throwing shoulder, surgery was thought necessary, and with rehabilitation Ellis was able to make it through 2005, 2006, 2007, and most of the 2008 season before finally having the labrum tear repaired on September 19, 2008.[29]

Ozzie Guillen

It is dangerous when two fielders are going for a batted ball lofted between them. This happened on April 21, 1992, in a game between the Chicago White Sox and the New York Yankees. In the ninth inning, Mel Hall lofted a fly ball between Chicago left fielder Tim Raines and shortstop Ozzie Guillen. It landed safely, a double for Hall, and there was a nasty collision between Raines and

Guillen. Raines' head, as he was diving to the ground, hit Guillen's right leg.[30] As a result, Guillen suffered torn anterior cruciate and medial collateral ligaments in his right knee.[31]

Chicago manager Gene Lamont said, "It was one of those in-between plays, where the ball gets up there like that, and you have to keep an eye on it. It may be the toughest play in all of baseball."[32]

All-Star Guillen had to have surgery on his knee to repair the ligaments, a three-hour procedure done by Dr. Scott Price. Guillen would miss the rest of the 1991 season.[33]

Guillen did fine in 1993, batting .280 in 134 games. He did well enough to get a $12 million extension for three years with a $4 million option for the fourth year.[34]

But Guillen may have lost a step after his knee surgery. He averaged 24 stolen bases per year from 1987 till 1991 but never stole more than six bases in a year after his injury. Guillen never won another Gold Glove after 1990. Or, was Guillen just getting older?

ALFREDO EDMEAD

Research revealed only one death in professional baseball from a fielder-to-fielder collision in the last 60 years. It involved a minor league player, Afredo Edmead, and represents the worst possible outcome from any collision.[35]

Edmead started and ended his brief baseball career in 1974 after signing a contract with the Pittsburgh Pirates at age 17. His first and only professional year started at Pittsburgh's Single-A affiliate, the Salem, Virginia, Pirates.

On August 22, Edmead was batting .318 with seven home runs and 59 stolen bases. He had just been chosen to the Carolina League All-Star team. There was speculation that he might move up to the Pirates' Triple-A team the next year.

All Dominicans, Pablo Cruz was playing second base, Alfredo Edmead was in right field, and future major leaguer and good friend of Edmead, Miguel Dilone, was in center field. It was a home game in Salem against Rocky Mount.

A routine fly ball was hit to short right field. Cruz raced out from second base and Edmead raced in from right field. At the last minute, Edmead dove for the ball. His head collided with Cruz's knee. Edmead was knocked unconscious and was not breathing. He was revived and then transferred to the local hospital, Lewis-Gale, but very soon thereafter he was pronounced dead. Edmead died of massive brain injuries.[36]

It was a very sad day in Salem, Virginia. Baseball was robbed of a very young, potential future star. He died in a fielder-to-fielder collision, the most severe collision injury in baseball history.

Chapter 12

Collisions with Objects on Field

Collision with a Wall

PETE REISER

There are other types of collisions. A player can also run into a wall that surrounds the field, infield or outfield. These can result in head concussions or other traumatic injuries. Fortunately in today's stadiums there are "warning tracks" and padding on the walls. These were not common till the 1950s, initiated about the same time as the use of hard plastic batting helmets. The first to add padding to outfield walls was General Manager Branch Rickey of the Brooklyn Dodgers. He had one-inch rubber padding added to Ebbets Field's outfield walls in 1948 to protect oft-injured Pete Reiser.[1]

In *Pete Reiser: The Rough-and-Tumble Career of the Perfect*

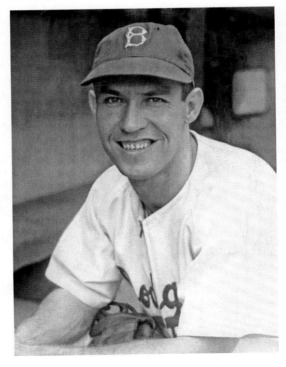

Pete Reiser of the Brooklyn Dodgers circa 1946 (National Baseball Hall of Fame Library, Cooperstown, New York).

185

Ballplayer, Sidney Jacobson documents Pete Reiser's collisions with the outfield wall that occurred several times from 1941 to 1947. In the section called "The Aftermath," Jacobson summarizes Reiser's injuries. "Pete Reiser collided with outfield walls seven times in his career, collapsing unconscious after five of them. The other collisions resulted in a dislocation of his ... shoulder and a fracture of his collarbone."[2]

The most severe injuries for Reiser were his head concussions in 1942 and 1947. Both injuries were crashes into concrete walls that he sustained while chasing fly balls. The first severe injury came when he ran into the concrete wall of the old Sportsman's Park in St. Louis.[3] The second was against concrete in Ebbets Field in Brooklyn.[4] The first time, he suffered a skull fracture. The second time he had a head concussion so severe a Catholic priest was called in to give Reiser his last rites.

In between the head concussions, he had a significant injury against a wooden outfield wall in 1945. Reiser was playing outfield for the Army at Camp Lee, Virginia. Yes, they had baseball teams in the Army during World War II. He crashed into the wooden wall, which gave way. He then rolled 25 feet down a hill[5] and dislocated his right shoulder, which continued to bother him for four more years, making his throws from the outfield difficult and painful. The shoulder finally improved after Reiser had surgery on it after the 1946 season, a surgery done by his personal physician and surgeon, Dr. Robert Hyland.[6]

To keep things symmetrical, Reiser injured his left shoulder crashing into a concrete wall in July of 1947. This injury was not as severe as the one he sustained to his right shoulder. He was only out a week and didn't need any further treatment, though at this point, the accumulated effects of all the injuries sustained by Pete Reiser were beginning to take their toll on his body.[7]

KEN GRIFFEY JR. — WRIST

Today's fences are padded, correct? That does not mean a player can't get injured running into the wall.

Previously mentioned is Ken Griffey Jr.'s hamstring injury (muscle and tendon stains and tears). He also had a traumatic wrist injury in May of 1995 after running into the fence trying to catch a batted ball. As opposed to Griffey's post–2000 injuries, his pre–2000 injuries never put him on the disabled list for more than a month at a time — except for his ill-fated wrist fracture in 1995.[8]

Ken Griffey Jr. won Gold Gloves ten years in a row (1990–1999). He was known for his outstanding outfield play while manning center field for the Seattle Mariners, but playing good defense sometimes involves taking risks.

On May 26, 1995, during a game at the Kingdome that the Mariners won, 8 to 3, Griffey injured his wrist. He made one of his great catches that typified his Gold Glove ability. On a drive off the bat of Baltimore's Kevin Bass, Griffey crashed into the right center field fence while making a spectacular backhand catch to rob Bass of a hit, preserving a one-run lead for Mariners pitcher Randy Johnson.[9]

Griffey, a left-hander, smashed the palm of his left hand into the padding of the fence while making his impressive catch. He fell down on the warning track. Realizing he had a severe injury, he immediately took himself out of the game. As he trotted off the field holding his left hand, he told Mariners trainer Rick Griffin he thought he had broken the wrist. X-rays confirmed that Griffey had fractured his forearm radius and ulnar bones close to his wrist.

This was not a simple fracture. The wrist was shattered into six pieces — three larger, three smaller. It took a three-hour operation by Seattle hand specialist Dr. Ed Almquist, with assistance from Seattle team physician Dr. Larry Pedegana, to put the wrist back together. A T-shaped metal plate and seven screws were needed to put all those pieces back together, restoring the bones to their original anatomic position.[10]

At age 25 Griffey made an almost miraculous recovery. He was on the DL only from May 27 to August 15. Research revealed no evidence to indicate he had any further problems with this left wrist, nor is there any indication that the metal plate and screws in Griffey's wrist were ever removed. It should be noted that Griffey acquired more metal screws when he tore his right hamstring severely in 2004 (previously mentioned). This sounds like a lot of metal, but it is probably not enough metal in one's body to set off those airport metal detectors.

Though Griffey played only 72 games in 1995, in 1996 he played 140 games, hitting 49 home runs with 140 RBI and a .303 average, finishing fourth in the MVP voting. One would call that a remarkable recovery from a potentially significant, career-altering injury.

Falling into Dugout

Mo Vaughn

It is uncertain why this type of injury does not occur more often. You see it all the time. A player plays aggressively and goes into the stands or dugout trying to catch a foul ball. This happened to Mo Vaughn in 1999. Mo Vaughn did not miss many games as he ended up playing 139 games. His stats were good with 33 home runs and 108 RBI. His injury did not result in any long-term problems. Why mention this injury at all? Because it is a classic example of an injury that can occur in a particular manner.

On April 6, 1999, in the Angels' home opener against the Cleveland Indians, on only the 12th pitch of the game Vaughn chased a foul popup off the bat of Omar Vizquel near the Indians dugout. He slipped on the "top step and slid down the short flight feet first, injuring his left ankle."[11] He played on with the ankle taped but had to be removed in the sixth inning.

The next day an MRI revealed a bone bruise and sprained ligaments. Vaughn missed three weeks on the DL.[12]

Not a great debut for a player who had just signed an $80 million, six-year contract with the Anaheim Angels in November 1998.[13] Where has this been heard before?

Collision with Ground

TONY OLIVA

Colliding with the walls surrounding the baseball field can cause an injury. Colliding with other players on the field can result in injuries. Simple gravity can indeed have an adverse effect on a body, as an encounter with the ground underneath the baseball player's feet can lead to injury. Whether the surface is synthetic turf, real grass, dirt, or some other composite material, hitting the ground on the fly can be hazardous. Such injuries occur rather frequently. Brain concussions caused in this manner make the biggest headlines, but injuries to any body part can occur. In some cases, these injuries have been career-altering.

One of the classic cases of a career-altering injury due to a collision with the ground happened to Minnesota right fielder Tony Oliva. At the time of his injury, Oliva possessed a career .313 average. He appeared to be a certain future Hall of Fame inductee. He had been Rookie of the Year in 1964 and had already won two batting titles. On June 29, 1971, all that changed for Oliva (only 31).

Oliva injured himself diving for a batted ball during the ninth inning of a 5 to 3 victory over the Oakland A's at the Oakland–Alameda County Coliseum. As Oliva dove for a sinking line drive off the bat of Joe Rudi, he landed in an awkward fashion, twisting his right knee. He had to be immediately removed from the game. As he left the field of play, he was noticeably limping. To add insult to injury, he missed making the catch.[14]

Recovery was slow. Several days after the injury, Oliva was called on to pinch-hit against the Milwaukee Brewers. Reality set in. After hitting a grounder, he wasn't able even to run out of the batter's box.[15]

In 1971 Oliva was nominated to his eighth All-Star team. But on the date of the All-Star Game, July 13, he was still unable to play due to his injury. He finally did return to the team after the All-Star break, but his level of play was significantly diminished from prior to the injury. His season finally ended on September 22, when he had surgery on the problematic right knee. A torn lateral cartilage (probably meniscus) of the knee was noted at the time of this surgery.[16]

Ironically in 1971 Oliva won his last batting title at .337 (he had been hitting .375 at the time of his injury on June 29). He barely qualified for the title with 518 total plate appearances (487 at bats plus 25 walks, two HBP, and four sacrifice flies, with 502 required to qualify for the batting title).

In 1972, things were not much better for Oliva. He played only ten games, mostly playing left field instead of his normal right field position, before going back on the DL. When conservative measures didn't lead to recovery, Oliva underwent yet another right knee operation on July 5. This surgery, lasting one hour, removed roughly 100 cartilage fragments floating in the knee. Also during the procedure, cartilage in the knee was shaved or "refashioned" and two bone spurs were removed. After surgery, Oliva missed the rest of the 1972 season.[17]

The 1973 season was historic. It marked the beginning of the American League's designated hitter rule. What better player to be a DH than Oliva, who at the time was continuing to have trouble with his bad right knee? In fact, after 1972 Oliva didn't do anything but DH until his retirement in 1976 at age 37.

Plate appearances and averages gradually declined from 1973 to Oliva's last year as a player in 1976 (1973: 571 official at-bats with .291 average; 1974: 459 at-bats with .285 average; 1975: 455 at-bats with .270 average; and 1976: only 123 plate appearances with a .211 average).

Despite the declining statistics, Oliva did end up with a final .304 average for his 15-year career, with 1,917 hits and 947 RBI in 6,301 at-bats. His knee injury may have prevented an even better career and possible induction into the Baseball Hall of Fame.

He has received some recognition in other forms despite his misfortune. In 1991 the Twins officially had Oliva's number six retired. In 2000 he was inducted into the Minnesota Twins Hall of Fame. Previous to that (1981) he was included as one of the truly greatest players ever in Lawrence Ritter and Donald Honig's book *The 100 Greatest Baseball Players of All Time*.[18]

JOE WOOD

"Smoky" Joe Wood is mainly remembered for his one great season in 1912 when he finished with 34 wins and only 5 losses. He had 258 strikeouts in 344 innings with an ERA of 1.91 and ten shutouts. To top off the season, he won three games and lost one in the World Series to lead the Boston Red Sox over the New York Giants in eight games (one game was suspended because of darkness as a tie). At one point during the 1912 season Wood had 16 straight victories.

During his early career Joe Wood was thought to have a blazing fastball, thus the name Smoky (also spelled Smokey). Walter Johnson, the other flame thrower at the time, thought "Smoky" Joe Wood threw harder than he. In an interview in 1912, Johnson said so. "Can anyone throw harder than Joe Wood? Listen, my friend, there's no man alive can throw harder than Joe Wood."[19]

There were great expectations for Joe Wood for 1913. It wasn't to be. During spring training on March 8, playing third base in practice, he sprained his ankle taking a wide throw to the bag.[20]

Wood struggled for some time with this ankle. But the career-changing injury occurred during a relief appearance at Tiger Stadium on May 12, 1913. He was trying to field a ground ball when he slipped on the wet grass and fell on his right thumb, his pitching hand thumb.

Ritter, in *The Glory of Their Times*, quotes Joe Wood, who says, "Broke it. The thumb on my pitching hand. It was in a cast for three weeks. I don't know if I tried to pitch too soon after that, or whether maybe something happened to my shoulder at the same time. But whatever it was, I never pitched again without a terrific pain in my right shoulder. Never again."[21]

A unique story found only in Glenn Stout and Richard Johnson's book, *Red Sox Century*, maintains that Wood broke this same thumb again during a game later in the 1913 season. He injured himself trying to chase future Hall of Famer Sam Crawford in a rundown on the basepaths.[22] This second injury basically ended Wood's season with only 11 wins and five losses. Subsequently, Wood was never the same pitcher again. He won ten games in 1914 and 15 games in 1915 for the Red Sox, but never won another game after 1915, none after the very young age of 25.

In 1918 he made a comeback with the Cleveland Indians, not as a pitcher, but as an outfielder, playing a few games at first base and second base along the way. His comeback as a position player was mainly in a part-time capacity. For instance, in 1921 for Cleveland he had a great .366 average, but played in only 66 games. In his final major league season, 1922, at age 32, Wood finally approached a more full-time status when he played in 142 games for Cleveland, batting .297 with 92 RBI and 150 hits in 505 at-bats. But this was Wood's last major league season. Wood ended up with a respectable .283 career batting average.

In 1922 Joe Wood retired from major league baseball to become baseball coach for Yale University, a position he would hold for 20 years. He lived to be 95, dying in 1985.

In 1981 Lawrence Ritter and Donald Honig jointly authored a book called *The 100 Greatest Baseball Players of All Time*. Joe Wood's name was included in the book. The authors coined the phrase "Smoky Joe Wood Syndrome," a term for a gifted and exceptional baseball player whose career was unfortunately cut short by injury.[23] Even though his career statistics did not get him into the Hall of Fame, Wood is included in Ritter and Honig's book as one of the greatest baseball players of all time, and for one season, he truly was.

Chapter 13

Getting Hit by a Bat

Impact by Bat or Bat Piece

Getting hit by a bat on the field or in the stands happens occasionally. Sometimes the catcher is hit by the backswing of the batter. Even the umpire can occasionally get hit. It is dangerous when the batter lets go of the bat during a swing, for whatever reason; also when the ball shatters the bat, the bat splinters into pieces, and the pieces fly into the air. This seems to be occurring more and more often in recent years. A bat being released or shattered can be especially dangerous to the fans in the stands. Almost everyone can remember at some point watching a baseball game on TV or from the stands where the batter either lets go of the bat or the bat shatters, and the whole bat or pieces of the bat go flying on the field or into the stands. It is amazing that serious injuries to fans and players don't occur more often.

Noted below are two players who were injured when an ash bat shattered: Larry Jackson, who was pitching for the St Louis Cardinals in 1961, and Steve Yeager, a catcher for the Los Angeles Dodgers in 1976. A brief discussion of recent concerns about shattered bats — maple versus ash bats — leads to discussion of two incidents where the bat has been used as a weapon (Juan Marichal in 1965 and Jose Offerman in 2007).

LARRY JACKSON

Larry Jackson pitched in the majors from 1955 to 1968, mostly with the St. Louis Cardinals (eight years) and the Chicago Cubs (four years). His career record was 194 wins and 183 losses with a respectable ERA of 3.40. His best season was 1964, when he won 24 games against 11 losses for the Cubs.

On March 27, 1961, during a spring training game, he suffered an unfortunate impact injury caused by a shattered ash wood bat, the barrel of the broken bat hitting him squarely in the jaw, breaking it. The shattered bat belonged to none other than Los Angeles Dodgers center fielder and future Hall of Famer Duke Snider. Subsequently, Jackson missed a whole month, subsisting on liquids and soft food the whole time. He finally came off the DL and pitched his first game of the regular season on April 25 against the Milwaukee Braves.[1]

Jackson did rebound from this injury, winning 11 of his last 12 games for the Cubs to end up the season with 14 wins and 11 losses. He started a surprising number of games in 1961 (33) considering he missed the first month of the season.

Jackson's broken jaw was not a career-altering injury, but illustrates the possible danger to the pitcher from a broken bat. Usually with a shattered bat, there is a little more time to get out of the way than would be the case with a batted ball — a few more milliseconds. But if the pitcher, as in this case, isn't paying very close attention, there may not be enough time to avoid the bat fragment. The pitcher, as the closest infielder to the batter, is the most likely to be hit by a piece of a shattered bat. The poor batter on deck is even closer than the pitcher to the action (see Yeager). The umpire (wearing protective gear) is also at risk. It is very fortunate that this type of injury does not occur more often (see discussion of maple bats).

STEVE YEAGER

Steve Yeager was a major league catcher for 15 seasons from 1972 to 1986, all with the Los Angeles Dodgers, except for his last year with the Seattle Mariners. His career batting average was only .228; he was mainly known for his excellent defensive skills.

He suffered a rather unusual traumatic injury on September 6, 1976. Shortstop Bill Russell of the Dodgers was batting. Yeager was standing in the on-deck circle, waiting his turn to bat. Russell swung at a pitch and hit it; the pitch shattered his ash bat. The jagged end of the bat went into foul territory and struck Yeager in the neck piercing his neck and esophagus. He needed emergency surgery which took over an hour and a half to remove all the bat fragments.[2]

Surprisingly, Yeager missed only two weeks of play after his injury. Luckily, the bat didn't pierce a major artery in his neck, such as the carotid artery, as this could have resulted in Yeager's almost immediate death.[3]

Even though the injury did not occur while Yeager was catching, the injury did inspire his invention of the "Billy goat" neck guard, a protector flap that is attached to the bottom of the catcher's mask. The device protects the catcher's throat from any errant foul ball, or possible piece of shattered bat, traveling straight back from the batter's bat that might cause injury. The device is presently used by many catchers in both major leagues and by some umpires, a popular protective device indeed.[4]

Maple vs. Ash Bats

Both Steve Yeager and Larry Jackson were hit by fragments of bats composed of white ash wood. In the last few years, the majority of major league players have used maple bats.

In 2008 there were a number of articles written on the dangers of maple bats. One by Tom Verducci was posted at SI.com.[5] It appeared to be a hot subject of discussion.[6]

For much of the history of major league baseball, northern white ash has been the primary wood used to make baseball bats, mainly from the states of New York and Pennsylvania. Previously, around the turn of the twentieth century, some bats were made of hickory. Babe Ruth used hickory. Later it was found that bat speed was a more important factor in generating power than the bat's weight. One can swing a lighter bat much faster than a heavier bat. Hickory bats of the same dimensions as ash bats are considerably heavier. Thus, hickory bats fell into disfavor even though at the same time, the wood was found to be harder.[7]

All bats have to have round barrels (this since 1893) no larger than 2¾ inches, and a composition made from a single piece of solid wood. The length allowed for bats is no longer than 42 inches. There are no official rules listed for weight of bat. Tom Verducci at SI.com notes a minimum diameter for the bat handle of ¹⁶⁄₁₉ inch. This diameter is not listed at MLB.com under official rules.[8]

The longest recorded bat ever used was one by Hall of Famer Al Simmons that was 38 inches long. The shortest bat ever used was only 30½ inches long, used by Hall of Famer "Wee" Willie Keeler. Also, the heaviest bat ever used was a 48-ounce hunk of lumber used by Edd Roush of the Cincinnati Reds. Several players have used a 30-ounce bat, including Hall of Famer Joe Morgan.[9]

Maple bats are thought to have been introduced in the early 1990s by Toronto outfielder Joe Carter. They became very popular after Barry Bonds broke the major league home run record in 2001 with his 73 dingers. Articles estimate the usage of maple bats in 2011 at 55 to 60 percent of total bats used.[10]

Although many feel that the ball travels farther when hit with a maple bat, there is very little objective evidence to support this. True, maple is a harder and denser wood than ash. Maple bats don't flake like ash bats. As long as they don't break with use, they tend to maintain their hardness longer than ash. On the downside when maple bats break they tend to explode, sending large, sharp, jagged fragments through the air up to a distance of 100 feet. Ash bats, when they break, more often than not just crack.[11]

There have been several injuries of significance with maple bats. On April 15, 2008, Pittsburgh Pirate Nate McLouth's bat shattered as he hit a double in the eighth inning. At that exact moment, Pittsburgh's hitting coach, Don Long, was quietly sitting in the visitors' dugout at Dodger Stadium. When McLouth hit the ball, Long looked up to follow the path of the ball. Unfortunately he did not see the fragment of the bat spinning rapidly directly towards him, as a large splinter struck him below the left eye, opening a large gash in his left cheek that ultimately required ten stitches to close. He initially showed signs of possible nerve damage, but this problem improved with time.[12]

Ten days after this incident a fan, also at Dodger Stadium, was struck by the barrel of a maple bat used by Todd Helton. Susan Rhoads was sitting in the box seats four rows behind the visitor's dugout when she was struck by a large piece of the bat, with the fragment shattering her jaw.[13]

On June 24, 2008, at Royals Stadium, home plate umpire Brian O'Nora was hit on the head by a piece of a bat. Miguel Olivo's bat shattered after a simple ground ball to shortstop. O'Nora suffered a cut on his forehead and a mild concussion, and for the latter problem he was admitted overnight to a Kansas City hospital. He did not work the game the following day.[14]

The article by Tom Verducci in 2008 notes that previously a minor league right-handed pitcher, Rick Heeling, was impaled in the left arm by a "15-inch shard" from a broken maple bat.[15]

An even more recent maple bat injury occurred September 19, 2010. Tyler Colvin of the Chicago Cubs was having a very successful rookie year (20 home runs in 394 official at-bats with 56 RBI) when his year ended abruptly due to an injury on the field. He was impaled with the sharp broken end of a maple bat.

Colvin was on third when Welington Castillo doubled during the second inning of an eventual Cubs 13–3 victory over the Florida Marlins. He was watching the flight of the ball, not noticing the sharp end of the broken bat coming right at him. The flying sharp point of the broken bat "hit him in the (left) chest, only inches from his heart and jugular vein." The bat fragment did not stick, but did penetrate far enough that Colvin was taken to the hospital for evaluation.[16] It was decided that the bat fragment penetrated the chest wall enough that a chest tube had to be inserted to prevent a collapsed lung. The wound was sutured shut.

Colvin had some trouble breathing for a few days. Once the chest tube was removed, his breathing improved. Despite this improvement Colvin still had to miss the rest of the season.

When asked about maple bats and the danger of them breaking, Colvin expressed confidence that major league officials were dealing adequately with the issue of excessive broken bats. He added, "I can't say much about it (broken maple bats), because I use a maple bat."[17]

From all this information, it is easy to see that there is the potential for even more serious injuries from broken maple bats.

What to do? On June 24, 2008, the same day umpire O'Nora was injured, there was a meeting of baseball's safety and advisory committee. Representatives from the commissioner's office, players' union, and teams planned to "consult with bat experts and bat manufacturers, conduct field and laboratory tests, and gather information about protective measures that could be instituted at ballparks."[18]

Sam Holman, the founder of the Original Maple Bat Corporation, speculated that part of the problem with the shattering maple bats has to do with some companies using inferior wood. To protect fans at ballparks, he suggested major league stadiums have extended netting from directly behind the plate all the way to the first base and third base dugouts. As an added precaution, the netting would have smaller holes than in the netting presently used. There are no uniform rules concerning netting at present.[19]

Another concern is the thickness of the bat handles. If the bat handles are too thin, bats are more likely to break. At present there is only a $^{15}\!/_{19}$-inch minimum diameter. It could be increased to make maple bats less likely to break.[20]

Replacing the maple bats with ash bats would be difficult. Many batters prefer maple bats. They have developed the habit of using maple bats. Habits are hard to break. It may be difficult to get players to switch to ash bats, and any changes made would have to be approved by the players' union. In addition, most bat manufacturers insist a change back to using all ash bats would be difficult. It would take a major shift in the present manufacturing process as well as an effort to find more sources of ash wood. The process of making ash bats takes time and involves picking out the tree, cutting the tree, drying the wood, and then cutting the bats on a lathe. The entire process takes over 30 days for each bat. New bats aren't made overnight.

Often when a problem presents itself, a study is done and this was no different. On December 9, 2008, results were released. In the study, 2,232 broken bats were collected (both ash and maple), of which 756 bats shattered into multiple pieces. Also included in the study were many bats that cracked, but remained in one piece.[21]

Maple bats were found to be three times more likely to break than ash. Experts insisted this should not be the case. Problems with the slope of the grain of the bat were thought to be a major contributor to maple bat breakage. The grain of wood must run straight on the handle of the bat. Even a deviation of 3 percent can be a problem.

Based on the study, new recommendations were made. Starting in 2009, manufacturers were to be held to a higher standard. Bats were to conform to new slope of wood grading techniques. These techniques included putting an ink dot before finishing on sugar maple and yellow birch bats to detect more accurately the slope of the grain.

A continuing system of monitoring bat quality was initiated. All bats from the 32 manufacturers were to be certified with conformity to a new list of standards related to the bat's manufacturing. Bats are to have serial numbers and ink marks to track breakage rates from each manufacturer.

A committee was organized in 2009 to monitor changes. The committee was to look for other contributing factors to bat breakage: shape related to barrel size to handle size ratios, and bat drying methods.

None of this comes cheap. The administrative fee charged to each manufacturer increased to $10,000 from the previous $5,000. Insurance requirements charged to each company making bats were raised (probably to cover possible liability due to bat breakage).[22]

Other changes have been proposed. More recently there has been a proposal to add a thin layer of plastic to the handles of bats called a "Bat Glove." This product, which would cost about $5 per bat, would help to keep pieces of the bat together when they break. Major league baseball is not sure about this idea.[23]

In 2011 two inventors proposed freezing bats before their use as a way to increase wood strength and thus decrease breakage. Jim Cortez and Greg Kendra came up with the idea of cryogenically freezing bats at minus 310 degrees Fahrenheit for up to 24 hours and then gradually allowing the bats to return to ambient temperature. They cite an independent university study that shows the bats using their process are then 26 percent stronger. An MLB spokesman declined to comment on this.[24]

Changes were made in 2010 concerning which bats could be used in the minor leagues. It was ruled that low-density, ultra-light maple bats could no longer be used. Subsequently in November of 2011 this ban on low-density maple bats was extended to the major leagues as part of the major league collective bargaining agreement (CBA). Starting with the 2012 baseball season players new to the major leagues cannot use low density maple bats. Players in the major leagues prior to 2012, though, can continue to use low-density maple bats. There is no ban on high density maple bats.

After all these changes have been made, including studying maple bats, comes concern about the source of the more commonly used ash bats. There is a bug infestation of northern white ash trees by the Emerald Ash borer that is killing millions of these ash trees. This non-native Asian pest first appeared near the Detroit area around 2002 and has since spread from Michigan to parts of Ohio, Indiana, Illinois, and Pennsylvania.[25]

The adult insect feeds on ash leaves but is not the problem. It is the larvae of this bug that are killing the trees. They infest the tree just under the bark, impairing transportation of nutrients and water up the tree trunk to the limbs and leaves, leading if unchecked to the tree's eventual death.[26]

Player Hit by Bat Held by Another Player

On only two occasions, research revealed, has the bat been used as a weapon during a game. In hockey the use of a hockey stick as a weapon happens frequently, which should not be a surprise as all the players on the ice have a stick. On the field in baseball, only the batter at the plate and the batter on deck have a bat in their hands. Thus hitting someone with a bat on purpose is rare.

JOHN ROSEBORO HIT BY BAT SWUNG BY MARICHAL

One instance of a bat usage is very famous, the two players forever remembered for their involvement in this scuffle. It happened on August 22, 1965, at Candlestick Park between future Hall of Famer, Giants pitcher Juan Marichal, and Dodgers catcher John Roseboro.[27]

Early in the game Marichal knocked down Dodgers Maury Wills and Ron Fairly with brushback pitches. Marichal came to bat in the third inning. Roseboro apparently wanted Sandy Koufax to throw a brushback pitch at Marichal. Koufax would not. So, after Koufax's second pitch, Roseboro returned the ball to Koufax by throwing the ball dangerously close to Marichal's nose. Some heated words were exchanged. Roseboro went to punch Marichal. Then the unexpected happened — Marichal hit Roseboro over the head with his bat, hitting him just above his mask on the left side of his head. He had swung the bat three times at Roseboro, connecting only once.[28]

The dugouts cleared and a 14-minute brawl resulted before order was finally restored. The Dodgers and Giants were already intense rivals; they didn't need this incident to spark even greater animosity between the two teams.

Roseboro had blood pouring down his head and left eye. He had to leave the game. Some sources note he had to have stitches to close the two-inch gash, but in his book *Glory Days with the Dodgers* he states he only needed butterfly bandages to close the gash above his left eye.[29] Tommy Davis's *Tales from the Dugout* states Roseboro needed 14 stitches to close his wound.[30]

NL President Warren Giles suspended Marichal for eight games and fined him $1,750. He was forbidden to travel to Dodger Stadium for the crucial two-game series between the Giants and Dodgers at the end of the season.

The Dodgers and Giants fought tooth and nail down to the wire for the National League pennant after this incident in 1965, with the Dodgers finally

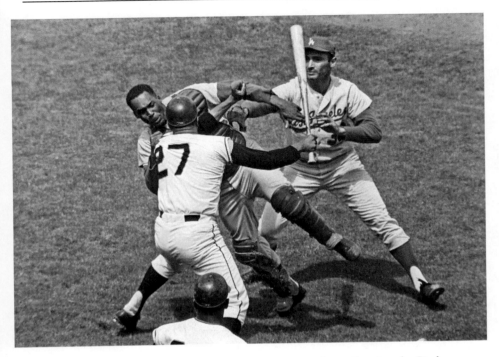

San Francisco Giants pitcher Juan Marichal (27) swings a bat at Los Angeles Dodgers catcher John Roseboro in the third inning at Candlestick Park in San Francisco, California, on August 22, 1965, apparently feeling Roseboro had thrown too close to his head. Los Angeles pitcher Sandy Koufax, rear, tries to break up the fight. Marichal was ejected and Roseboro was treated for head and facial cuts after the incident (AP Photo/Robert H. Houston).

coming out on top and winning the World Series in seven games over the Minnesota Twins.

Roseboro admits throwing the ball dangerously close to Marichal's face, but contends this did not justify Marichal swinging the bat at him. After their careers were over, Roseboro and Marichal became close friends, this after many years of being bitter rivals.

Jose Offerman Swings Bat

The other instance of a batter using a bat as a weapon happened in 2007. It did not occur at the major league level, but did involve a former major league player, Jose Offerman. Offerman, the two-time All-Star, was making an attempt to return to the major leagues by playing for the Long Island Ducks of the Atlantic Independent League. He had not played in the major leagues since 2005, when he was with the New York Mets.

In a game against the Bridgeport Bluefish in Bridgeport, Connecticut, on August 14, 2007, Offerman went ballistic after being hit in the calf by a fastball. Offerman felt he was being thrown at on purpose because of the home run he had hit in his first at-bat. He charged the mound, swinging his bat twice at the opposing pitcher. The pitcher was hit on the hand and the catcher, who had followed Offerman to the mound, was hit in the head by Offerman's back-swing. The Bridgeport catcher, John Nathans, sustained a concussion and had to be taken to the hospital. The pitcher, Matt Beech, wound up with a broken middle finger on his glove hand.[31]

After an on-field delay of 20 minutes, several players were ejected from the game: pitcher Beech, Offerman, and Bridgeport manager and former major leaguer Tommy John.

Things got worse for Offerman. After the game as he was arrested by the city police for second-degree assault. The police had been providing security at the game. He was later freed on $10,000 bond. To add insult to injury, the whole incident was caught on video and played on YouTube for a long time.[32]

In the end, Offerman did not have to go to jail, but got "two years probation with the possibility of having the case expunged from his record in October of 2009 if he stays out of trouble." In 2008 and 2009, Offerman played in the Mexican league. In 2009 and 2010 he was involved in the Caribbean Series as player and then player-manager.[33]

After the incident in 2007, a suit was filed by Bridgeport Bluefish catcher John Nathans in U.S. district court in Bridgeport, seeking $4.8 million in damages related to Offerman's bat-wielding attack. Nathan said he was hit in the head by "Offerman's bat, causing a brain concussion, inner ear damage, vertigo, headaches, and post-concussion syndrome." The suit maintains that the attack left him with permanent career-ending injuries. "I have a ton of headaches every day, vomiting every week," Nathans said. "There is not a day that I don't have symptoms. There's days I'm completely debilitated."[34]

Apparently Offerman didn't learn how to control his anger. The next time, in 2010, he did not hit anyone with a bat. Offerman, the interim manager of the Dominican Licey Tigers, took a swing with his fist at an American umpire in a playoff game in the Dominican Winter League on January 16, 2010. For his efforts he received a lifetime ban from managing in the Dominican League.[35] It is unknown at the time of this writing if Offerman appealed this ban or not.

Chapter 14

Traumatic, Bizarre, Unusual Injuries

Equipment injury

VINCE COLEMAN

Another injury mechanism is that a player can run into or get hit by equipment used on the field. In a very rare event, one that might have affected the outcome of the 1985 World Series, left fielder Vince Coleman of the St. Louis Cardinals had a bizarre equipment injury just before the start of the fourth game of the NLCS between the Los Angeles Dodgers and the Cardinals. In most ballparks, the tarp that covers the field when it is raining is simply stored on a cylinder sitting next to the first base dugout. It is manually rolled onto and off of the field. At Busch Stadium on October 13, 1985, there was an electronically operated tarp system. The tarp cylinder was stored beneath the field. When needed, the cylinder, with or without the tarp, was mechanically raised to field level and then rolled in or out.

On October 13, the tarp covered the field during pre-game warm-ups because of light rain. The crew was preparing to roll up the tarp. The tarp cylinder was elevated and rolled onto the field of play. The crew had not noticed that Vince Coleman, who had set a rookie record with 110 stolen bases that year, was standing on the first base side of the tarp cylinder. Before anything could be done to stop it, the cylinder rolled over Coleman's left ankle and up his left leg all the way to his knee. Coleman screamed for help; he was trapped for at least 30 seconds before assistance came. Coleman had to be removed from the field on a stretcher.[1]

Tests revealed that he had sustained a bone chip fracture in his left knee and a bruised leg. He missed the rest of the NLCS. Fortunately, in the NLCS at least, the Cardinals went on to win in six games, the last two games coming in rather dramatic fashion, decided by home runs in Games 5 and 6 by Ozzie Smith and Jack Clark respectively.

The World Series, though, did not go as well for the Cardinals. They were up three games to one against the Kansas City Royals, but the Royals rallied to win the last three games and the World Series. Who knows what would have happened if Vince Coleman had not been injured by the tarp cylinder collision? This was an unusual traumatic equipment injury.

MICKEY MANTLE — SPRINKLER HEAD INJURY, KNEE

Another bizarre equipment injury happened to Mickey Mantle. Mantle needs very little introduction. The Hall of Famer played his entire 18-year career with the New York Yankees. He was a three-time MVP with a career .298 batting average and 536 home runs.

Most research information concerning Mantle's injury comes from Tony Castro's book, *Mickey Mantle: America's Prodigal Son.*[2] David Falkner's book, *The Last Hero: The Life of Mickey Mantle*, briefly covers this injury.[3]

His bizarre accident happened during the sixth inning of the second game of the 1951 World Series between the New York Yankees and the New York Giants. Mantle was playing right field with an aging Joe DiMaggio in center field.

In the sixth inning, Willie Mays hit a short fly ball to right center. Casey Stengel had instructed Mantle to be aggressive in going for fly balls as DiMaggio was not as fast as he used to be. Therefore Mantle took off thinking that DiMaggio had little chance to get the fly ball. As Mantle neared the ball, he saw DiMaggio camped under the ball calling, "I got it." Mantle had to slam on the brakes to avoid a collision with DiMaggio, and as he did he caught the spikes on his right shoe on the rubber cover of the drainage hole just beneath the outfield grass (part of the sprinkler system). *The Sporting News* says the cover was wooden.[4] A Mantle interview available on youtube.com says the cover was rubber, as does Falkner's book.[5]

Mantle felt a loud pop and his right knee gave way. He fell to the ground in pain and had to be carried off the field on a stretcher. A splint was placed on the knee, and the next day Mantle was taken to Lenox Hill Hospital. The injury was severe enough to require surgery. The exact extent of the injury is unclear. Book and newspaper sources are often incomplete in describing injuries in clear medical terms. Tony Castro's book indicates Mantle had two torn ligaments in his knee, but does not mention which ones.[6] The nature of the injury, the knee swelling up to twice its normal size, would indicate at least one of the torn ligaments could be the anterior cruciate ligament. Another source indicated Mantle also had cartilage damage in his right knee.[7] *The Sporting News* of October 17, 1951, said nothing about possible cartilage damage.[8]

In 1951 the treatment of ligament tears and cartilage tears was primitive compared to today, and it is unknown whether this had anything to do with Mantle's persistent problems with his right knee after this injury. It is reported that after Mantle's recovery, his speed was never quite as blazing as it had been before the injury.

DUKE SNIDER

Duke Snider of the Brooklyn Dodgers also suffered a knee injury caused by the infamous Yankee Stadium sprinkler system. Glenn Stout, in his book, *The Dodgers: 120 Years of Dodgers History*, describes the incident.[9] In the sixth game of the 1955 World Series, future Hall of Famer Duke Snider, in center field for the Dodgers, caught his foot on the head of one of the sprinklers and wrenched his knee. He had to be pulled from the game and was pinch-hit for by Don Zimmer.

The knee hobbled Snider, but he, unlike Mantle, was able to play the next day. It was the World Series, and the injury had to be pretty severe to keep a determined Snider out the seventh game. In fact, in the sixth inning Snider was able to run fast enough to beat out a very important bunt. On the play, the throw from Tommy Byrne, the pitcher, to Bill "Moose" Skowron, the Yankees' first baseman, was dropped by Skowron as he attempted to tag Snider running down the first base line. The ball simply popped out of Skowron's glove, and Snider was safe. Eventually an important run scored in the inning.[10]

The Dodgers went on to win the 1955 World Series, and the injured Snider played an important role in the seventh game, a 2 to 0 Brooklyn victory. The next season (1956), Snider suffered no ill effects of his injury as he was able to play 151 games. There were no serious long-term, detrimental effects from Duke Snider's injury. Still, Snider's injury is a good example of a traumatic equipment injury, an injury that easily could have been much worse. Duke Snider in 1955 was luckier than Mickey Mantle had been in 1951.

CARL FURILLO'S HAND INJURY

Another unusual injury happened to Dodger Carl Furillo. He broke a bone in his hand in an unusual fashion on September 6, 1953. The injury occurred during an altercation between Furillo and Leo Durocher at the Polo Grounds in New York, the home of the New York Giants.

Furillo spent his entire 15-year career with the Dodgers, both in Brooklyn and after the Dodgers moved to Los Angeles in 1958. He ended up with a respectable .299 lifetime average and played mainly right field for the Dodgers.

Leo Durocher was Furillo's manager in 1946 and part of 1948. Afterwards Durocher managed the rival New York Giants from the middle of 1948 to 1955.

While Durocher managed the Dodgers, Furillo and others noticed that Durocher was often quick to tell his pitchers to purposely throw at batters. Furillo knew this.[11]

When Durocher managed the Giants in 1950, Giants pitcher Sheldon Jones hit Furillo in the head, sending Furillo to the hospital overnight.[12] Only the protective lining in Furillo's cap prevented a more serious injury.[13] Furillo accused Durocher of saying "Make him eat it" at the time the pitch was thrown by Jones.[14] After this injury, Furillo did not keep his future plan a secret. As long as Durocher was manager of the Giants, if any other Giants pitcher ever hit him with a pitch again he was going "to get" Durocher.[15]

Well, on September 6, 1953, when Furillo was leading the league in hitting at .344, Giants pitcher Ruben Gomez hit him on the wrist with a waist-high pitch.

Immediately Furillo walked a little bit towards the mound, but when Gomez walked away from him, Furillo proceeded to first base. After Gomez made two more pitches, Furillo made a beeline to the dugout to get Durocher, not even bothering to ask the umpire at first base for time out.[16] Furillo reported that Durocher made a "beckoning gesture" to him before he left first base.[17] Durocher, never one to turn away from a challenge, came out of the dugout to meet him face to face. They grappled. Furillo missed a roundhouse punch as they both fell to the ground. Then, and it certainly was no surprise to the fans who were present, the benches cleared, with players on the field and pouring from the dugouts joining in the melee.[18]

When the smoke cleared, Furillo had injured his left hand. He was the only one injured. X-rays revealed that he had broken the fifth metacarpal in his hand[19] (the bone just proximal to the little finger). The exact way the injury occurred is unclear. Furillo was out of the lineup until the World Series, if the Dodgers made it that far, which they did.

The whole scene is played out in much detail, even including a couple of revealing pictures, in the September 16, 1953, issue of *The Sporting News* under the caption "Pull 'Em Apart Party at the Polo Grounds punchbowl." There are six articles in this issue concerned with the scuffle, giving many different angles to the story line of the fight.[20]

In one article Furillo is quoted as saying he didn't hear anything Durocher said.[21] Furillo said whatever gestures Durocher made to him, he just assumed were a challenge to him. In the article by Roscoe McGowen, Durocher denied making a beckoning gesture. He said, "he's a blankety-blank liar. I never said a word to him and I didn't make any gestures to him."[22]

Surprisingly, no one was suspended. National League president Warren Giles said Furillo had withdrawn his threat to "get" Leo. As far as Giles was concerned, the matter was ended. Giles stated, "I have talked with Furillo and told him I am convinced there was no intent on the part of Gomez to hit him with a pitched ball in last Sunday's game. I also told him that he was wrong in leaving first base to rush towards the Giants' dugout, but his tussle with Durocher, in itself, did not require any action by our office."[23]

In the end, Furillo suffered a fifth metacarpal fracture of his left hand. One *Sporting News* article suggested that someone stepped on Furillo's hand during the melee following the instigating pitch.[24] The doctors examining Furillo suggested the same possibility. In an interview Furillo gave in Flushing, NY, in 1970, he stated this was not possible. Furillo said if his hand had been stepped on, he would have had cleat marks on his hand, and there were none.[25] But would it not be possible to trample on the hand without spikes?[26] Could someone have fallen on the hand with a knee or shoulder? *The Sporting News* suggested that Furillo could have suffered the injury while hitting Durocher.[27] The very nature of this common fifth metacarpal hand fracture, often called a boxer's fracture, might suggest this as a possibility. Furillo denied hitting Durocher.[28] In 1970 Furillo suggested a fourth possible mechanism. He said, "I knew Durocher had grabbed my finger and twisted it when we were wrestling, so as to put me out for the year."[29]

Furillo still ended up with a batting crown in 1953, as he had sufficient at bats to qualify for the batting crown with his final .344 average. He recovered in time to play in the World Series against the New York Yankees. His fine performance in the six-game World Series, eight hits in 24 at-bats with two doubles, one home run, and four RBI, was not sufficient to secure a victory for the Dodgers.

A bizarre accident on the field indeed, fortunately with no long-term consequences for Carl Furillo, was just another incident in the long-standing rivalry between the Giants and the Dodgers.

MILTON BRADLEY'S KNEE INJURY

In 2007 San Diego player Milton Bradley suffered a rather unusual knee injury. The left fielder had been obtained earlier in the year in a trade from the Oakland A's.

The injury occurred during an argument between Bradley and first base umpire Mike Winters in the eighth inning of a game between the Colorado Rockies and Padres at Petco Park on September 23.[30]

Prior to Bradley's eighth inning at-bat, home plate umpire Brian Runge had issued a warning to Bradley. Earlier, in the fifth inning, Bradley had allegedly flipped his bat in the direction of Runge. Runge had not seen this but apparently first base umpire Winters did and informed Runge of the incident.

When Bradley arrived at first base after his eighth inning single, Winters told Bradley it was he who had informed Runge about the bat-flipping episode.

Tulowitzki did recover from this injury in time to finish with a .263 average in the 101 games he played. It didn't help the Rockies, though, who ended up with only 74 wins against 88 losses for the year.

CARLOS QUENTIN — WRIST INJURY

Carlos Quentin of the White Sox had a similarly nasty run-in with his bat on September 1, 2008, but unlike with Tulowitzki, Quentin's bat did not shatter.[37]

Carlos Quentin was in the middle of an MVP-caliber year (100 RBI and 36 homers in only 130 games) when he broke his wrist in a rather unusual fashion. Quentin states that he often misses or fouls a pitch off. He deliberately holds onto his bat in the left hand and hits down on the bat head with his right hand with a closed fist to show his frustration. He had done this a thousand times before, since he was a kid, and no damage had ever resulted. This time there was damage. After fouling off a pitch on September 1 against Cliff Lee, he did the same thing he had always done, except this time he came down awkwardly and hit the end of the bat on the wrist instead of his closed hand. He felt nothing after the initial incident, but 40 minutes later, he realized something was wrong. By the next morning he knew he had a significant problem, and x-rays confirmed that Quentin had fractured his wrist (the exact bone is not mentioned). The fracture was severe enough to require a pin inserted to stabilize the fracture site, essentially ending Quentin's 2008 season. Sadly, he ended up fifth in the American League MVP voting, not receiving a single first-place vote.[38]

KHALIL GREENE — HAND INJURY

Khalil Greene was already having a bad season when he suffered a hand fracture on July 30, 2008. Frustrated after recording his 100th strikeout of the season, Greene punched a Petco Park storage cabinet. Not a good idea! Greene broke the fifth metacarpal bone on his left hand. As a result of his anger, he then missed the rest of the season.[39]

Greene was in his sixth season with the San Diego Padres. He signed a two-year contract in February 2008 after turning down a four-year contract extension for $29 million. He had a breakout season in 2007, finishing with 155 hits, 27 home runs, and 97 RBI with 611 at-bats in 153 games. Hopes were high for 2008. It was not to be. At the time of his injury, he was batting a career-low .213 with only 83 hits, 35 RBI, 10 home runs, and 100 strikeouts in 389 at-bats, production considerably decreased from Greene's 2007 highs.

Greene was traded by the Padres to the St. Louis Cardinals before the 2009 season. He had recurring anxiety problems in 2009. He subsequently was signed as a free agent by the Texas Rangers in 2010, but was let go when problems with anxiety once again became an issue.[40] He has not played in the major leagues since.

RANDY MESSENGER — HAND INJURY

Almost a carbon copy of the injury to Khalil Greene was the injury to San Francisco Giants reliever Randy Messenger. Mad about having just given up a game-ending double to Atlanta's Chipper Jones, he punched an unnamed plastic object in the dugout. The accident in Atlanta resulted in a broken fifth metacarpal in his left (non-pitching) hand. The specific injury to the knuckle attached to the little finger is called a boxer's fracture. The injury was severe enough that Messenger required surgery.[41]

Whether or not the injury had anything to do with it, Messenger found himself pitching relief for the Seattle Mariners in 2008, instead of the Giants.

KEVIN BROWN — HAND INJURY

Kevin Brown, a right-handed pitcher with a respectable career record of 211 wins and 144 losses, pitched for 19 years in the majors, mostly for the Texas Rangers (eight years) and Los Angeles Dodgers (five years). The last two years of Brown's career were spent with the New York Yankees, where he achieved a mediocre record of 14 wins and 13 losses. On September 3, Brown punched the wall out of frustration during a game. He was on the losing end of a 3 to 1 score against Baltimore. He broke two bones in his non-pitching hand, badly enough to require surgery. Two pins were inserted in the hand at Columbia Presbyterian Medical Center. Brown's 2004 season was over.[42]

JASON ISRINGHAUSEN — WRIST INJURY

Why do players punch immovable objects when they are upset? The history of this type of injury just goes on and on.

Jason Isringhausen, whose career is discussed under his Tommy John surgery, also suffered such an injury. In a fit of anger, the 24-year-old pitcher, while on a rehab assignment for the Mets organization at Triple-A Norfolk, punched a clubhouse trash can on April 11, 1997, fracturing two small bones in his right wrist.[43] His rehab, after arthroscopic surgery on his shoulder and elbow the previous year, had not been going well. In two starts at Norfolk he had allowed seven runs, 15 hits, and seven walks in 13 innings.

So take it out on the trash can! Isringhausen ended up in a cast for four weeks. He could have at least used his non-pitching hand to hit the trash can. There is no indication that Isringhausen suffered any long-term problems from the fractured bones. He did go on to have a long career and is the all-time saves leader in St. Louis Cardinals history. There is also no indication he ever suffered a similar injury again. Live and learn!

RYAN MADSON — TOE INJURY

Each year adds another player who has taken his frustrations out on a somewhat immovable object. The 2010 season was no different. On Wednesday, April 28, in an extra-inning game, the Phillies' Ryan Madson gave up a run in the bottom of the 11th inning against San Francisco at AT&T Park. He blew his second save of the year. In his frustration he tried to kick over a metal chair, but caught his big toe underneath the chair, fracturing the right big toe in the process. He was placed on the DL on April 30. A CT scan on Monday, May 3, revealed the damage was worse than expected, and Madson had surgery. He was on the DL until July 8 and actually pitched better after he came off the DL than before he went on the DL.[44]

Madson was actually named the winning pitcher in the game on April 28. The Phillies came up with two runs in the top of the 11th inning to win the game. Nelson Figueroa, though he gave up a run to San Francisco in the bottom of the 11th, picked up his first save of the year.[45]

KENDRYS MORALES — ANKLE INJURY IN CELEBRATION

Even more recent is the bizarre injury to Kendrys Morales of the Los Angeles Angels. Morales hit a walk-off grand slam home run in the tenth inning of the 5 to 1 Angels victory over the Seattle Mariners in Anaheim on May 29, 2010. When arriving at home plate to cheering, waiting teammates, he took a double jump or hop, landing awkwardly as he hit the plate with his left ankle. He had to be taken off the field in a mobile vehicle. Tests revealed the ankle was fractured. The fibula, the bone near the ankle on the outside, was fractured.[46]

Apparently the fracture was severe enough that surgery was deemed necessary. It was not operated on immediately, as time had to pass for the swelling in the ankle to go down. Morales was not able to put weight on the ankle for six weeks after the fracture surgery. Surgery was done by Dr. Phil Kwong, a foot and ankle specialist at the Kerlan-Jobe Clinic. Morales missed not only the rest of the 2010 season but all of 2011 as well. He did not play again in the major leagues until March 22, 2012.

Chapter 15

Impact Injuries by Baseball

Yadier Molina

Another important injury mechanism occurs when a player is hit by the baseball, either thrown (by pitcher or fielder) or hit (called impact injuries). For example, Yadier Molina in 2005 and 2007 had two impact injuries by each of these two mechanisms. On July 7, 2005, he was hit on the left hand by a pitched ball that fractured the fifth metacarpal bone in his left hand.[1]

Two years later, in May 2007, he was hit on the left wrist by a different mechanism: he was catching and the batter foul-tipped the ball.[2] The ball deflected ever so slightly, hitting Molina's wrist. Both times Molina was placed on the DL, missing more than two weeks before returning to play. Molina's injuries are examples of the two main types of impact injuries, hit by pitch/throw or hit by batted ball.

Most of the examples to follow involve more serious injuries than the ones sustained by Yadier Molina. Molina's later injury illustrates why being a catcher is a risky and difficult job, always at risk for deflected pitches.

Pitched Impact Injuries — Beanings

The next major cause of impact injuries is beanings, players hit in the head by a pitched ball. There are several well-known beanings and even more not-so-well-known beanings. There is considerable discussion of this subject noted by myself on internet sites and in books.

Tony Conigliaro

One well-known impact injury clearly shortened a potentially great career and encouraged the use of the batting helmet with the addition of the earflap. The injured player was Tony Conigliaro.

Tony Conigliaro broke into the major leagues for the Boston Red Sox at the age of 19 in 1964. In his rookie season, he hit .290 with 24 home runs, and 52 RBI. He could have been Rookie of the Year, except his wrist was broken by a pitch from Moe Drabowsky in August. If that wasn't enough, Conigliaro was also hit that year on the forearm by Pedro Ramos, missing even more time due to that impact injury. The result: Conigliaro's season was limited to 111 games by the injuries, hurting his chance to win ROY.[3] Tony Oliva, playing in 161 games with 217 hits, 32 home runs, a .323 average, and 94 RBI, won the American League honor that year.

In his sophomore year, 1965, Conigliaro hit 32 home runs to become the youngest ever to lead the league in that category. In his third season, 1966, he hit 28 home runs and had 93 RBI. At age 22, he became the youngest player ever in the American League to reach the milestone of 100 home runs.

The 1967 season marked triumph for the Boston Red Sox. They won the American League pennant for the first time since 1946. They made it to the World Series. Carl Yastrzemski became the last player to win the Triple Crown.

Conigliaro contributed to the team's success. He was nominated to his first All-Star Game in 1967. By the middle of August he was hitting .287 with 20 home runs and 67 RBI. But on August 18, all that changed for Tony Conigliaro.

It was well known that Conigliaro crowded the plate, far more than most hitters, almost daring the pitcher to throw inside. At Fenway Park, Jack Hamilton, a pitcher known to thrown inside occasionally, was pitching for the California Angels in the fourth inning. He threw a fastball on the inside part of the plate, high and tight. Conigliaro, with his head held over the plate as he usually did, was unable to get out of the way. The ball smacked Conigliaro hard on the left cheek just below the temple (he was a right-handed batter). He sustained a broken cheekbone and a more severe injury to his left eye. He was batting with a hard plastic helmet, but it didn't have a protective earflap. It is thought the earflap might have prevented the severity of Conigliaro's eye injury. Conigliaro fell to the ground in agony. Though he never lost consciousness, his injury was severe enough that he had to be removed from the field on a stretcher.[4]

Conigliaro missed the rest of the 1967 season. He also missed the entire 1968 season except for limited participation in spring training. Early on it was apparent he had significant eye problems. David Cataneo, in his book *Tony C: The Triumph and Tragedy of Tony Conigliaro*, documents Conigliaro's eye problems very well.[5]

His injuries in 1967 made it dangerous for him to play in 1968. Dr. Charles Regan of Retinal Associates of Boston oversaw the recovery of Conigliaro from his eye injury. He had damage to central part of the retina (the macula), the most important area for sharp visual acuity and depth perception.

Conigliaro played in spring training in 1968 but after he hit only .125 with 22 strikeouts in 66 at-bats, it was obvious that something was still wrong with his vision. There was a need to step back and reassess the eye problem. Dr. Regan noted Conigliaro had 20/10 vision in his right eye, but only 20/300 in his left eye. Conigliaro was legally blind in the left eye. No glasses were going to improve retinal damage. Dr. Regan determined that the retinal damage was so severe that if Conigliaro attempted to play baseball in 1968, he risked

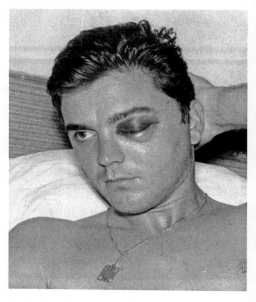

Boston Red Sox star outfielder Tony Conigliaro sports a shiner at Santa Maria Hospital in Cambridge, Massachusetts, on August 19, 1967, being treated for a fractured left cheekbone. Conigliaro was hit by a fastball thrown by California pitcher Jack Hamilton the day before at Fenway Park (AP Photo/files).

bodily harm. It was dangerous enough to judge 90 mile per hour fastballs with good vision. He also risked a retinal detachment which could result in loss of all eyesight in the left eye.[6] This assessment ended his 1968 season in spring training.

There was some concern by Dr. Regan that Conigliaro might never play again. Conigliaro shifted to plan B. If he couldn't come back as a hitter, he might try pitching. Thus, in the spring of 1969, he made an attempt to come back as a pitcher.[7] He met with only mild success, being roughed up in several outings. As there wasn't a DH in 1969, pitchers had to bat for themselves. In hitting, Conigliaro had some encouraging results, both during the game and in batting practice. He gradually worked into playing some outfield in between pitching assignments, with continued success batting.

It was time to reassess the situation again. Dr. Regan determined that Conigliaro now had 20/20 vision in his left eye, though he still had some central visual deficits.[8] While batting, he found that if he turned his head slightly to the side instead of staring straight at the pitched ball, he could compensate for his central vision difficulty.

Through hard work and determination, he came back in 1969 and, after hitting 20 home runs and driving in 82 runs, he was named "Comeback Player of the Year." In 1970, he hit even better, with 36 home runs and 116 RBI. Even though he was successful, Conigliaro admitted he was still having some trouble seeing the ball. He was also dealing with frequent headaches that started after his injury.[9] This didn't make life any easier.

The next difficulty Conigliaro had to confront was in 1971. He was traded by his beloved Red Sox to the California Angels. It was difficult enough for Conigliaro, a native New Englander, to play with his eye problems, but now he had to adjust to a new team, a new environment, and new expectations.

The 1971 season didn't go well. By the All-Star break, he was hitting only .229 with four home runs. Out of frustration, he left the Angels to have his eyes examined once again. The results: he was seeing 20/30 in his left eye overall, but his central vision was only 20/300.[10] This visual acuity was measured with him looking straight ahead, not turning his head slightly to the side. He left the Angels and quit baseball completely instead of reporting back after a brief absence. He decided to shift gears and concentrate on other business matters, including managing his own restaurant, Tony C's.

But the will to play never left Conigliaro. After several years off, he made another comeback attempt for his hometown Red Sox in 1975. Even though his vision had improved and the defect in his central vision deficit had decreased in size, he still had a rough time. He was now 30 years old. He was older and had to deal with nagging injuries he hadn't experienced when younger. He had hamstring and neck injuries, limiting his ability to practice and improve.

Conigliaro also had the numbers game to deal with. The Red Sox had a very good team in 1975, one that would play in the World Series at year's end, losing to Cincinnati in seven games. The Red Sox had new players like Freddy Lynn (Rookie of the Year and MVP in 1975) and future Hall of Famer Jim Rice on the team. Then there were veterans Dwight Evans and Juan Beniquez. The outfield positions were full and there were many, including Carl Yastrzemski, who could probably fill the role of DH better than Conigliaro could. There was considerable question as to whether Conigliaro would make the team during spring training.

He made the team, but after more hamstring problems and after hitting only .123 in limited action, he was optioned to Boston's Triple-A affiliate, Pawtucket, on June 14, 1975. He hit only slightly better in the minor leagues, batting .203 with three home runs and 12 RBI. With a week left before the Triple-A season was over, Conigliaro quit the team.[11] He admitted that even though his vision had improved slightly since 1971, it still wasn't good enough to hit major league pitching. That, poor hitting, injuries, and decreased motivation to put in the work to be successful again, especially with the prospect of playing more time in the minors, all went into his decision to hang the cleats up once and for all.

Tragedy followed Conigliaro's life after baseball. On January 3, 1982, at age 37, on his way to Boston's Logan Airport with his brother Billy driving, Tony suffered a heart attack.[12] The heart attack was severe. Tony suffered significant brain damage from a prolonged episode of shock depriving his brain of much-needed oxygen. The anoxia spell lasted too long. He never fully recovered and died eight years later at the young age of 45, a sad ending to a career cut short by an impact injury from a beaning.

MICKEY COCHRANE

Another impact injury from a pitched ball happened to catcher Mickey Cochrane. Research information presented here on Cochrane's injury is gleaned from *Baseball Hall of Fame, Cooperstown: Where Legends Live Forever*, by Reidenbaugh, Hoppel and editors of *The Sporting News*, and *Mickey Cochrane: The Life of a Baseball Hall of Fame Catcher*, by Charlie Bevis.[13]

Mickey Cochrane, a left-handed batter, was a catcher for the Philadelphia Athletics and Detroit Tigers. His major league career spanned 13 years starting in 1925. He played on three American League pennant winners for the Athletics (1929–1931) and two for the Tigers (1934–1935). Three of these teams won the World Series (1929, 1930, and 1935). For Detroit, 1935 brought their first World Series win ever. In addition to being a player for the Detroit Tigers, Cochrane was also their manager. He was named AL MVP in 1928 with Philadelphia and in 1934 with Detroit

Cochrane's best year was 1930, when he hit .357 with ten home runs, 85 RBI, and 110 runs scored. For his career he batted .320, best among all retired or deceased major league catchers. He caught at least 110 games each year from 1925 through 1935. His on-base percentage of .419 ranks among the top 20 players of any position all-time. For his career he struck out only once every 24 plate appearances.

His career as a player came to an end on May 25, 1937. He was hit in the head on the right temple (beaned) by a pitch from Yankees pitcher Bump Hadley. Cochrane was not wearing a batting helmet, as they were not mandatory until 1971 (more on that later). He did not even have the plastic cap inserts which were used by some players in the early 1940s and 1950s. He suffered a fractured skull. He was unconscious and close to death for two days and hospitalized for ten days. He never played another game in the field. He did come back to manage in 1938, but he was replaced on August 6 of that year. He went on to manage a baseball team for the navy during World War II, but he never managed at the major league level after the war.

Although his playing career was cut short by his beaning in 1937 at age

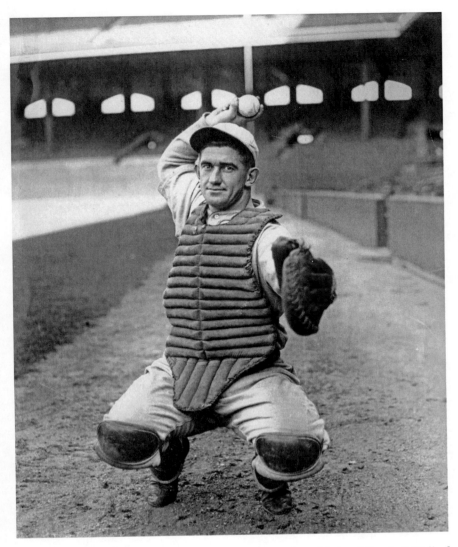

Mickey Cochrane of the Detroit Tigers on unknown date (National Baseball Hall of Fame Library, Cooperstown, New York).

34, his career as a player and manager was impressive enough to earn election to the Hall of Fame in 1947.

JOE MEDWICK

Joe Medwick's career is described well in *The Fierce Fun of Ducky Medwick*, by Thomas Barthel.[14] Medwick was a Hall of Famer who in his 17-year major league career hit .324.

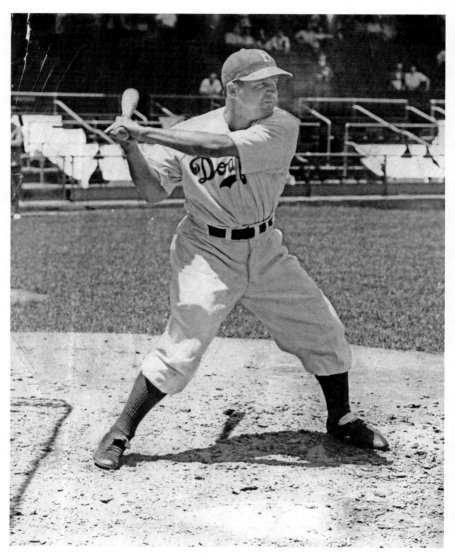

Joe Medwick, Brooklyn Dodgers, during batting practice, 1942, showing typical batting stance (National Baseball Hall of Fame Library, Cooperstown, New York).

Medwick was the unfortunate recipient of a beanball on June 18, 1940. Ironic as it may seem, Medwick had just been traded on June 13 from the St. Louis Cardinals to the Brooklyn Dodgers, and the beanball was delivered by none other than St. Louis Cardinals pitcher Bob Bowman.[15]

Stories revolve around such historical events. First, there is the story of how Medwick and Dodgers player/manager Leo Durocher had bumped into Bowman on the elevator. Medwick had told Bowman that he would be knocked out of the game early. Bowman replied he would take care of both Medwick and Durocher in his own way.[16]

Then there are stories surrounding Medwick's at-bat about how he came to be beaned, and whether he was hit deliberately or not. It is said that Dodgers coach Charlie Dressen was stealing signs by watching how Bowman held the ball before he threw. If Bowman twisted his glove, it meant he was going to throw a curve, and then Dressen would whistle. The Cardinal catcher, Don Padgett, noted this, went out to the mound, and informed Bowman about this sign stealing. The two decided to cross things up by having Bowman hold the ball in his glove like he was going to throw a curve, but then cut loose a fast-ball.[17] This decision was made as Medwick stood at the plate, and on the very first pitch Bowman threw to Medwick, it happened.

Dressen whistled. Medwick leaned over to hit a curve and the fastball came in high and tight, hitting him on the left side of the head, where the button on his cap was, just above his left ear. Medwick wore no protective head gear; nobody did in 1940. Medwick had no protection; he just had on his regular old playing cap.

Medwick was taken off the field on a stretcher. Though it was uncertain if he lost consciousness, Medwick related he didn't remember anything about getting hit. He talked to his wife after being taken to the clubhouse and then was whisked away to Caledonian Hospital in Brooklyn.

Fortunately, Medwick was not found to have a skull fracture.[18] He was discharged from the hospital at 7 pm that night despite having a throbbing headache and blurred vision. He was told to take at least a week off.[19]

Despite having persistent double vision and dizzy spells, Medwick insisted on returning to the lineup. Durocher allowed it. Medwick pinch-hit in a game on June 22, just four days after his beaning on June 18.

Initially Medwick did okay, going 9 for 32 in his first few games, and he was 39 for 134 for a .291 average and 24 runs batted in July. He really didn't hit stride until late August, when he started a 16-game hit streak, all of this despite having persistent problems with double vision, though this bothersome symptom gradually improved as the season progressed. He ended up hitting .300 for the Dodgers in 106 games in 1940.

Did Medwick come back too soon? His teammate, Pee Wee Reese, had been beaned on June 1 and was out three full weeks. Robert Creamer, in *Baseball and Other Matters in 1941*, notes that shortstop Billy Jurges of the Giants missed the entire season after being beaned in 1940, just two weeks after Medwick was beaned.[20] Shouldn't Medwick have stayed out at least as long as Reese? With today's level of care for concussions he would have stayed away longer than he did, especially with his complaints of double vision and dizziness. His stats after the injury, as mentioned, were not bad, though not as good as Medwick had had in the past, especially not like 1937 when he was the National

League MVP and the last National Leaguer to win the Triple Crown, batting .374 with 154 RBI and 31 home runs.

Did the beaning initiate a decline in Medwick's ability? Was his stance altered by his beaning? Did he involuntarily start pulling away from pitches intermittently after this injury? This is difficult to say, as it has been noted that Medwick always had an unusual batting stance, a right-handed hitter who stepped in the bucket, and swung while stepping backward.[21] He had always hit that way.

Bill James, the guru of baseball statistical analysis, in *Politics of Glory*, points out that many Hall of Fame players had their best years before age 28, and Medwick's stats did gradually decline after age 28.[22]

Barthel, in *The Fierce Fun of Ducky Medwick*, shows a steady decline in extra-base hits with Medwick's peak of 99 in 1937, and then a decline to 76 in 1938, 70 in 1939, and 59 in 1940.[23] The declines in 1938 and 1939 were prior to Medwick's injury. Referring to baseball-reference.com for stats, it is rather obvious that Medwick did not drive in more than 100 runs in any year after age 27 (1939), nor did he hit 20 or more home runs after age 26 (1938), even though he played until age 36. (It makes one wonder why the Yankees gave a ten-year contract at $27.5 million a year to Alex Rodriguez at age 32, an age when his best years should be behind him.)

It is common to look at a single event that changes a baseball player's career, but Medwick's decline in batting could easily be attributed just to advancing age. This author found no other reference indicating Medwick had any problems with double vision or dizzy spells after 1940, the year he was beaned.

DON ZIMMER

Most of the information obtained about Don Zimmer comes from his book, *Zim: A Baseball Life*. Don Zimmer was hit three times in the head in his career: two times on pitched balls and once on a foul ball. He states, "the most defining moments of my career have involved my head."[24]

On the cover of his book he is wearing an army helmet to protect his head, something he wore in the dugout of the Yankees just after the last time he was hit on the head. The picture gives an exclamation mark to his quotation.

The first time Don Zimmer was hit on the head he almost died. He was working his way up the Dodgers' farm system when the injury occurred. On July 7, 1953, while playing for the Dodgers' Triple-A affiliate, he was hit in the head by right-handed pitcher Jim Kirk.[25]

There were apparently some unfortunate circumstances that led to the beaning and the severity of the beaning. It was a twilight game, making the ball difficult to see. The hitter's background was bad. There were trees in the outfield that made the ball difficult to pick up. Finally, there were no batting helmets (more on this later).

Zimmer was drilled on the left side of his head, fracturing his skull. He was briefly alert after the accident but was unconscious for six days. His injury was so severe he had clots form in his head. These had to be drained to decrease the pressure on his brain. Three holes were drilled in the left side of his skull and one on the right side.[26]

He remained in the hospital for some time. After he woke up, his speech was impaired. He had decreased sensation in the right side of his body (the left side of the brain controls the right side of the body). His eyesight remained blurred for some time. Even after his speech returned, he continued to stutter for several weeks. He lost a lot of weight (dropping from 174 to 124 lbs). He had headaches and continued to have migraines for a year after the injury.[27]

He was away from baseball till the next year. By then his recovery was rather complete, with resolution of all symptoms except the headaches. By the way, the holes drilled in his head were covered with tantalum buttons.

As a result of the injury, the Dodgers were one of the first teams to use protective inserts under their caps when they batted. These were not the true helmets that were later adopted.

Zimmer's second beaning occurred on June 23, 1956.[28] He had made it to the majors and was playing for the Dodgers. He is not sure if the beaning was deliberate or not. Hal Jeffcoat threw the ball that was just a little too far inside. It hit him in the left side of the face, fracturing his cheekbone (Zim was a right-handed batter). Zim was only unconscious for a brief time. Once again he was taken to surgery, to repair the injury.

Other than the cheekbone fracture, the major concern was that he might have a retinal detachment and might lose his eyesight. The equipment available to evaluate such a problem then was not as sophisticated as it is now. Then again, any blood noted in the eye chamber during any simple ophthalmologic exam (looking with a light at the back of the eye) would make one suspect that there could be a detached retina.

Zimmer was given pinhole glasses for six weeks, with gradual improvement in his eyesight. He stated that after this he didn't think he was ever the same batter, although his statistics aren't much different before or after the injury. Much later he noted that occasionally when he would move his head, he would note a black spot in his field of vision in his right eye.[29]

The third injury, the least severe, was not a beaning, but a batted foul ball. The injury occurred during the first game of the division series in 1999 between the Yankees and the Texas Rangers. Zimmer, the bench coach, was sitting in the Yankees dugout when Chuck Knoblauch hit a foul ball that nailed Zim in the side of the head. He reports he was only half-looking at the field and half-looking at the batter at the time.[30]

This time Zimmer was not knocked unconscious, but he was bleeding profusely. This was mainly due to the injury to his ear, which does bleed easily. After bandaging the injury, he remained in the game. The next day, as something of a joke, someone presented Zimmer with an old army helmet, and he did wear it in the Yankees dugout.

DICKIE THON

A more serious beaning was the one that felled Dickie Thon, a 25-year-old shortstop for the Houston Astros. In 1983 he had his best year in the majors, hitting .286 with 20 home runs, 177 hits, 79 RBI, 81 runs scored, and 34 stolen bases. The sky appeared to be the limit for this young player. In 1983 he had even represented Houston in the All-Star Game. Big things were predicted for his career.

Only five games into the 1984 season, all that changed. On April 8, Thon's bright future went south. In the first inning of the game between the New York Mets and Astros at the Astrodome in Houston, Mike Torrez, the Mets' pitcher, struck Thon out on a low and away fastball. When Thon came up again in the third inning, he crowded the plate, looking for another outside pitch. With the count two balls and one strike, Torrez let go a fastball that ran high and tight. Torrez thought the pitch sailed on him a bit. Thon quickly ducked, but he ducked right into the beanball. The ball glanced off Thon's earflap, hitting him just above the left eye. Thon dropped to the ground and lay semi-conscious while being carried off the field on a stretcher. Astros team physician Dr. William Bryan called for an ambulance.[31]

Thon was rushed to Houston's Methodist Hospital, where X-rays revealed a fracture of the orbital rim, the bones just above the left eye. The injury necessitated surgery, and Thon underwent successful surgery on April 11 to repair what was classified as a tripod fracture near his left eye.[32]

The fracture was not Thon's most significant injury. Unfortunately, he had suffered damage to the retina of his left eye. Soon after the injury, the vision in the left eye was noted to be 20/150. By June 1, Thon's left eye vision had improved to 20/50. But this was not a correctible deficit. Wearing glasses was not going to make Thon's vision any better, as he had damage to the retina. Only over time would his vision ever get better, and this was not a certainty. By March of 1985, Thon's vision had improved somewhat to 20/40. By the end of the 1986 season, Thon's vision in the left eye was 20/30. This is good enough to drive a car, but a very significant deficit when one talks about hitting a 90 mile an hour fastball or about catching a hard-hit ball off the bat to the shortstop.[33]

Sometimes it is not clear if a beaning leads to a significant change in a player's career. A noticeable shift in statistics or in playing time after an injury is a good indication. This has been noted with both Don Zimmer and Joe Medwick. Objective changes, such as an altered visual acuity or complaints of visual blurring, persistent headaches, and dizziness, present after the injury, and not present prior to the injury, are also good indications of a possible career-changing injury, especially when combined with decreased performance in the field and at bat.

A significant statistical difference in Thon's batting before and after his injury is noted. Thon had his best year at age 25. At that age he should have had similar or better years to follow. He did not. He had only one similar year, in 1989 while playing with the Phillies. That year he had 60 RBI, a .271 average, and 15 home runs. Other than 1989, he never had more than nine home runs or 48 RBI. In the year prior to his injury (1983) he hit .286. He never hit better than .271 after that.

Thon played no more games that whole 1984 season. While struggling in 1985 with continued visual problems, he played only 84 games. He did manage 106 games in 1986, though only as a platoon player.

In Astros spring training in 1987, he walked out of camp after going hitless in eight at-bats and making three errors in the field. He left due to continued visual problems. He rejoined the Astros on May 8 after a short minor league stint. But after only 66 at-bats, he again left the team on July 3, missing the rest of the season.[34]

Thon signed with San Diego in 1988, citing improved vision as a reason for optimism. He was able to play in a part-time role in 1988. He went on to have three better years —1989–1991— as the full-time shortstop for the Philadelphia Phillies, averaging 509 at-bats those three years. He even had 15 home runs and 60 RBI in 1989, but those are not the stats of an All-Star. He hit .271 in 1989 but his average fell off to .255 and .252 in 1990 and 1991 respectively. He resumed his part-time role for Texas in 1992 and Milwaukee in 1993.

Finally, in 1994 after signing with the Oakland A's, he called it quits at age 35, noting recurring visual problems as the main reason. He said he could see to hit, but defensively the visual problems were causing significant impairment. Apparently after his beaning, Thon continued to have severe headaches intermittently.[35]

RAY CHAPMAN

The most severe beaning, and the only one to result in the death of a major league player in a game, happened to Raymond Chapman on August 16, 1920, on a pitch thrown by Carl Mays. *The Pitch That Killed: The Story of Carl Mays, Ray Chapman, and the Pennant Race of 1920,* by Mike Sowell, documents Chapman's death.[36]

Ray Chapman, a shortstop, began his major league career with the Cleveland Indians in 1912. In 1918 he led the American League in runs scored and walks. He was a good fielding shortstop who led the league in putouts three times and assists once. He batted better than .300 three times and led the Indians in stolen bases three times. When he died, he was having one of his best seasons, batting .303 with 97 runs scored, and the Cleveland Indians were in the middle of the American League pennant race (which they won).

Carl Mays of the New York Yankees threw the pitch that killed Chapman. Mays threw with an unusual submarine style, and had a very successful 15-year career doing so, winning 207 games against only 126 losses (26–11 record in 1920). It was often difficult for batters to pick up the ball on his pitches (especially right-handers), as he often appeared to throw the ball almost off the top of his shoes. He can't be accused of being excessively wild, walking only 734 batters in 3,021 innings. He did hit 89 batters, not an excessive number considering the number of innings he pitched. However, 49 of those 89 were prior to 1920, during the first five years of Mays' career. He was accused of deliberately throwing at batters' heads.[37] Ty Cobb accused him of this.[38] Mays never admitted to throwing at batters deliberately.

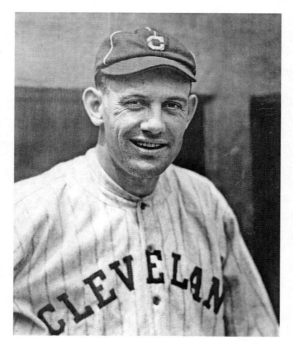

Raymond Johnson "Ray" Chapman of the Cleveland Indians in a road uniform, c. 1917/18 (National Baseball Hall of Fame Library, Cooperstown, New York).

Mays had also been accused of doctoring the ball to give it extra movement, though by 1920 the rules on doctoring the baseball had changed. Prior to 1920 baseballs were left in the game despite whatever appearance they had during the game. In the winter before 1920, many ways of altering the ball were banned. When the ball was dirty or appeared altered in any way, the umpire was to remove it from the game. Mays actually accused the home plate umpire, Tommy Connolly, of not properly removing the ball that hit Chapman. He stated the ball had a rough spot which caused the ball to sail on him.[39] Connolly, Mays stated, should have removed the ball from the game prior to his infamous pitch to Chapman.[40]

The Yankees were playing Cleveland in an afternoon game

at the Polo Grounds in New York (Yankee Stadium became home to the Yankees in 1923). It was overcast and gray, and a light rain had fallen during the first four innings.[41] The beaning happened in the fifth inning.

Chapman had bunted the first two times up, the first and third innings, both to advance runners. He was well known for sacrifice bunts and bunting for hits to take advantage of his great speed. Chapman led off the inning. Mays thought Chapman squared slightly to bunt, so at the last minute made a decision to throw the ball high and tight to make bunting difficult.[42] Chapman, a right-handed batter who often leaned a little over the plate, was hit on the left temple. The prevailing opinion is that Chapman didn't see the ball clearly if at all, as he did not appear to make any effort to get out of the way. After the impact, the ball came directly back to Mays, who threw to first base, thinking the ball had hit Chapman's bat.[43] But the ball had bounced off Chapman's skull.

Chapman did not lose consciousness initially. In fact, though a little dazed, he walked on his own as far as second base on the way to the center field clubhouse. He stumbled then and had to be carried by two teammates, his arms over their shoulders. He was talking some before he was taken by ambulance to St. Lawrence Hospital in New York City, but shortly thereafter became unconscious. At 9:30 P.M., x-rays revealed a depressed fracture to the left temple extending three and one-half inches to the base of Chapman's skull.[44]

When Chapman's condition deteriorated with a falling pulse rate, surgery was initiated at 12:29 am. Some of the depressed bone was removed as well as blood clots during the 75-minute procedure. Initially Chapman improved with rising pulse and improved breathing. But he then took a quick turn for the worse and died at 4:40 A.M. on Tuesday August 17.[45] (Note: Artificial respirators were not available in 1920. Iron lungs — the first form of artificial respiration and mainly used for polio victims — were not even present until 1927. If a patient's breathing slowed sufficiently in 1920, he/she died.)

The death was unfortunate. Chapman might not have died had he been wearing a batting helmet. Yet despite this, no reliable form of head protection was initiated until the 1940s and none was mandatory until 1956. There was some discussion briefly in 1921 of using leather helmets like the ones football players wore, but the idea never caught on.

OTHER BEANINGS

There have been numerous other significant beanings: Paul Blair in 1970, Terry Steinbach in 1991, Robbie Thompson in 1996, J.T. Snow in 1998, and Joe Girardi in 2000.[46]

Dan Schlossberg, in *Baseball Gold*, mentions two others: Jim Ray Hart in 1963 and Kirby Puckett in 1995.[47]

Rick Swaine also mentions Giants rookie Jim Ray Hart. In his first day in the majors, Hart was hit in the shoulder blade by Bob Gibson, and missed the rest of the season after a beaning in August by Curt Simmons.[48] Welcome to the big leagues.

Batting Helmets

Batting Helmets: Peter Morris, in *A Game of Inches: The Game on the Field*, cites some obscure cases of head protection used. For instance, the inventor of shin protectors, Roger Bresnahan, used some form of "Head Protector" after a beaning as early as 1907 (Morris's book is a good reference on the absolute earliest forms of head protection). Negro Leagues star Willie Wells was reported to have used a modified construction worker's hat in 1937.[49]

These were isolated cases of batting helmet or head protector use. Use by a group of players (team), as opposed to an individual, started in 1941. Their use was initiated by Brooklyn Dodgers General Manager Larry MacPhail. The stimulus: in 1940 there were severe beanings of Dodgers Joe Medwick and Pee Wee Reese. These helmets were not actually helmets as we would think of today, but just plastic inserts that zippered in under the regular baseball cap, similar to what horse jockeys were wearing at the time. The inserts were designed by Johns Hopkins surgeons Dr. George E. Bennett and Dr. Walter Dandy.

They probably helped. In 1941 Pete Reiser of the Dodgers had a significant beaning, but it is thought that the "plastic insert" he was using helped avert more severe damage.[50]

Other players began to use the plastic inserts in the early 1950s. After Don Zimmer's severe beaning in 1953 (no insert used), the Dodgers were the first to require *all* their players at *all* levels of their organization, minor and major leagues, to use the plastic inserts, by order of General Manager Buzzie Bavasi.[51]

The Pittsburgh Pirates in 1952 and 1953 were the first team to use the hard plastic helmets similar to the ones used today. It should not be surprising that the General Manager of the Pirates at the time was Branch Rickey, the owner of the American Baseball Cap, Inc., the company that first designed the hard plastic helmets. The company was under the direction of Charlie Muse, a later executive for the same Pirates.[52]

At first the Pirates used the hard helmets *at all times* while batting, on the bases, and even in the field. Soon thereafter the Pirates quit using the helmets except when batting and running the bases.[53]

The hard-shelled plastic helmets were more widely used after some severe beanings, such as the 1954 beaning of the Braves' Joe Adcock by the Dodgers'

Clem Labine. Adcock was wearing the new plastic helmet. He was knocked unconscious for 15 minutes by the smack on the helmet. It was quickly recognized that he would have been much more severely injured had he not been wearing the new plastic helmet.[54]

Adcock was beaned on August 1, 1954. The day before — July 31 — Adcock hit four home runs against the same Dodgers.[55] Do you think Labine beaned Adcock on purpose?

RON SANTO

Ron Santo was one of the first to use an earflap on his hard plastic helmet. He had a severe beaning on June 26, 1966, on a pitch thrown by the Mets' Jack Fisher. The pitch fractured Santo's left cheekbone, which had to be surgically wired together during Santo's three-day hospitalization.[56]

After returning from the DL on July 4, Santo started using the earflap on his batting helmet to protect his face from re-injury.[57] The earflap did not catch on right away, and it was not until 1983 that earflaps were made mandatory on all batting helmets.[58] The earflap is required on the side of the helmet that faces the pitcher. Switch-hitters often wear helmets with two earflaps; either that or they have to keep two helmets on hand, one for batting on each side of the plate.

Ron Santo's trip to the DL ended a steak of 390 consecutive games played and occurred during an extended hitting streak. Santo had hit in 26 straight games when he was beaned on June 26. On July 4 he hit in both ends of a doubleheader to set a career high, hitting in 28 straight games, a Cubs record that stood until Jerome Walton hit in 30 straight in 1989.[59]

Active players in 1971 and 1983 were not required to follow the regulations put into effect if they chose not to. All new players entering the majors were required to follow the mandatory rules. Only a very few active players in 1971 and 1983 chose to follow their previous habits in not using a plastic helmet (1971) or a plastic helmet with an ear flap (1983).

As noted by Rudy Marzano in *The Brooklyn Dodgers of the 1940s*, some lives may have been saved by hard plastic batting helmets. He notes a particularly severe beaning of Mike Piazza by Roger Clemens on July 8, 2000, as an example.[60]

There have been many more head injuries in baseball, and not just beanings. Helmets are used by runners on the basepaths. Rudy Marzano notes one situation in the 1950s where a pitcher running from first to second standing up was hit square in the head, in the middle of the "P" on his helmet, splitting his helmet. It should be of no surprise the pitcher running the bases was playing for Branch Rickey's team, the Pittsburgh Pirates, the first team using the hard plastic helmets.[61]

On the defensive side of the game, only a catcher wears a helmet as part of his protective gear. Very rarely does any other position player on the field wear a protective helmet (John Olerud did because of previous brain aneurysm surgery).[62] On the field, major league batboys and batgirls are required to use helmets. In 2008 there was a ruling that coaches on the field were required to wear batting helmets.[63]

A rash of beanings in 2009 speeded up the possible major league adoption of a new helmet by Rawlings Company called the S100. The S100 is thicker and vented. It features a composite insert and an expanded liner made of polypropylene. The material is similar to some industrial and bicycle helmets.

Scott Rolen ended up on the DL with a concussion after being hit in the head on August 2 by Colorado's Jason Marquis.[64] Then David Wright went on the DL after being beaned by a 94 mile an hour heater from San Francisco's Matt Cain.[65] Earlier in the year, Padres infielder Edgar Gonzalez was hit in the head by a ball thrown by Colorado's Jason Hammel.[66]

There has been some criticism of the new helmet, as one would expect with any new baseball innovation. Cubs pitcher Ryan Dempster is quoted as saying that wearing the helmet made him feel like he was having "my own bobblehead day."[67]

The new Rawlings S100 helmet was required at the minor league level in 2010. In late 2009 six of the helmets were sent to each major league team for trial use.[68] A modified version became required for all major league batters in 2013. Smaller and lighter, the new helmet, the S100 Pro Comp, has a carbon fiber composite shell and is said to protect a batter from a 100 mph pitch.[69]

Runners Hit by Throw

GROVER CLEVELAND ALEXANDER

Not all throwing impact injuries occur to the batter. Sometimes runners on the bases are hit by baseballs, especially if they are unfortunate enough to get in the path of the thrown ball. In *Who is the Greatest Pitcher?*, Jeff Kisseloff discusses just such a case.[70] The injury almost ended a career before it started. Future Hall of Fame pitcher Grover Cleveland Alexander was hit in the head during a minor league game in 1909, while running from first to second base. The throw from the shortstop hit him square in the head. He collapsed on the spot. The injury was so severe that he was bleeding and choking on the blood pouring down his throat. Another player on the field may have saved his life from the choking. He survived the initial part of the injury, but remained unconscious for a week. After waking up, he suffered from double vision for several months. Rick Swaine, in *Beating the Breaks: Major League Ballplayers Who*

Overcame Disabilities, contends that this same impact injury is what initiated Alexander's subsequent long-standing epilepsy, a disorder greatly misunderstood in the early twentieth century, and a malady Alexander may have tried to mask with excessive drinking.[71]

Who would take a chance on such a severely injured player? Well, the Philadelphia Phillies were the only team to take that risk on Alexander. It paid off, as during Alexander's 19-year career (1911–1930) he won 373 games with only 208 losses. His 28 wins in his rookie season of 1911 still stands as a record. Alexander averaged 27 wins a year in his first seven years, winning 30-plus games each season from 1915 to 1917.

Despite his injury, Grover Cleveland Alexander was known for his great control. He recovered from his 1909 problem with double vision and averaged only 1.6 walks per game in his career. It was a good thing that the Phillies took a chance on this injured pitcher. And it cost only $500 to sign him.

Chapter 16

Impact Injuries
Caused by Batted Ball

Impact by Batted Ball — Pitchers

Injuries can also be severe from a batted ball, and certainly the pitcher, as the closest fielder, other than the catcher, is very prone to impact injuries from a batted ball. These can be especially severe if the pitcher is hit in the face, and can put him on the disabled list for some time or even end his career.

BOB GIBSON

A famous impact injury was suffered in 1967 by Bob Gibson, the Hall of Fame pitcher for the St. Louis Cardinals. The injury is described well in Gibson's autobiography, *Stranger to the Game*.[1] The injury occurred on July 15 on Gibson's first start after the All-Star Game. Roberto Clemente hit a line drive off Gibson's right shin, breaking Gibson's fibula bone just above his ankle. Gibson subsequently missed two full months of the season, not pitching again in the majors until September 7. Because of the injury and trip to the DL, Gibson was only able to win 13 games during the regular season in 1967. More important, Gibson recovered well enough to pitch in the 1967 World Series and led the Cardinals to the championship with three complete-game victories in this seven-game series against the Boston Red Sox. For his effort, he was named the 1967 World Series MVP.

By 1968 Gibson was fully recovered and pitched as if he had never been injured by setting a record for the lowest ERA (1.12) in modern baseball history. In the process he won 22 games, with 28 complete games and 13 shutouts. Thereafter, Gibson suffered no further more problems from this right ankle (fibula) injury.

Knee problems were actually Gibson's biggest problem in the later part of his career, ultimately leading to his retirement in 1975 after 17 years in the major leagues. His knee problems started with an injury in August 1973 where Gibson twisted his right knee, causing cartilage damage, as he attempted to dive back to first base to avoid being doubled up after a line drive by Ted Sizemore to a New York Mets third baseman.

DIZZY DEAN

Dizzy Dean was not as lucky with his impact injury as Gibson was — at least on the surface it would appear that way. Dean had three 20-win seasons

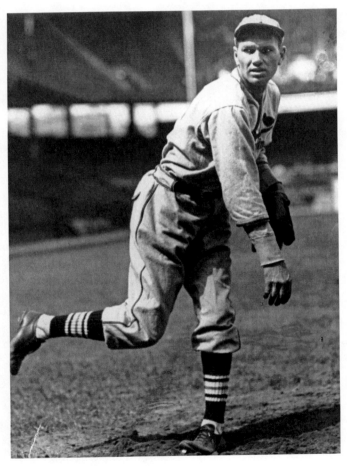

Dizzy Dean of the St. Louis Cardinals on unknown date (National Baseball Hall of Fame Library, Cooperstown, New York).

and one 30-win season from 1933 to 1936. His 1934 season was stellar with 30 wins and only 7 losses, the last National Leaguer to win 30 games in a season. But while pitching in the third inning of the 1937 All-Star Game, Dean suffered a broken toe from a line drive up the middle off the bat of Earl Averill. After the 1937 All-Star Game, Dean won only one more game before his season was over. He was never the same after his injury. The legend is that the broken toe altered his pitching motion and led to shoulder problems.

Branch Rickey, the brilliant GM of the Cardinals in 1937, apparently sensing Dean was through after the 1937 season, traded him to the Cubs. He pitched for the Cubs from 1938 to 1941, and even pitched once for the St. Louis Browns in 1947, but he never pitched more than 100 innings in a major league season after 1937 and never won more than seven games in one season.

Whether a longer period of time off after the toe injury would have helped (to let it heal better) is not known. Whether modern medicine would have helped the shoulder problems he developed is pure speculation. It is held to this day by most sources that the fractured toe from this baseball impact injury ended what could have been an even greater career for Dizzy Dean.[2]

Vince Staten, in *Ol' Diz*, presents a different spin on Dean's arm problems. He notes that Dean started off 1937 5–0, but thereafter went only 7–7 after that great start leading up to the All-Star Game. This would appear to indicate that possibly he was having some problems before the infamous All-Star Game injury. Staten in particular notes an Associated Press article published just before the All-Star Game. In it, Dean is quoted as saying his decreased performance leading up to the All-Star Game was due to his right arm. "It was just not quite right," he said, "but I'm going to pitch in the All-Star game anyway."[3]

Staten's suggestion is that Dean, who had pitched 1,531 innings in the five years leading up to the 1937 All-Star Game (tops in the majors), was already beginning to have arm troubles from his heavy workload. Maybe the toe injury was just the straw that broke the camel's back, so to speak. Yes, it changed his delivery, but it mainly aggravated arm problems that were already there.

Either way you look at it, the impact injury marked a change in fortunes for Dean. After the injury he was never the same, whether the injury was a significant factor in the development of his arm problems or not.

WALTER JOHNSON

Another not-so-lucky pitcher was Walter "The Big Train" Johnson. Walter Johnson's career ended in 1927 with 417 wins, 279 losses and an ERA of 2.17. He was one of the first five players inducted into the Baseball Hall of Fame. Johnson was injured during spring training in 1927, when he was forty years old. Hard to believe, but Johnson might have pitched more years if not for a fractured leg sustained on a line drive hit while he was pitching. He tried to come back after that injury, but without much success. One source mentioned he may have even tried to pitch with a leg brace for a period of time.[4] It didn't work. This impact injury from a batted ball basically ended Walter Johnson's career.

HERB SCORE

Herb Score was born on June 7, 1933. In high school he was a phenom, often striking out 17 or 18 batters in a seven-inning game. He was also very wild. The left-hander possessed a blazing fastball and a great slider. He was so good, he signed with the Indians for an almost unheard-of amount of $60,000.

He went through the Cleveland minor league system very rapidly, arriving in the big leagues in 1955. In his first year with the Cleveland Indians, he finished with a 16–10 record and 245 strikeouts in 227 innings. This rookie strikeout record eventually was broken in 1984 by Dwight Gooden. Score's stats were so good he was named the 1955 American League Rookie of the Year.

In 1956 he did even better. He finished with 20 wins and 9 losses, an ERA of 2.53, and 263 strikeouts in 249 innings.

In 1957 he appeared to be cruising along with 39 strikeouts in 33 innings when an event occurred that changed his life. On May 7, he was pitching against the New York Yankees. Gil McDougald was at the plate. He apparently anticipated that Score might throw him a low fastball. He hit it very hard up the middle, hitting Herb Score in the face and the right eye. Score was not knocked unconscious, but he experienced considerable bleeding and immediate marked swelling around the right eye. He was injured severely enough that he had to be carried off the field on a stretcher.

With the swelling around Score's eye, there was considerable concern that his vision might be permanently impaired. But as the 1957 season progressed, his vision returned to normal.

After Score's impact injury, he missed the rest of the 1957 season. He returned to play in 1958. There were periods when he appeared close to returning to his previous greatness, but he was never really the same. Score only won two games in limited pitching in 1958, and for the remainder of his career he won only 17 more games against 26 losses before pitching his last game for the Chicago White Sox in 1962 at the age of 29.

Why did Score's career end the way it did? The common opinion is that Score, fearful of being hit in the face, again altered his delivery, which made him a less effective pitcher. The altered delivery also resulted in an elbow injury that curtailed any further greatness he might have achieved.

This common opinion is perpetuated by many, including veteran Cleveland broadcaster Jimmy Dudley (1948 to 1967). Terry Pluto, in *The Curse of*

Rocky Colavito, interviewed Jimmy Dudley, who states, "I still insist Herb never got over the blow to his eye, and compensated for it and ended up with some bad habits."[5]

Terry Pluto also interviewed Herb Score. He gives a different spin on the story, saying, "The reason my motion changed was because of my elbow (in the spring of 1958), and I compensated for it and ended up with some bad habits."[6]

The elbow injury Score speaks of occurred in April of 1958. On a cold, windy night, while pitching against Washington, he began to experience forearm discomfort early in the game. The soreness in the left elbow became very severe by the seventh inning and Score had to be removed from the game.[7] With continued pain, he ended up on the disabled list for 30 days. When he returned later in 1958, he again experienced soreness in his arm, especially when he threw his fastball.

In 1959 Score felt better, but according to observers his normal motion had been altered. He was noted to be "stiff arming it" and dragging his foot.[8] As a result Score was now throwing a flat fastball with very little movement to it, and he now had less control of his curveball.

It could be speculated from the history that Score might have suffered a torn ulnar collateral ligament in his pitching elbow and maybe even had a torn flexor muscle. But there were no MRIs in 1958 to make a diagnosis of a torn UCL, and certainly no treatment in 1958 even if Score did have a torn ulnar ligament or flexor muscle.

In Terry Pluto's book, Score said the elbow injury was a more significant factor in his altered pitching motion and poor performance after 1957.[9] The more common belief is that Score was fearful of getting hit in the face again by a batted ball. Did this fear lead to bad habits and then to elbow problems, or was it the elbow problem that came first? We may never know the answer.

There have been other less publicized but more recent impact injuries to a pitcher's face. Dick Pole and Bryce Florie injuries are classic examples.

DICK POLE

The story of Dick Pole's impact injury is told best in the book, *'75: The Red Sox Team That Saved Baseball*.[10]

Pole was signed by the Red Sox as a free agent in 1969. He made it to the major league with the Red Sox in August of 1973 after several good years in the minor leagues. He appeared in 12 games with seven starts in 1973 and 15 games in 1974, spending part of the 1974 season in the minor leagues at Pawtucket, the Red Sox's Triple-A affiliate.

He was with the Red Sox from the beginning of the season in 1975 and started six games in June of 1975, the last on June 30. It was during Pole's last start in June that he suffered a significant impact injury to his face. The game was at Fenway Park against the Orioles, and Pole was pitching one of his best games of the season. He had thrown eight shutout innings leading up to the ninth inning.

In the ninth, Pole struck out the first batter. Jim Northrup, Brooks Robinson, and Ken Singleton followed with singles to load the bases. Up stepped Tony Muser. He lined the ball right up the middle. The ball smashed into Pole's right cheekbone just below the eye. The ball was hit so hard that after hitting Pole, it bounced over the third baseman Rico Petrocelli's head and into the outfield for a double, with two runs scoring. Pole had to be removed from the game.

Pole was taken to Hannemann Hospital. X-rays revealed a fractured right cheekbone, but more significantly, Pole had an injury to his eye. Surgery to correct the cheekbone fracture was a given. Pole's impaired eyesight was another whole issue. An article in *The Sporting News* by Peter Gammons noted Pole's vision before the injury wasn't very good, adding to the concern about possible future visual difficulties.[11]

Pole missed two full months before returning on September 1, just in time to make four more starts. He even pitched once in relief during the 1975 World Series, won by the Cincinnati Reds in seven games.

At this point history is not clear. Numerous internet articles mention that Pole developed significant problems with the vision in his right eye.[12] *'75: The Red Sox Team That Saved Baseball* says the injury changed Pole's life forever, but gives no information to substantiate this claim.[13]

In 1976 Pole pitched well for the Red Sox. At age 25 he appeared in 31 games, including 15 starts, with a 6–5 record and an ERA of 4.33. He went in the expansion draft to the Seattle Mariners, the seventh player drafted overall, which suggests that the Mariners were not very concerned about his vision. That Pole had two rather mediocre seasons for the Mariners, before being released by their organization in 1979, is not attributed to visual problems in any source researched.

One might expect a visual problem to impair a player's fielding (as it did with Tony Conigliaro), but Pole in his six-year career made only four errors, one each in 1974, 1975, 1976 and 1977: two errors probably before his injury and two after his injury.

We also can't judge the eye injury affecting Pole's batting. With the DH rule, Pole had only one recorded major league at-bat, and that was in 1976. Pole grounded out to Oakland A's pitcher Stan Bahnsen. Not enough data is here to make a conclusion.

After being released by the Mariners in 1979, Pole went on to play a year in the Pittsburgh minor league system, one year in the Tigers' minor league system, and finally part of 1981 and the 1982 in the Mexican League before calling it quits as a player.

Despite whatever visual problems he has had, he was hired as a pitching coach by the Cubs from 1988 to 1993. He went on to serve as a pitching coach for the Giants, Red Sox, Angels, Indians, and most recently the Cincinnati Reds.

An attempt was made to contact Dick Pole in 2008 via mail. An attempt was made to try to clear up the issue concerning his visual problems. Did his visual difficulties have anything to do with his declining success for the Mariners in 1977 and 1978, and his subsequent release by the Mariners in 1979? This attempt was unsuccessful.

Even though the nature of Pole's injury was severe, one cannot say emphatically that his visual problems caused him significant difficulty in pitching at the major league level after his impact injury on June 30, 1975.

BRYCE FLORIE

Bryce Florie's major league career before his impact injury was unremarkable, but the injury he sustained was very noteworthy: he was hit by a line drive off a bat.

Florie was drafted in the fifth round of the 1988 draft by the San Diego Padres. He made his major league debut in July of 1994, six years later.

He pitched mostly in relief, though he did start eight games in 1997 and 16 in 1998. He was traded several times, twice at the trading deadline. He played for the San Diego Padres 1994–1996, Milwaukee Brewers 1996–1997, Detroit Tigers 1998–1999, and Boston Red Sox from 1999–2001. His career ERA was 4.47 and he only won 20 games, losing 24, in his eight-year major league career.

On September 8, 2000, while pitching for the Boston Red Sox, he suffered his severe impact injury in the ninth inning. Ryan Thompson hit a line drive that smashed into the right eye socket of Florie. The ball caromed off Florie to third baseman Lou Merloni, who threw out Thompson for the final out of the inning.[14]

Florie immediately fell to the ground, blood gushing from his nose and around his eye. He never lost consciousness. He was transported by ambulance to the Massachusetts Eye and Ear Infirmary.

He was diagnosed with fractures around his right socket as well as his nose. He had surgery on September 9 to relieve some of the swelling around the eye.[15]

Once the swelling went down, Florie had surgery again on September 18. Several small plates were used to fuse the fractured bone fragments around his right eye. For correct function of the eye, the position of the fragments around the eye had to be very close to perfect. At the same time as Florie's eye socket surgery, his nasal fracture was put back into place (reduced).[16]

Visual impairment was noted very early and thought to be due to retinal damage, blood behind the retina. In early September Florie's vision in the right eye was 20/200, and by October it was noted to be 20/125.[17]

Florie came back in 2001, still having visual impairment. As late as February of 2002, his vision in his right eye was only 20/50, not correctable with eye glasses. His vision in his left eye, corrected by a contact lens, was 20/20.[18]

Florie pitched in the minors in early 2001, but finally returned to the major leagues on June 28, almost nine months after his eye injury. He entered with two outs in the second inning of a game against the Devil Rays, when Boston starter Frank Castillo left with a muscle strain in his right side. The crowd's response to Florie's appearance was very positive as they realized his comeback had taken considerable effort in overcoming a possible career-ending injury. He ended up pitching two and one-third innings, giving up one run.[19]

Florie's comeback was short-lived. At age 31 he pitched only six more games in the major leagues, giving up 11 runs in eight and two-thirds innings before Boston released him. He never again pitched in the majors.[20]

After his release, he pitched a few Triple-A games for the Tigers' Toledo team before the Tigers released him in October. During the off-season he had arthroscopic surgery on his pitching elbow to remove some bone chips. In 2002, after being a non-roster invitee to spring training for the Oakland A's, he pitched for Sacramento, their Triple-A affiliate.[21]

Florie was out of baseball completely in 2003. He attempted a comeback in 2004 with the Florida Marlins but was cut during spring training.[22]

OTHERS

There have been several recent near misses, such as Mike Mussina (May 14, 1998 — laceration above left eye and nasal fracture off line drive by Sandy Alomar Jr.), Chris Carpenter (September 16, 2000 — laceration inside mouth requiring 18 stitches off line drive by Jose Valentin), and Matt Clement (July 26, 2005 — mild concussion from impact behind right ear off bat of Tampa Bay Rays batter Carl Crawford).[23]

In 2008 there was an impact injury to San Diego pitcher Chris Young. He was hit by a line drive up the middle off the bat of Cardinal Albert Pujols on May 21, 2008. Young sustained a lacerated, fractured nose, facial fractures, and a small crack in his skull in addition to a concussion, though he never lost consciousness. Only the nasal fracture required surgery, an operation on June 30 that also corrected a deviated nasal septum. He was out of the lineup from May 22 to July 29 on a San Diego team that desperately needed his presence.[24]

In 2009 Hiroki Kuroda of the Dodgers was hit in the head by a line drive on August 15 off the bat of Arizona Diamondbacks rookie Rusty Ryan at Chase Field in Phoenix. Kuroda didn't suffer any broken bones, but wound up on the disabled list with post-concussion syndrome.[25]

In 2010 St. Louis pitcher Blake Hawksworth sustained a significant impact injury to his face. On September 25 he was struck by a line drive in the fifth inning of a game between the Cardinals and Cubs at Wrigley Field. The injury required 30 stitches to his mouth and upper lip and he needed some dental surgery. He missed the rest of the season.[26]

It seems almost every year there is an injury to a pitcher from a batted ball. Some are near misses, some are not. Twenty-four-year-old Rockies pitcher Juan Nicasio's injury was not a near miss; he was hit square in the right temple by a line drive off the bat of the Washington Nationals' Ian Desmond on August 5, 2011, at Coors Field.

Nicasio immediately fell to the ground. The ball bounced over the first base line into foul territory. Nicasio did not lose consciousness. When he complained of neck pain, a stabilizing board was put on his neck and he was carted off the field and subsequently taken to Denver Health Medical Center, where tests were done. MRI and CT scans revealed a fractured C-1 vertebra and some internal bleeding. Surgery was deemed necessary, and neurosurgeon Dr. Peter Witt inserted two screws into the C-1 fractured vertebra and placed a small metal plate to stabilize the broken bone.[27]

It is unknown if the impact of the ball or the fall after the injury caused the fractured vertebra. A fractured C-1 vertebra is very unusual in baseball. This fracture is more typical of a car accident or with someone diving into a pool where the water is too shallow.[28]

Apparently Nicasio had a neck brace for at least six weeks prior to rehabilitation. There was optimism expressed for his return to the majors in the spring of 2012.[29] Nicasio did end up returning in 2012 but made only 11 starts (58 innings) before injuring his knee, which led to season-ending surgery. In 2013 he was at spring training and appeared to be fully healthy again for the first time since the neck injury.

In 2012 two pitchers sustained impact injuries from batted balls: Brandon McCarthy and Doug Fister. Fister's impact injury during the World Series did not result in any significant damage. Oakland pitcher McCarthy, though, suffered a concussion and skull fracture on September 5 and had to have surgery the same day to evacuate an epidural hemorrhage and stabilize the fracture. He missed the rest of the season and playoffs.

These injuries subseqently stimulated discussion of how to protect the pitcher against further such events. Bulky batting helmets have not been considered practical, but inserts that would fit inside the pitcher's cap, using "military grade composite" material "fortified with Kevlar,"[30] have been considered, as have other ideas.

The pitcher who is just 60 feet 6 inches away before propelling himself forward to deliver the ball to the plate just doesn't have time to get out of the way. Pitchers whose follow-throughs are less balanced are at even greater risk.

Impact by Batted Ball — Position Players

NICK JOHNSON

One of Nick Johnson's many injuries was a classic bad-hop injury, a fractured right cheekbone. It is a surprise that bad-hop ground balls don't cause more injuries. Often the ball hits the fielder in the chest, goes under him, or hops over him. If it does approach the face, most often the fielder pulls his head out of the way or puts his glove in front of his face.

Johnson, a 25-year-old first baseman for the Montreal Expos, was injured Friday, August 20, 2004, at Coors Field during a game between the Expos and the Rockies. In the third inning, Colorado's Royce Clayton hit a wicked shot towards first base. The ground ball took an odd bounce and hit Johnson between the right cheek and jaw.[31] Johnson went down face-first in the dirt in obvious pain, "kicking his feet up and down." He lay on the field for ten minutes before being carted off on a stretcher. He never lost consciousness. X-rays at the hospital revealed a fractured cheekbone. Research revealed no information that he ever required surgery. He initially was placed on the 15-day DL, but later was moved to the 60-day DL on September 15.[32]

He apparently suffered no long-term effects as the Nationals (the Montreal Expos moved to Washington in 2005) signed him to a $1.45 million contract on January 14, 2005. Apparently a back injury Johnson sustained in early 2004 created more concern for the Nationals than his cheekbone injury. But an exam of his back cleared him to be signed to a new contract.[33]

JUAN ENCARNACION

Juan Encarnacion suffered an impact injury caused by a foul ball that hit his left eye socket. He was simply in the wrong place at the wrong time.

Encarnacion had an 11-year major league career, good though not outstanding, breaking into the majors with the Detroit Tigers in 1997 at the age of 21. He had a lifetime average of .270 with career highs of 80 runs scored and 94 RBI. He averaged 14 home runs, hitting as many as 24 in 2002 while splitting his season between Cincinnati and Florida of the NL.

On August 31, 2007, he was hit by a foul ball in the left eye. An article by the Associated Press appearing at SI.com on September 1 describes the events well. Encarnacion was in the on-deck circle, waiting to pinch-hit in the sixth inning. Aaron Miles, batting right-handed, hit an outside pitch thrown by Cincinnati left-hander Jon Coutlangus into foul territory. The ball hit Encarnacion squarely in the left eye. He was not knocked unconscious, just dazed. He was taken to the hospital and stayed overnight for observation.[34]

Very soon after the injury, a retinal surgeon noted the injury was very serious with significant damage to the optic nerve and retina which could ultimately cause complete loss of vision.[35]

Encarnacion subsequently underwent surgery in Boston to repair the eye socket fractures sometime during September. By early October Encarnacion had regained some of his vision, but it was no better than 20/400 in his injured left eye. He is thought to have permanent retinal damage.[36]

Encarnacion did not play at all in 2008. That November he filed for free agency as his contract with the Cardinals had run out. A report said he "had not yet recovered enough vision in his left eye to be able to drive, let alone attempt to play baseball."[37] Encarnacion has not played in the major leagues since his injury in 2007.

LUIS SALAZAR

Spring training of 2010 brought about a severe impact injury to a member of the Atlanta Braves organization.

Luis Salazar, a minor league coach helping at the major league level during spring training, was hit on the left side of his face by a foul ball as he stood at the top step of the Braves dugout on March 9, 2010. The line drive came off the bat of the Braves' left-handed-hitting catcher, Brian McCann.

It was obvious the injury was severe. Salazar was knocked out immediately; he had tumbled several feet and landed face-first on the dugout floor. He was bleeding extensively from the left side of his face, his mouth, and his nose.[38] He initially wasn't breathing, though by the time he was airlifted by helicopter, he had resumed breathing. Salazar was unconscious at least 20 minutes.[39]

Salazar had surgery Wednesday night, March 9, on his facial fractures and again had surgery Thursday, March 10. The second surgery concentrated on treatment for his left eye, which was crushed by the impact injury.[40] At the time of the second surgery, there was fear Salazar might not regain vision in his left eye.

After a few days and evaluation by Orlando area eye specialists, it was apparent that not only was Salazar not going to regain vision, he was going to lose the eye. Surgery to remove the eye was done March 15 at Orlando Regional Medical Center. The surgeon in charge was not mentioned.[41]

Salazar returned to the Atlanta Braves' minor league camp on March 23 after spending a week at his home in Boca Raton, Fla. He reflected a good attitude about his recovery. He said, "Nothing is wrong with my brain; that is the greatest news that I have heard. I'm very fortunate to be alive. God gave me a second chance in this life, and I'm going to take advantage of it."[42]

At the time of this writing, Salazar was to resume his minor league managing duties, managing the high Class-A Lynchburg Hillcats for the Atlanta Braves organization.

MIKE COOLBAUGH

In the news in 2007 was an even more severe impact injury. Here, not a pitcher, but a first base coach, was fatally injured.

On July 22, 2007, Tulsa Drillers hitting coach Mike Coolbaugh died less than an hour after being hit below the left ear by a foul line drive off the bat of Tulsa designated hitter Tino Sanchez. The severe injury to Coolbaugh's head and neck occurred in the ninth inning of a game between the Arkansas Travelers and Tulsa Drillers in Little Rock, Arkansas. Coolbaugh was coaching first base. He probably wasn't paying any attention to the batter, but rather to the Tulsa runner at first base who had led off the inning with a single.

Immediately following the injury, all attempts at resuscitation by coaches and then by paramedics were unsuccessful. Coolbaugh never regained consciousness after being hit. The autopsy revealed a ruptured artery in Coolbaugh's neck just below the left ear. The artery was the left vertebral artery that travels against the left spinal column and supplies blood to the brain.[43]

Coolbaugh played in the minor leagues for almost 16 years with nine organizations. At the major league level he played only 39 games for the Milwaukee Brewers in 2001 and five games for the St. Louis Cardinals in 2002.[44]

After a long minor league career and a very brief major league career, Coolbaugh moved into coaching. He had just joined the Drillers as hitting coach on July 3, 2007. This event shows how severe impact injuries off a batted ball can be, especially if the injured person is hit in the neck or head.[45]

Ironically, a pitcher for the same minor league Tulsa Drillers suffered a severe head injury off a batted ball on April 23, 2007, at the same Dickey-Stephens Stadium in Little Rock, Arkansas. Jonathan Asahina was struck by a line drive near his left temple. He suffered a fractured skull and a ruptured eardrum. His injuries were so severe he was hospitalized for nearly a week, but he later rejoined the team.[46]

The Tulsa Drillers are the Double-A affiliate of the Colorado Rockies.

As a result of Coolbaugh's fatal injury a new rule was instituted in November of 2007. Beginning in spring training in 2008 it was mandatory for coaches on the field in the major leagues to wear batting helmets.[47]

Conclusion

Fortunately impact injuries by a batted ball are rare events. When one estimates with good wood on the ball, the ball can leave the bat at speeds approaching 100 mph (bat exit speed), the potential for serious injuries can be easily appreciated.[48] And, for a position player without any protective gear the pitcher is at greatest risk for more serious injury because of his close distance to home plate. This gives him a very short reaction time to get out of the way of a ball hit up the middle. At present it seems unlikely in the near future major league pitchers will be required to wear any type of protective gear, certainly not helmets like coaches and base runners are required to wear.

The catcher does wear protective gear, but is still at risk for injury from impact from fouled balls. He is especially at risk for foul balls off the mask causing concussions.

Chapter 17

Head Concussions

There are several possible results from a head concussion, singular or multiple in nature.

The first outcome is that following the concussion, however severe, the injured person completely recovers with no short-term or long-term side-effects ever noted.

A second situation is that symptoms persist for weeks, months, or years after the injury or injuries, though eventually with resolution of symptoms and any neurologic deficits.

The third situation is that the injured person suffers permanent deficits in neurologic functioning. These deficits may be apparent immediately or may not manifest until much later. For example, Mohammad Ali presented with permanent damage manifesting in Parkinson's Disease many years after his multiple head concussions from boxing.[1]

A fourth situation is death immediately or soon after the initial injury. "Second impact syndrome" needs to be included here: a second head injury following soon after an initial injury, with devastating results.[2]

The etiology of concussions in baseball is varied. The most common cause at *any level* of the sport, as noted by an article in *Sports Medicine* in 2005, is impact injuries caused by the baseball itself,[3] either a thrown ball or a batted ball.

Less commonly, players can run into each other either while pursuing a batted ball or while running the bases. The catcher is especially prone to this type of injury with collisions at home plate, a reason for catchers to wear protective gear. Lastly, players can run into walls on the sides of the field, fall into the stands or dugout, or simply land hard on the grass or other playing surface after diving for a ball (this is especially bad with artificial turf, and it is fortunate that few ballparks have artificial turf now).

The increased interest in sports-related concussions has led to intense discussions and even to national meetings on head concussions. One was held in March of 2007 by the Sports Concussion Institute in Marina Del Rey, California. There has been a considerable proliferation in scientific and lay articles written on head concussions.[4]

There is no exact definition of a head concussion, but one used by many sources is an "immediate and transient impairment in the neurologic function (e.g., alteration of consciousness, mental status changes, disturbance of vision, vertigo) due to mechanical acceleration and deceleration forces acting on the brain."[5]

An article in the journal *Brain Injury* in 2001 agrees with this definition, adding only that the symptoms are due to nerve cell injury and brain chemical changes.[6]

The First International Symposium on Concussion in Sports defined concussions in a similar manner. A concussion is defined, in part, as "a complex pathophysiologic process affecting the brain, induced by traumatic biomechanical forces."[7] This is a very technical but concise definition.

An article at www.medcoathletics.com/education/head_concussions/print _out.htm gives a good summary of methods to grade injuries and discusses recommendations for return to action. Even though most of their recommendations concern football players, the same would apply to baseball players.[8]

They recommend the Glasgow Coma Scale in doing an initial evaluation of the athlete (one of several methods to evaluate concussions). This involves a numerical scale based on three parameters: (1) eye opening, (2) motor responses, and (3) verbal responses. Motor responses include coordination (the ability to walk). Verbal responses would cover amnesia for events recent and remote, for example. Based on all three points of evaluation, a scale from 3 to 15 is derived, with 3 being the worst impairment and 15 indicating very little if any impairment.[9]

After this Glasgow Coma Scale, concussions are graded I to III, with III being the worst.

> Grade I or mild concussion is characterized by no retrograde amnesia and no to slight mental confusion with no loss of coordination or tinnitus. Grade II or moderate concussion is characterized by less than five minutes of loss of consciousness, retrograde amnesia (recent memory), noticeable loss of coordination, and moderate dizziness. Grade III or a severe concussion is characterized by greater than five minutes of loss of consciousness and possible anterograde amnesia. Also, severe mental confusion and profound loss of coordination is present.[10]

Anterograde amnesia, also called antegrade amnesia, is a form of memory loss in which events are not transferred from short-term memory to long-term memory. Sufferers have no memory for any new events when questioned only moments after the event.

Once the severity of the injury is assessed and the athlete's symptoms improve, there needs to be a decision concerning when he/she can return to play. Generally, in order to return to play, any symptoms or mental status deficits must completely resolve within 15 minutes after the injury.[11] This includes headaches, which unfortunately are often a discarded symptom when making these decisions. The athlete must be asymptomatic at rest and with exertion, because some symptoms will appear in a delayed manner.

In baseball it is impossible to hold up a game for 15 minutes to assess if the player can return. Once out of the game, he cannot be re-inserted back into the game. Thus, to be cautious, a baseball player with even a slight concussion should be taken out of the game.

In football or hockey, the player can be taken out of the game, have his condition assessed on the sidelines, and if a very mild concussion is apparent (certainly not worse than a grade I) with quick resolution of symptoms, he can return to action in the ongoing game. The only time a baseball player could play the same day of the head injury would be in the occasional doubleheader.

As in other sports, it is unfortunate that baseball players with mild concussions and mild symptoms sometimes do not report them. One reason: they don't want to be removed from the game as it reflects a lack of toughness or machismo. The failure to report MTBIs (mild traumatic brain injuries) can result in bad consequences in the long term. Education to make coaches and players aware of the possible consequences of not reporting even mild concussions is now being stressed to all major league teams and players. Part of that education is provided by organizations that specifically deal with concussions, such as the Sports Concussion Institute in Marina Del Rey, California. It was founded to treat, evaluate, and educate on issues especially related to sports concussions. In recent years the University of Pittsburgh Medical Center started a concussion program, also with education and research on head concussions. This medical center also came up with a computer software program called ImPACT. It helps team trainers better evaluate a player's brain function, recall, processing speed, and reaction time. More specifically, ImPACT is a neuropsychological testing program consisting of eight cognitive tasks and a 21-system inventory.[12] This is an alternative testing system to the Glasgow Coma scale. A number of MLB teams, including the St. Louis Cardinals, have started using the computer software. The NFL, NHL, and professional boxing began using the computer software before baseball.

A baseball player cannot be re-inserted into the lineup after being taken out. Can he play the next game? If symptoms or mental status deficits resolve in 15 minutes or less, he probably can play the next game. If symptoms last longer than 15 minutes, and the head injury is graded a Class II in severity, then the player should be removed from play for at least one week, and return to play only after the mental deficits and symptoms are gone for one week.

During this week he needs to have day-to-day assessment of symptoms and cognitive skills. Progressive symptoms or persistent symptoms and cognitive deficits require referral and possible diagnostic imaging studies (MRI).

Multiple injuries, MTBIs, require ongoing assessment of memory retention and mental processing and the careful assessment of persistent symptoms. Some teams have started doing baseline mental studies at the beginning of the season to assess this possibility (such as ImPACT). Deviations from the baseline studies indicate a problem.

It should be noted that once a player has sustained "a concussion in a season he is three times more likely to sustain a second concussion compared with uninjured players." In other words, it takes less head trauma to cause the same problem.

Susceptibility to another concussion after the first or second may be due to changes at the nerve cell level. The journal *Progressive Brain Research* in 2007 notes there are changes at the cellular level by MTBIs.[13] There are disturbances in ionic homeostasis, disturbances of acute metabolic function, and alterations in cerebral blood flow at the cellular level, resulting in increased extracellular calcium. This extra calcium makes the cells more susceptible to further damage. Disruption of nerve cells' function makes the neurons more susceptible to re-injury, and if re-injured the cell may take longer and longer to return to a normal state of functioning.[14] Further trauma can result in irreversible neuron cell changes leading to the death of nerve cells. It should be noted that you don't grow new nerve cells once the cells die. Other cells in the body regenerate (like stomach cells), but not neuron brain cells. Once a nerve cell is dead, it is not replaced by another nerve cell.[15]

To summarize: the acute changes to nerve cells' function are thought to be responsible for signs and symptoms of a concussion. Repeated concussions typically delay the eventual recovery of nerve cells' function and thus can result in persistent symptoms. Repeated concussions and severe concussions can result in long-term cognitive deficits (memory loss, etc.) most often due to nerve cell death.

Under impact injuries, concussions have already been discussed. One noteworthy case was Don Zimmer's injury. His first severe concussion in 1953 from a beaning resulted in the complication of migraine headaches that persisted for one year after the initial injury.[16]

It could be argued that the headaches, representing persistent symptoms, indicated he maybe should not have returned to play when he did. It can also be argued that persistent symptoms (headaches), by themselves, according to present literature, should not be the only determining factor in any decision made for a player to return to play. Baseline ImPACT testing would have been beneficial before and after his injury. This would more accurately assess any cognitive deficits. ImPACT testing would have more accurately determined whether Zimmer should have returned to play when he did. Despite continuing headaches, there was Zimmer in 1954, during spring training, playing baseball again. Fortunately for Zimmer, he had no additional concussions in 1954 while he was still having headaches. He did have another rather severe concussion in 1956, but by that time his symptoms from the 1953 injury (headaches) had resolved. Research revealed no information that would indicate Zimmer had any significant memory (cognitive) problems as a result of his beanings in 1953 and 1956.

Head concussions in baseball are common, though as stated earlier, many are not reported. The simple "ding" or "bell-ringer" often is overlooked. In an article by Marcia C. Smith on June 19, 2007, she notes a series of reported concussions in major league baseball just in May and June of 2007. Several players missed at least a day or more because of their injury. These are the reported concussions[17]:

1. June 16, 2007 — Angel Casey Kotchman, sliding into second base, hit in the back of the head
2. June 2, 2007 — Yankee Doug Mientkiewicz at first base, knocked in the head by the knee of runner Mike Lowell
3. June 1, 2007 — Ranger Mark Teixeira sliding into home plate when hit by throw from outfielder Ichiro Suzuki
4. May 28, 2007 — Cincinnati outfielder Ryan Freel smacked in the head by elbow of teammate Norris Hopper. Freel reports this is the ninth or tenth concussion he had but the only one with lingering effects
5. May 27, 2007 — Cardinal Scott Rolen, trying to beat out an infield hit, collided with first baseball Dmitri Young
6. May 24, 2007 — Phillies batter Abraham Nunez was accidentally punched in the jaw by catcher Miguel Olivo as he was trying to throw out a runner.

This is just a small list of concussions that were recognized. Who knows how many were unrecognized or not reported?

Another special head concussion symptom complex in the news lately is a condition called "post-concussion syndrome," or PCS for short.[18] Noted symptoms of concussion are headache, dizziness, decreased concentration, memory problems, irritability, fatigue, visual disturbances, sensitivity to noise (or light), judgment problems, depression, and anxiety. Most of these symptoms resolve within two weeks. When symptoms persist, the condition is called post-concussion syndrome. The exact amount of time that must pass before one gets PCS is not clear. The lay press often says that anything beyond a few days is post-concussion syndrome. Scientific articles say symptoms of concussion that do not resolve within one month give the diagnosis. Some say six weeks. At three months, you definitely have PCS, although many articles use another name for symptoms that last this long: persistent PCS. Symptoms present early after a concussion do vary somewhat from symptoms noted months after the original injury. Later symptoms of depression and anxiety become a larger and larger problem. This should not be a surprise as symptoms of anxiety and depression often become apparent with the passage of time for any chronic illness.

PCS can start after a major brain concussion. Or symptoms can develop after either a single minor concussion or after many minor head concussions over a period of time (Minor or Mild Traumatic Brain Injury — concussion — is also abbreviated MTBI, or mTBI). It is often difficult to understand why symptoms should persist after relatively isolated minor traumatic events.

The exact reason for persistent concussion symptoms is not clear. Most say there is an organic reason. With a severe concussion or multiple minor concussions, this is easier to understand. A severe concussion causes more damage (example: Don Zimmer). Multiple minor concussions cause much more damage than would occur by just adding each individual injury. Damage with a second concussion might be four times worse instead of two times worse with each single episode. With a third concussion, there might be eight times more damage instead of three times more damage. More damage takes longer to heal because the damage from the previous concussion may have not completely resolved. What is difficult to understand is when a single injury, what would be minor concussion (grade 1 or maybe mild grade II), gives persistent symptoms beyond six weeks, sometimes lasting for months and even years. The symptoms in some cases can even become permanent. The journal *International Review of Psychiatry* in 2003 states, "Most investigators now believe that a variety of pre-morbid, injury-related, and post-morbid neuropathological and psychological factors contribute to the development and continuation of these symptoms in those sustaining mild traumatic brain injury (MTBI)."[19] In other words, people are different before a concussion; people react differently to the same or similar injury. Some get over it quickly, and others do not. Why that is, is not clear.

What follows is a presentation of several cases of post-concussion problems.

Jim Edmonds

Jim Edmonds played 17 productive years in the major leagues, mostly for the Anaheim (California) Angels (seven years) and the St. Louis Cardinals (eight years).

Edmonds sustained a head concussion on June 21, 2006, slamming into the left-center field fence as he tried to reel in a home run by Joe Crede of the White Sox. He fell backwards, hitting the back of his head on the turf. The injury occurred at U.S. Cellular Field in Chicago, in an interleague game between the White Sox and Cardinals.[20]

Edmonds missed three days after this injury. He reported feeling dizzy and having a headache. Then in mid–August, almost two months after the initial injury, he began feeling the same way as he had in June. He could not exactly pin down a specific injury, though he did note the recurrence of symptoms after diving for a couple of balls in the outfield. He also reported just not feeling normal (clueless). This symptom began after a game around August 11, in which he had some difficulty catching a couple of fly balls. He had dizzy spells and complained of blurred vision. Because of the recurrence of his symptoms, he had an MRI of his head which was reported as normal. He also had some blood tests that were also normal.[21]

Edmonds went on the disabled list in late August and missed a month before returning. He played in only four games in the season's final six weeks. There was some question whether he would get better by the playoffs, but he did. In the 2006 post-season he contributed ten RBI in 16 games. He seemed well enough that the Cardinals offered him a two-year extension on his contract.[22]

Edmonds was lucky. He apparently had no further problems from his 2006 concussion. He played four more seasons before announcing his retirement from baseball on February 18, 2011.[23] There was no indication given that post-concussion symptoms had anything to do with Edmonds' retirement.

Corey Koskie

Both Corey Koskie of the Milwaukee Brewers and Mike Matheny of the San Francisco Giants had prolonged episodes of "post-concussion syndrome" lasting much longer than Jim Edmonds'. Both Koskie's and Matheny's symptoms eventually led to their retirement from major league baseball.

In the last few years, almost any general discussion of concussions in baseball touches on Koskie's post-concussion problems. This is probably because of the very persistent nature of Koskie's symptoms over a long period of time, caused by a baseball-related injury.[24]

Koskie's career spanned nine seasons — seven with the Twins, one with the Toronto Blue Jays, and one with the Milwaukee Brewers. His career stats are good, with a lifetime batting average of .275.

Koskie's post-concussion problems stem from a single incident of what would be classified as at most a grade one concussion. This is not the typical case with persistent post-concussion problems.

Koskie was playing third base on July 5, 2006, for the Brewers against the Reds. He was pursuing a pop fly off the bat of Felipe Lopez when he flipped awkwardly trying to catch the ball, landing on his back. The ball popped out of Koskie's glove and into shortstop Bill Hall's glove. If Koskie's head hit the turf at all, it was barely noticeable. Koskie's main problems were caused by a whiplash-type injury.[25]

Immediately after the play, Koskie was very dizzy and slightly nauseated. He did manage to hit against Cincinnati's Kent Mercker the next half-inning, but was removed after his at-bat as he was still dizzy.

When Koskie's symptoms did not improve, he was placed on the disabled list on July 15, 2006.[26] After the initial injury, Koskie couldn't get out of bed without being overwhelmed by feelings of nausea and dizziness. He had to take naps frequently because of feelings of exhaustion and sleepiness. Just watching any form of movement with his eyes, such as a ballgame live or on TV, caused him to be dizzy and feel ill.[27]

Koskie reports knocking over objects on the dinner table when he reached for them, as his depth perception was bad. Just walking into a room, he would often run into the door frame.

He had memory problems. For instance, when he would drive his car to a location and then drive back, he often couldn't remember the trips. Soon after a conversation, he would forget what he talked about.[28]

CT scans and MRIs were normal as is the case often with post-concussion syndrome. These tests had been part of Koskie's evaluation at the University of Pittsburgh Medical Center and their head concussion program.

A later evaluation at the University of Buffalo led to the institution of a graded exercise program where exercise intensity is gradually increased over a period of time, depending on the individual's response to each step in the program. Though often helpful in post-concussion cases, this was only mildly helpful in Koskie's case. Any exertion getting Koskie's heart rate up brought on dizziness and nausea.[29]

Many of Koskie's treatments weren't helping much. Finally, Koskie reported that symptoms began to improve in December of 2008 after he began to concentrate much of his treatment, with the help of physical therapist Dr. John Groves, on the muscles in his neck.[30] These were the muscles aggravated by Koskie's whiplash injury.

Koskie missed the remainder of the 2006 season after going on the DL for his injury. He missed all of the 2007 and 2008 seasons. With improved symptoms over the off-season in 2008–2009, he made an aborted attempt to play baseball again in 2009. He signed a minor league contract with the Chicago Cubs and actually had a few at-bats before he decided it just wasn't worth risking the return of post-concussion symptoms. After those few at-bats, he formally announced his retirement from baseball.[31]

Mike Matheny

Mike Matheny was a four-time Gold Glove winner. He played in 1,305 games for Milwaukee (1994–1998), Toronto (1999), St. Louis (2000–2004), and San Francisco (2005–2007). Mike Matheny was one tough catcher. He played through several injuries, including a cracked rib and a beaning. In contrast to Matheny's other injuries, his post-concussion symptoms were something else altogether. Mike Matheny's post-concussion syndrome ultimately led to his retirement from major league baseball.

Matheny's problems were the result of multiple minor concussions (MTBIs) during a short period of time. Several foul balls smacked into his catcher's mask as he squatted behind home plate. The last ball careened off his mask on May 31, 2006, during a game against the Florida Marlins. He had a very similar foul ball off the bat of Miguel Cabrera of the Marlins just two days prior to the last injury. There had been yet another "bell ringer" just the week before.[32]

Matheny, when he didn't recover right away from the last MTBI on May 31, was placed on the disabled list on June 2. He never got off the disabled list in 2006.[33]

Matheny announced his retirement on February 1, 2007. Prior to his retirement Matheny, like Corey Koskie, was evaluated by the Dr. Michael Collins at the University of Pittsburgh Medical Center head concussion program. Like Koskie, Matheny had significant symptoms whenever his heart rate became elevated to any extent. Matheny became fatigued easily, had memory problems, had trouble focusing, and had trouble seeing straight. When his symptoms didn't improve over the 2006–2007 off-season, doctors recommended retirement instead of his risking more permanent damage from further concussions.[34]

Justin Morneau and Jason Bay

No season in baseball is without some significant concussion injuries. In 2010 it was injuries to Justin Morneau and Jason Bay that made the news, both season-ending injuries.

Minnesota Twins first baseman Morneau was in the middle of another MVP-like season in 2010, similar to the MVP year he had 2006, when he suffered a concussion on July 7. Sliding into second base, trying to break up a potential double play, he sustained an inadvertent knee to the head by Toronto infielder John McDonald. He did not return in 2010, missing the Twins' play-offs for the second year in a row[35] (having been out of action in 2009 due to a stress fracture in his spine).

Morneau had suffered a previous concussion in 2005 courtesy of a beanball by Seattle's Ron Villone, but this injury had only put him on the disabled list in 2005 for the minimum 15 days (April 7 to 21).

There was hope for recovery for Morneau, but when he was still having daily symptoms of "headaches, dizziness, and general aches and pains" as of the middle of August, some 30 days after his injury, his rehab was put on hold.[36] The Twins were fortunate to do well enough in Morneau's absence to make the playoffs without him. Michael Cuddyer, Morneau's replacement at first base, performed admirably.

The Twins were initially cautious with Morneau in 2011. But he played nine spring games without difficulty and appeared ready for opening day.[37] Unfortunately, other injuries followed in 2011, including another concussion on August 29 which ended Morneau's season. This concussion was milder, and Morneau came back in 2012 to compile a solid season, playing in 136 games and batting .267 with 19 home runs and 77 RBI.

Left fielder Jason Bay of the New York Mets, who had just signed a four-year, $66 million contract before the 2010 season, suffered a head concussion when he ran into the wall at Dodger Stadium on July 23. He made one of the better defensive plays of the year when he collided with the padded wall but managed to hold onto the ball.

Oddly, Bay didn't start suffering significant concussion symptoms till two days later when he started to experience "a dull, boring headache" during the flight back to New York following a dismal 2–9 road trip for the Mets.[38]

A specialist saw Bay soon after the road trip and concluded Bay's main problems stemmed from his head snapping back on the wall collision, suffering a whiplash injury.[39]

Bay's main persistent symptoms were almost daily headaches that lasted until late September. As with other cases, exercising, such as riding an exercise bike, to raise Bay's heart rate was tried, with mixed success. Full rehab excluding baseball activities was not started till after his headaches had subsided.[40]

By spring training 2011, Bay was having no problems with post-concussion symptoms.[41] Spring went well and all looked good for 2011 until Bay experienced some left rib-cage discomfort (oblique?) during batting practice.[42] He was on the DL until April 21. The following year was marked by a broken rib in an April 23 game, then another concussion on June 15 in a collision with the left field wall at Citi Field. This concussion put Bay on the DL until July 17. His shortened season concluded with a .165 batting average, 8 home runs and 20 RBI. At this writing, Bay has not regained his pre-concussion form.

Conclusion

Careers Resisting Injury

Cal Ripken Jr.

After going through the list of baseball injuries, one is amazed at what "Iron Man" Cal Ripken Jr. achieved. He played in 2,632 consecutive games over 16 seasons. The odds of a similar streak are close to the odds of winning a multi-state lottery. One certainly would be smart to bet against the possibility that Ripken's record will ever be broken.

There have to be many things going right for one to set such a record. You have to have a body that resists injury. If one is injured, one has to recover quickly. There has to be a big element of luck involved. There has to be motivation to play every day even with minor aches and pains. Your manager has to let you play every day, which many managers don't believe in. One has to avoid suffering any significant illnesses not related to injuries. The streak is a combination of many factors, amazing to achieve.

Setting aside the consecutive game streak and looking at the rest of Ripken's career, one has to be impressed. His lifetime average is only .276, but he had 3,184 hits with 431 home runs and 1695 RBI. The number of hits alone would get him in the Hall of Fame (he was elected in 2007). He

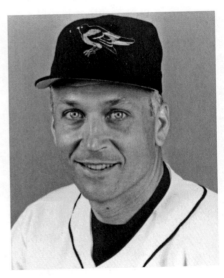

Cal Ripken of the Baltimore Orioles, date unknown (National Baseball Hall of Fame Library, Cooperstown, New York).

won the Rookie of the Year award in 1982 and was voted MVP in 1983 and 1991. He was twice named MVP of an All-Star Game. He was on the All-Star team 19 consecutive years. Amazing!

This book is about baseball injuries, and Ripken is mentioned as an example of someone who was seldom injured until the last three years of his 21-year career. He had few trips to the DL. His relatively DL-free career serves as a contrast to injury-plagued careers of many other players.

He came into the American League in 1981 at the age of 20. On May 30, 1982, he started his streak of consecutive games played. He did not miss another game until September 20, 1998, 2,632 games later. His first trip to the DL was on April 20, 1999, for back pain.[1]

There were injuries along the way. Noted in an article in *The* (Baltimore) *Sun* in 2001 and in Ripken's biography, *The Only Way I Know,* by Cal Ripken and Mike Bryan, several specific injuries threatened to end "the streak" by putting Ripken on the DL.[2]

On April 10, 1985, Ripken sprained his left ankle taking a pickoff throw at second base in the third inning of a game between the Orioles and Rangers. There was an exhibition game the next day, but by the next night in a regular season game, there was Ripken again.[3]

On September 11, 1992, he sprained his right ankle running out a double against the Brewers.[4] He did not come out of the game, and missed no further games.

The injury that came closest to ending the streak occurred in 1993. Ripken describes events on June 6 at Camden Yards:

> Although Seattle's Chris Bosio had thrown behind a couple of our batters, it hadn't occurred to me that retaliation was in order. But with two outs, Mike Mussina plunked Bill Haselman with a fastball on the shoulder in the seventh inning. Haselman charged the mound. I was running towards the mound from shortstop to help protect our pitcher when my foot slipped as I turned to face the wave of Mariners arriving at the scene from their dugout. I heard the pop in my right knee, and then I ended up on the bottom of the pile with a couple thousand players on top of me.[5]

Ripken wasn't too worried about his ankles. He had learned to tape them up well to treat the acute sprains and prevent recurrences. He had had a sore shoulder in 1983 and required a cortisone shot, but the knee injury was quite a different problem altogether.

When he got up the next day, Ripken could barely walk. At the trainer's recommendation, he iced it at home. Three to four hours before the game, the trainer tried "cold whirlpools, muscle stimulation, and ultrasound."[6]

Ripken tried testing the knee before the game, hoping the treatments he had received before the night game might help. He walked a little, took batting practice and infield, ran some quick starts and stops, and only then made the decision to play. He did just fine. The injury could have been worse. He could have torn his cruciate ligament like Milton Bradley did in 2007, instead of having a simple sprain.

Then there were the back problems. Ripken states in his 1997 book that he had had intermittent problems with his back almost every season. The trainer had to "manipulate his back three or four times a season."[7]

Newspaper articles written after the publication of Ripken's book reveal more serious back problems starting in July of 1997 during a West Coast trip to Oakland and Anaheim. No specific, inciting injury is mentioned. For a while, Ripken's occasional treatment for his back became a daily routine of therapy before each game. Ripken was having biting pain in his back and left leg with associated numbness. Pain was not only present during the day, but was affecting Ripken's sleep. Despite back problems that persisted the last two months of the 1997 season, Ripken's streak continued through the end of the season.[8]

The 1998 season was relatively pain-free when compared to 1997. That season Ripken ended his streak on his own terms on September 20, 1998, long after he had beaten Lou Gehrig's 2,130-game streak.

The year after the streak was broken, 1999, was full of injuries. In spring training and in the early part of the year, it was obvious that there was a very significant back problem. Ripken was even having trouble walking.[9] That Ripken's father died of cancer during spring training probably didn't help matters. Certainly such an event would make it difficult to cope with chronic pain.

Cal Ripken went on the DL for the first time in his career on April 18, 1999.

He improved well enough to come off the DL on May 13, but when the back pain recurred he went back on the DL a second time from August 1 until September 1.[10] He had received a cortisone shot in his lower back in early August.[11] This apparently didn't help much, and with the return of back problems in September, he finally succumbed to season-ending surgery on September 23.[12]

With all the back pain, it was rather surprising that Ripken had as good a year at the plate as he had in 1999. He ended up batting .340, the highest average in his career, but he did not qualify for a batting title as he had only 354 plate appearances.

What was the nature of Ripken's back problem? Spinal stenosis was mentioned. This could indicate either a narrowing of a nerve root as the nerve exits the spinal column, or a narrowing of the spinal cord itself within the spinal canal. The cause: a herniated disc is mentioned most often, but a possible bone spur is also mentioned.[13]

With continued problems as previously stated, surgery was done on September 23, 1999, by well-known spinal surgeon Dr. Henry H. Bohlman at

Case Western Reserve University Hospital in Cleveland, Ohio, witnessed by Baltimore's orthopedic team physician, Michael Jacobs. The surgery was described as "decompression" to relieve pressure from a nerve root. Exact details of the procedure and the exact nature of Ripken's problems were not revealed, at the family's request.[14]

The year 2000 was again a difficult one for Cal Ripken because of recurrent back discomfort. On May 15, Ripken again received a cortisone shot in his lower back from Dr. Bohlman. Tests prior to the injection revealed nothing surgically correctible, and Ripken was just thought to have scar tissue and a small piece of disc material where his previous surgery had been performed.[15]

When Ripken continued to have problems with his back, he once again went on the DL (third time in his career) on June 28, 2000.[16] Results of an MRI taken at the time were not revealed. He remained on the DL until the Orioles roster was expanded on September 1.[17]

Ripken had few problems with his back in 2001 and stayed off the DL that year. He did have a fractured rib in the spring, but this did not impair his play during the season. He announced his retirement on June 19, insisting he was not retiring because of his back problems. That injury had simply taken away some of the fun of playing the game and made it more difficult to cope. He was retiring on his own terms at his own time.[18]

Ripken's streak of games played is amazing after noting all the significant baseball injuries in this book. His streak will more than likely never be broken. What a fitting way to end a book about injuries — to contrast these many injuries with an individual who escaped significant injuries and trips to the DL until late in his career.

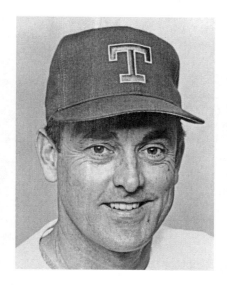

Nolan Ryan

Two other prominent players lasted a long time with relatively few injuries. The first is Nolan Ryan, the Hall of Fame pitcher who escaped trips to the DL for a quarter-century, until his last season.

Nolan Ryan needs very little introduction. He had the second-longest major league career, lasting 27 years in which he pitched for the New York Mets (1966–1971), California Angels (1972–1979), Houston Astros

The Texas Rangers' Nolan Ryan, date unknown (National Baseball Hall of Fame Library, Cooperstown, New York).

(1980–1988), and Texas Rangers (1989–1993). (His career is the longest in more modern times. Cap Anson played 27 consecutive years, 1871–1897.) Ryan's career record was 324 wins and 292 losses with 5,714 strikeouts in 5,386 innings. He tossed 61 shutouts and seven no-hitters. He struck out 19 batters in a game three times. In 1973 Ryan struck out 383 batters, breaking Sandy Koufax's record of 382.

He often threw 100 mph fastballs and was clocked at 100.9 on August 20, 1974, a record that stood for many years.[19]

The reason to mention Nolan Ryan is that he threw his fastball at a high velocity for a long time (27 years). Many hard-throwing major league pitchers' careers end very early because of injuries and subsequent wear on the joints, muscles, tendons, and ligaments that occur when throwing the baseball at 95+ miles per hour (e.g., Koufax).

The extra velocity and torque taxes the body to the limit. Some hard-throwing pitchers, if injured frequently, are converted to relief pitchers in an effort to prolong their careers (e.g., Kerry Wood and John Smoltz for a brief period of time).

Most pitchers, if they do last to their late 30s and 40s, suffer injuries that gradually reduce the speed on their fastball. If they are not injured, the simple aging process slows down the velocity on the baseball significantly. Often such pitchers come to rely more on finesse than power (e.g., Frank Tanana).

Nolan Ryan's injuries, up until his last year, were relatively minor (except 1967), with few trips to the DL until Ryan's body basically fell apart during the last year of his career.

He had some type of forearm problem in 1967 while making a transition from the minor leagues to the major leagues. This injury sounds much like a medial collateral ligament problem, as Ryan felt a pop in his forearm while throwing.[20] He missed much of 1967, but he pitched thereafter without disabling forearm problems until 1986, 19 years later. The injury could have been a partially torn UCL or maybe even a strained or partially torn elbow flexor muscle tear that healed with rest.

In 1968 Ryan had some problems with recurrent blisters on his fingers. He used pickle brine on his fingers to toughen up the skin. Later on Ryan learned to shave the calluses that built up on his fingers.[21] Research revealed no mention of a blister problem after 1968.

The first year Ryan needed surgery was 1975. He pitched most of the year with elbow pain and a series of muscle pulls (strains). Though he missed the last five weeks of the season, he still ended up pitching 198 innings in 28 starts.

Despite elbow problems in 1975, Ryan pitched his fourth career no-hitter to tie Sandy Koufax's career record. Ryan's 1975 season ended with his first surgery of any kind; four bone chips were removed from his elbow on August

23.[22] This would be one of only two baseball-related surgeries Ryan would have during his career.

Ryan was on the DL nine times in his first 22 seasons, but only once during that time span did he need surgery. Other than this 1975 surgery and the 1967 injury, Ryan's most significant trips to the DL were in 1986, when he was on the DL twice due to elbow soreness.[23]

Surgery in 1986 was recommended by Dr. Frank Jobe for possible damage to the right elbow medial collateral ligament, but Ryan decided against surgery, saying at age 39 he was just too old to have the surgery done. He proceeded to pitch seven more seasons, despite having intermittent elbow discomfort every year after 1986.

Finally, in his last two years, 1992 and 1993, age caught up to Ryan. Most pitchers or position players have long retired before they get to age 45 or 46. In April 1992, Ryan missed 23 days because of a left calf-muscle strain and inflamed right Achilles' tendon.[24] He still went on to start 27 games that year.

In 1993, at age 46, the roof caved in. At the time Ryan was the oldest active player in the majors, and he was still throwing baseballs in the 95 mph range. He had only his second baseball-related surgery on April 15 when he had arthroscopic surgery to remove damaged parts of his medial and lateral menisci in his right knee.[25]

That was only the beginning of problems in 1993; Ryan missed 22 days because of the knee. Then he missed 72 days because of a strained hip muscle, 21 more days because of a ribcage injury, and finally a season-ending right elbow injury.

The elbow, which had had a probable partial tear of the medial collateral ligament in 1986, ripped completely through on September 22, 1993. It was a game against the Seattle Mariners in the Kingdome. Ryan had faced six batters in the first inning without getting an out. He felt the ligament give way on a 1–1 pitch to the Mariners' Dave Magadan. He said it felt like the ligament "popped like a rubber band."[26] He threw one more pitch and then he took himself out of the game.

Mariners team physician Dr. Larry Pedegana confirmed the injury was probably a torn medial collateral ligament, an injury that would require tendon-transplant surgery (Tommy John surgery). As Ryan was going to retire at the end of 1993 anyway, surgery wasn't considered. One can function just fine for most everyday activities with a torn ligament in the elbow: you just can't pitch, especially not at the major league level.

Considering that for most of his career Nolan Ryan threw an upper 90s to 100 mph fastball, to last until age 46 is very remarkable. It is a unique accomplishment for a pitcher, one that may not be soon repeated. He resisted many significant baseball injuries up until the end of a 27-year career, one of the two longest major league careers on record.

Lou Gehrig

Closing our discussion of baseball injuries is another player who played many games consecutively. That is not to say he was never injured. It was just deemed by himself and his manager that his injuries were not severe enough to miss a game, not in the 2,130 consecutive games he played. It is the "Iron Horse," Lou Gehrig.

Gehrig played for the New York Yankees from 1923 until 1939, when he was forced into early retirement by ALS, now called Lou Gehrig's Disease. He died in 1941.

In his career he had 2,721 hits, 493 home runs, and 1995 RBI with a career batting average of .340.

He had the streak of 2,130 consecutive games played. That said, it should be noted Gehrig had a few games after the first 1931 games played where he was removed after his first at-bat. He had injuries which few players today would have played through.

On August 5, 1936, in an extended interview with Sid C. Keener of the *St. Louis Star-Times*, he outlined some of the injuries he played with. He had fractured his little finger four times. "What's a broken finger when your ball club is fighting for a pennant?" he said.[27]

He busted toes a couple of times. He sprained his ankle half a dozen times. He suffered a severe beaning. More than once, he had a severe cold or lumbago that put him to bed, but he played the next day.

The most severe injury Gehrig suffered actually occurred during an exhibition game. Often in the 1930s, when a team had a day off during the season, they actually didn't have a day off. Instead, they played exhibition games against local teams, some of them minor league teams.

The severe beaning Gehrig suffered on June 29, 1934, was at the hands of the minor league Norfolk, Virginia, Tars. Ray White, a fellow Columbia University alumnus, had a particularly bad first inning against the Yankees, giving up three runs, including a home run by Gehrig. In the second inning Gehrig again came to bat. White, probably still upset about the previous inning, fired a high and inside pitch to Gehrig. The pitch hit him two inches above his right eye (no helmets in 1934).

"Gehrig collapsed like a rag doll."[28] Gehrig lay unconscious for five minutes at least. When he finally got up, dazed, he had to be helped to the dugout with arms over the strong shoulders of Yankees catcher Bill Dickey. "He wobbled toward the dugout."[29]

From there he went to the local hospital where x-rays revealed no fracture. His doctor, Dr. S. B. Whitlock, diagnosed Gehrig as having a "moderate concussion of the brain."[30]

The next day Gehrig had an enormous welt on his head. He had a terrible headache. Tests revealed his vision was normal. Because of the welt, x-rays were repeated and were once again negative for a fracture.

Despite the headache, and against the recommendation of his doctor, Gehrig insisted on playing the next day. Manager McCarthy wasn't going to stop him. He had to borrow one of Babe Ruth's hats and cut the seams, as his head was too swollen up to put his own cap on. Gehrig managed to hit three triples in the first five innings. The fine plate performance was washed away with the rain, the game being called before becoming official.[31]

No way in modern baseball would Gehrig have been allowed to play the next day with such a significant concussion after such a beaning. He might have been put on the DL.

Overall, 1934 was not a good year for injuries. No sooner had Gehrig recovered from his beaning than he faced another significant obstacle to his streak, a severe backache. On July 13 he had to be removed from the game in the first inning after hitting a single. He could barely straighten up and he "hobbled" off the field, replaced by a pinch-runner.[32] Gehrig's condition was described as a bad case of "lumbago."[33] The next day, with continued back problems, the streak was in jeopardy. His manager, Joe McCarthy, inserted him in the leadoff spot in the lineup. In the top of the first inning he "limped" to home plate, hit a single, and struggled to make it to first base.[34] He was immediately removed from the game for a pinch-runner. He never played in the field in the bottom of the first inning. The next day, Gehrig was described as moving "gingerly" but managed to play the whole game, hitting three doubles and a single to boot.[35]

Gehrig also had to be removed from a game on August 5, 1935, because of a backache.

A more serious injury had occurred earlier that year on June 8. Always a risk for a first baseman is a collision with a runner moving rapidly down the line trying to beat the throw to first base. An errant throw causing the first baseman to stretch out in an awkward manner to avoid letting the ball possibly sail over his head leaves the defender in a very vulnerable position. That is exactly what happened on June 8, in the first inning in a game against the Red Sox. The runner, Carl Reynolds, a big man, flattened Gehrig, once again knocking him unconscious briefly.[36]

Surprise! Gehrig stayed in the game. Not only that, he homered, singled, and stole a base before being removed in the eighth inning.

Even prior to all the talk of the streak, way back in 1928, injuries posed a threat to Gehrig's developing a consecutive game streak. During the last game of the regular season Gehrig hit his 27th home run of the season in the top of the seventh inning. In the bottom of the seventh, a grounder ran up his arm and smacked him in the face, knocking him unconscious though only briefly. He left the game. But there he was for the first game of the World Series despite having a very sore face.[37]

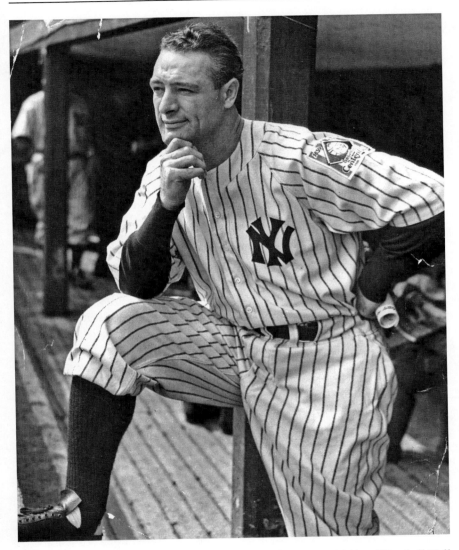

New York Yankees' Lou Gehrig in the dugout, date unknown (National Baseball Hall of Fame Library, Cooperstown, New York).

There were numerous other injuries that could have stopped the streak, such as when Gehrig played in June of 1931 with a chipped bone in his foot.

One injury occurred during an off-season tour of Japan in 1931. Gehrig was hit in the right hand by a pitch, breaking two bones.[38] That was it for the tour. Gehrig did not play another game. But it was not during the regular season or World Series.

Many of the injuries Gehrig suffered during his streak might have led to a trip to the DL today. He played through some significant injuries, including concussions and broken bones. Yet Gehrig could have had many more severe injuries than he experienced, both overuse and traumatic, any of which could have ended his consecutive game streak.

Conclusion

Every day, someone in the big leagues has an overuse or traumatic injury. Injuries are a fact of life in the big leagues and affect every aspect of the game. The player's career can be put on hold because of an injury, can be altered in an adverse manner, or can even be ended.

Teams' fortunes can be changed by injuries. Within a season a team's possible trip to the playoffs or World Series can be brushed aside by an injury to a key player. Often trades are made that simply would not have been made because of an injury to a key player. It is unknown how many careers today are prolonged by doctors' ability to diagnose and treat injuries. The ulnar collateral ligaments probably ended many a career before the advent of Tommy John surgery, just one innovation among the many made. How many, who knows? They were diagnosed with a bad arm and limped along for a few more years or were immediately sent back to the farm, never to pitch or play again. Ah, what a career Koufax might have had, if he had had Tommy John surgery and been able to pitch a few more years. What of Lefty Gomez and his bad arm?

Pitchers were also diagnosed as having a bad shoulder and sent packing. What might have happened if Don Drysdale had had a shoulder arthroscopy? What might have been found and treated? What of Smoky Joe Wood? And the list goes on and on.

All this speculation does not even include all the traumatic injuries that could not be diagnosed or treated optimally. What of the beanings that occurred before someone had sense enough to put a helmet on every batter? What if surgery on Ray Chapman's head had been done with techniques known today? Might not Chapman have lived despite his beaning while not wearing a helmet? Might he have lived if he had been put on a respirator post-op?

But we live in the present day. We are subject to what is presently known about diagnosis and treatment. What of the future? Who knows what diagnostic innovations and treatments are to come that will once again change the sport of baseball?

Appendix

Tommy John Surgery List

It is almost impossible to list everyone who has had Tommy John surgery. A partial list with references is given. The list gets bigger all the time. Also, the list of players with a history of two Tommy John surgeries keeps growing. From this list, it should be rather obvious that the vast majority of players having Tommy John surgery are pitchers.

1974 Tommy John[1]
1981 Tim Candiotti[2]
1985 David Wells[3]
1986 John Dayley[4]
1992 Mariano Rivera (didn't have) (several references list Rivera as having had Tommy John surgery, but in an interview Rivera denies it)[5]
1995 Al Reyes (again in 2005),[6] Darren Dreifort (again in 2001),[7] Jose Rijo[8]
1997 Billy Koch,[9] Eric Gagne[10] (not in 2005 as listed in many sources)
1998 Jason Isringhausen (again in 2009),[11] Matt Beech (again in 1999)[12]
1999 Matt Morris,[13] Kerry Lightenberg,[14] Paul Wilson,[15] Tom Gordon,[16] Kerry Wood,[17] Odalis Perez[18]
2000 John Smoltz,[19] Sterling Hitchcock[20]
2001 Kris Benson,[21] Xavier Nady (position player) (again in 2009),[22] Matt Mantei,[23] Doug Brocail (again in 2002)[24]
2002 John Leiber,[25] Jeff Zimmerman (again in 2004)[26]
2003 Rick Ankiel,[27] Ryan Dempster,[28] Joe Mays,[29] A. J. Burnett,[30] Andy Ashby,[31] Paul Byrd,[32] Denny Neagle[33]
2004 Rafael Soriano[34]
2005 Cezar Izturis (position player),[35] Brian Anderson (again in 2006),[36] Octavio Dotel,[37] Erubiel Durazo (position player),[38] Randy Wolf[39]
2006 Mike Hampton,[40] Francisco Liriano[41]
2007 Josh Kinney,[42] Chris Carpenter,[43] Carl Pavano,[44] Bruce Chen[45]

2008 Billy Wagner,[46] Josh Johnson,[47] Tim Hudson,[48] Shaun Marcum[49]

2009 Edinson Volquez,[50] Anthony Reyes,[51] Mike Aviles (position player),[52] Jordan Zimmermann[53]

2010 Joe Nathan,[54] Manuel Corpus,[55] Stephen Strasburg,[56] Jamie Moyer[57]

2011 Adam Wainwright,[58] Joba Chamberlain,[59] Jorge De La Rosa,[60] John Lackey[61]

2012 Joakim Soria (previously 2003),[62] Ryan Madson,[63] Joey Devine (previously in 2009),[64] Brian Wilson (previously in 2003)[65]

Notes

Preface

1. George A. Sheehan, *Dr. George Sheehan's Medical Advice for Runners* (Mountain View, CA: World Publications, 1978).

2. James R. Andrews, Bertram Zarins, and Kevin E. Wilk, *Injuries in Baseball* (Philadelphia, PA: Lippincott-Raven, 1998).

3. Jack O'Connell, "Mattingly: Does Back Pain Signal End?" *The Sporting News*, September 20, 1990.

4. "New York Yankees Team Review," *The Sporting News*, February 3, 1997.

5. Frank Deford, *The Old Ball Game: How John McGraw, Christy Mathewson, and the New York Giants Created Modern Baseball* (New York, NY: Atlantic Monthly Press, 2005).

6. Ray Robinson, *Matty: An American Hero, Christy Mathewson and the New York Giants* (New York, NY: Oxford University Press, 1993).

7. Jack Smiles, *Big Ed Walsh: The Life and Times of Spitballing Hall of Famer* (Jefferson, NC: McFarland, 2008), 156, 162, and 165.

8. Ibid., 182–183.

9. "Sports of the time: remembering players M.L.B. has forgotten" by Dave Anderson, *The New York Times* on March 13, 2004.

10. "Anabolic steroids: a review for the clinician" *Sports Medicine* 32.5 (2002): 285–296.

Introduction

1. Freddie H. Fu and David A. Stone, *Sports Injuries: Mechanisms, Prevention, Treatment* (Philadelphia, PA: Lippincott Williams & Wilkens, 2001).

2. Kannus and Josza, "Histopathological changes preceding spontaneous rupture of tendon: A controlled study of 891 cases," *The Journal of Bone and Joint Surgery* 73.10 (December 1991) 1507–1525.

3. Beck, Jason, "Zumaya to have surgery,"
MLB.com, May 7, 2007; Lowe, John. "Zumaya to miss three months. Right-hand finger has ruptured tendon," *Detroit Free Press*, May 8, 2007.

4. Marko Pecina and Ivan Bojanic, *Overuse Injuries of the Musculoskeletal System*. 2nd Ed. (Boca Rotan, FL: CRC Press, 2004).

PART I

Chapter 1

1. Meister, "Injuries to the shoulder in the throwing athlete: Part I," *The American Journal of Sports Medicine* 28.2, 265–275.

2. Henry Schulmann, "Giants closer calls it a career," *The San Francisco Chronicle*, February 20, 2005: "Giants closer to retire after another setback," an ESPN.com news service, February 20, 2005.

3. Henry Schulmann, "GIANT'S NOTEBOOK: Nen draws inspiration from Schilling," *The San Francisco Chronicle* on May 18, 2003; John Shea, "GIANT FANFEST: Nen is shouldering responsibility: S.F. closer trying to regain form after three surgeries," *The San Francisco Chronicle*, February 9, 2004; Josh Suchon, "Nen has questions about diagnosis," *The Oakland Tribune*, February 9, 2004.

4. Joe Strauss, "One bad series Mulder: We've got to find what's going on," *St. Louis Post-Dispatch*, June 23, 2006; Joe Strauss, "Mulder MRI shows problem," *St. Louis Post-Dispatch*, June 24, 2006.

5. W. Norman Scott, *Arthroscopy of the Knee: Diagnosis and Treatment* (Philadelphia, PA: W. B. Saunders, 1990), 1–10.

6. Derrick Goold, "Mulder has surgery on shoulder," *St. Louis Post-Dispatch*, September 13, 2006.

7. Derrick Goold, "Mulder is back on the sidelines," *St Louis Post-Dispatch*, May 8, 2008; Derrick Goold, "More surgery not an option," *St. Louis Post-Dispatch,* May 30, 2008.

8. "Sports," *The Boston Globe*, September 6, 2009.

9. David Lennon, "Surgery for Pedro torn rotator cuff to shelve Martinez for first half of '07 season," *Newsday* (Long Island, NY), October 1, 2006.

10. Mike DiGiovanna, "Colon to begin extensive rehab but no surgery planned," *Los Angeles Times,* August 12, 2006; Ben Shpigel, "Yankees hope Bartolo Colon can recapture old form," *The New York Times*, January 26, 2011.

11. Serge F. Kovaleski, "Pitcher's treatment draws scrutiny," *The New York Times*, May 11, 2011.

12. Ben Shpigel, "Yankees hope Bartolo Colon can recapture old form," *The New York Times*, January 26, 2011.

13. C.J. Nitkowski, "A firsthand experience with stem cell treatment in pitching arm," cnnsi.com, August 3, 2011.

14. Jack Etkin, "Saberhagen couldn't beat shoulder pain," *Rocky Mountain News* (CO), October 8, 1995.

15. Ibid.

16. Jerry Cresnick. "'Sabes' saves arm for next start," *The Denver Post*, August 20, 1995.

17. Jerry Cresnick, "Don't write off Saberhagen yet," *The Denver Post*, September 18, 1995.

18. Associated Press, "Surgery on sore shoulder should put Saberhagen back in Rockies rotation," *The Gazette* (Colorado Springs), October 25, 1995.

19. Tracy Ringolsby and Jack Etkin, "Saberhagen drops in on Rockies, Right-hander wants to pitch for club if he tries a comeback," *Rocky Mountain News*, June 25, 1996; Mike Klis, "Saberhagen: Rehab a waste," *The* (Colorado Springs, CO) *Gazette*, June 25, 1996.

20. A wire service article, "Rockies will let Saberhagen become off season free agent," *Sun-Sentinel* (South Florida), September 11, 1966; Sean McAdam, "Saberhagen, Red Sox close," *Daily News of Los Angeles* (CA), December 9, 1996.

21. Dan Shaughnessy, "Glory Days gone: Saberhagen back," *The Boston Globe*, August 23, 1997.

22. Larry Whiteside, "Saberhagen set free," *The Boston Globe*, October 29, 1997.

23. "The Sporting News American League comeback Player," at sportingnews.com; "Tony Conigliaro award," bostonbaseballwriters.com.

24. Michael Silverman, "Baseball: Sox get news on Saberhagen," *Boston Herald*, November 6, 1999.

25. Jack Thompson, "Saberhagen shuts down for season," *Chicago Tribune*, September 3, 2000.

26. "Saberhagen says he will retire," *San Jose Mercury News* (CA), August 9, 2001.

27. Ken Corbitt, "Sabes enters Royals Hall of Fame," *The Topeka Capital-Journal*, August 15, 2005.

28. Don Drysdale and Bob Verdi, *Once a Bum, Always a Dodger,* (New York, NY: Simon & Schuster, 2003).

29. Hal Bodley, "'Bird' Fidrych was workhorse in '76," usatoday.com, August 10, 2006.

30. Billy Bowles, "Clinic puts athletes back in action," *Detroit Fee Press*, May 21, 1986.

31. Ben Bolch, "Schmidt gets good odds on recovery," *Los Angeles Times*, June 21, 2007.

32. Paul Meyer, "Surgery successful for Cordova, Schmidt," *Pittsburgh Post-Gazette*, August 19, 2000.

33. Ken Gurnik, "Schmidt's shoulder worse than thought," MLB.com, June 21, 2007.

34. Dylan Hernandez, "Schmidt a 'longshot' to return to Dodgers this season," *Los Angeles Times*, August 7, 2008; Alden Gonzalez, "Schmidt, Zaun join open market," MLB.com, November 11, 2009.

35. *Post-Dispatch* staff, "Cards pitcher Carpenter's season over following more surgery," *St. Louis Post-Dispatch,* August 6, 2003.

36. Joe Strauss and Rick Hummel, "Club is unsure when Carpenter will pitch again," *St. Louis Post-Dispatch*, September 30, 2004.

37. Larry Whiteside, "Choice to be made: Clemens weighs possible surgery," *The Boston Globe*, August 24, 1985; Larry Whiteside, "Clemens to seek second opinion," *The Boston Globe*, August 25, 1985; Larry Whiteside. "Bad News for Clemens: surgery deemed a must," *The Boston Globe*, August 30, 1985; Larry Whiteside, "Armas hammering ball again," *The Boston Globe*, September 4, 1985; Roger Clemens with Peter Gammons. *Rocket Man: The Roger Clemens Story* (Lexington, Massachusetts: Stephen Greene Press, 1987).

38. Roger Clemens with Peter Gammons. *Rocket Man: The Roger Clemens Story*, 51.

39. Ibid., 52.

40. Larry Whiteside, "Choice to be made Clemens weighs possible surgery," *The Boston Globe*, August 24, 1985; Larry Whiteside, "Clemens to seek second opinion," *The Boston Globe*, August 25, 1985.

41. Larry Whiteside, "Armas hammering ball again," *The Boston Globe*, September 4, 1985.

42. Roger Clemens with Peter Gammons, *Rocket Man–The Roger Clemens Story*, 56.

43. Ken Dailey, "Hershizer may miss season-Dodgers ace faces surgery today," *Daily News of Los Angeles* (CA), April 27, 1990.

44. Ken Dailey, "Orel surgery results in optimism," *Daily News of Los Angeles* (CA), April 28, 1990; Phil Collier, "Hershizer's shoulder reconstructed: doctor optimistic," *The San Diego* (CA) *Union*, April 28, 1990.

45. David Falkner "That farewell to arms feeling," *The Sporting News*, May 20, 1996.

46. Ibid.

47. Ibid.

48. Jeff Passan, "Pristine mechanics caused Prior pain," sports.yahoo.com/mlb/news, May 12, 2009.

49. Gordon Whittenmyer, "Prior done with Cubs? Even if right-hander returns to mound in '08, his career on North Side probably over," *Chicago Sun-Times*, April 26, 2007.

50. Gordon Whittenmyer, "Prior done with Cubs? Even if right-hander returns to mound in '08, his career on North Side probably over," *Chicago Sun-Times*, April 26, 2007; Associated Press, "Prior out for season after shoulder surgery," ESPN.com, April 25, 2007; Bill Center, "Prior to injuries, he was it: Padres pitcher not ready to hang it up," *The San Diego* (CA) *Union Tribune*, May 9, 2009.

51. Bill Center, "Title: Padres the game center how they won," *The San Diego* (CA) *Union-Tribune*, June 6, 2008; Tom Krasovic, "Prior has shoulder tear, will have season-ending surgery again," *The San Diego* (CA) *Union-Tribune*, June 2, 2008.

52. Corey Brock, "Padres part ways with oft-injured Prior," MLB.com, August 1, 2009.

53. "mlb 2010 Free agent tracker," ESPN.com; Jerry Crasnick, "Source: Yanks ink Mark Prior for minors," ESPN.com, December 14, 2010; Alden Gonzalez, "Prior excited about possible return to majors," MLB.com, January 5, 2011.

54. Jeff Passan, "Pristine mechanics caused Prior pain," sports.yahoo.com/mlb/news, May 12, 2009; Bob Kelley, "High & Inside," *The Philadelphia* (PA) *Inquirer*, August 7, 2010.

55. Peter Gammons, "Gammons: 2010 Draft belongs to scouts," MLB.com, June 5, 2010.

56. Jeff Passan, "Pristine mechanics caused Prior pain," sports.yahoo.com/mlb/news, May 12, 2009.

57. Glen Macnow, "The pitcher in winter," *Detroit Free Press*, March 9, 1986.

58. Ibid.

59. Ibid.; Bob Finnigan, "Milt Wilcox ready to prove to M's he can still pitch," *The Seattle Times*, February 11, 1986.

60. United Press International article, "Tigers' Wilcox may need surgery to repair his sore right shoulder," *The Orlando Sentinel*, June 6, 1985.

61. Curt Sylvester, "Fantasy ending? Wilcox is impressing Mariners," *Detroit Free Press* on March 22, 1986.

62. "M's release Milt Wilcox," *The Seattle Times*, June 14, 1986.

63. Gerry Fraley, "Sutter returns looking more like himself," *The Atlanta Journal-Constitution* on September 4, 1985; Gerry Fraley, "Braves' notebook: Sutter's arthrogram scheduled," *The Atlanta Journal-Constitution* on September 24, 1985; Gerry Fraley, "Season over for Sutter, but no severe damage found in shoulder," *The Atlanta Journal-Constitution*, September 26, 1985.

64. Gerry Fraley, "Braves' Sutter has surgery on ailing shoulder," *The Atlanta Journal-Constitution*, December 12, 1985; Bud Shaw, "Sutter trying for his biggest save," *The Atlanta Journal-Constitution*, June 28, 1987.

65. Harold Klawans, *Why Michael Couldn't Hit: and Other Tales of the Neurology of Sports.* (Avon Books: New York NY, 1998), 177–181.

66. Ibid.

67. Ibid.

68. Gerry Fraley, "Tests reveal Sutter has damage to rotator cuff," *The Atlanta Journal-Constitution*, August 14, 1986.

69. Gerry Fraley, "Sutter realizes odds are low after surgery," *The Atlanta Journal-Constitution*, February 12, 1987.

70. Daryl Maxie, "Sutter has knee surgery," *The Atlanta Journal-Constitution*, September 27, 1987.

71. Joe Strauss "Sutter 99.9% sure career over: Medical exam reveals recurrence of shoulder injury," *The Atlanta Journal-Constitution*, March 28, 1989.

72. Ibid.

73. Ibid.

74. Joe Strauss, "Baseball: 3 pitchers released by Braves," *The Atlanta Journal-Constitution*, November 15, 1989.

75. Ray Ratto, "Don't blame the split-finger," *The San Francisco Chronicle*, August 5, 1989.

76. SP Ringel, M Treiharft, M Carry, R Fisher, and P Jacobs, "Suprascapular neuropathy in pitchers," *The American Journal of Sports Medicine* 18.1 (1990), 80–86.

77. JC Hsu, GA Paletta, RA Gambardella, and FW Jobe, "Musculocutaneous nerve injury in major league pitchers: A report of two cases," *The American Journal of Sports Medicine* 35.6 (June 2007), 1003–1006.

78. Joe Strauss, "Pitching plans for first round omit Carpenter," *St. Louis Post-Dispatch*, September 24, 2004; Joe Ostermeier, "Cards spring profiles: Carpenter is armed and ready for a repeat performance," *The* (IL) *Belleville News-Democrat*, March 13, 2005.

79. JC Hsu, GA Paletta, RA Gambardella, and FW Jobe, "Musculocutaneous nerve injury in major league pitchers: A report of two cases," *The American Journal of Sports Medicine* 35.6 (June 2007), 1003–1006.

80. Ibid.

81. Ibid.

Chapter 2

1. MJ Rohrer, PA Cardullo, AM Pappas, DA Phillips, and HB Wheeler "Axillary artery compression and thrombosis in throwing athlete," *Journal of Vascular Surgery* 11.6 (June 1990), 761–769.

2. Ibid.

3. GS DiFelice, GA Paletta Jr, BB Phillips, and RW Wright, "Effort thrombosis in elite throwing athlete," *American Journal of Sports Medicine* 30.5 (Sept.-Oct. 2002), 708–712.

4. MJ Rohrer, PA Cardullo, AM Pappas, DA

Phillips, and HB Wheeler "Axillary artery compression and thrombosis in throwing athlete," *Journal of Vascular Surgery* 11.6 (June 1990), 761–769.

5. AW Nichols, "The thoracic outlet syndrome in athletes," *Journal of the American Board of Family Practice* 9.5 (Sept.-Oct. 1996), 346–355.

6. Troy E. Renck, "Able to win without Walker: Shaky Cook undergoes tests," *Denver Post*, August 8, 2004; Mike Klis, "Cook's season over after scare. Blood clots in lungs sideline RHP," *Denver Post*, August 9, 2004; Mike Klis, "Cook's recovery outweighs return," *Denver Post*, August 18, 2004.

7. Troy E. Renck, "Changes a foot for Wilson: Cook's rehab slow," *Denver Post*, December 12, 2004; Irv Moss, "Nearly a year after he almost died there… Cook steps to mound," *Denver Post*, July 29, 2005.

8. Irv Moss, "Nearly a year after he almost died there… Cook steps to mound," *Denver Post*, July 29, 2005; Troy E. Renck, "Phils strike quick in win: Cook keeps perspective: PHILLIES 8, ROCKIES 7," *Denver Post*, July 31, 2005; Thomas Harding, "Heart of Order: Aaron Cook," MLB.com, October 22, 2007.

9. Ibid.

10. Jon Paul Morosi, "Bondo done in '08: Blood clot likely to sideline right-hander rest of season," *Detroit Free Press*, June 8, 2008.

11. Steve Kornacki, "Blood clot stops Bonderman: Detroit likely loses pitcher for the rest of season," *The Grand Rapids Press*, June 8, 2008.

12. Jon Paul Morosi, "Bondo done in '08: Blood clot likely to sideline right-hander rest of season," *Detroit Free Press*, June 8, 2008.

13. John Lowe, "Bonderman surgery goes as anticipated: necessary rehab will definitely end season," *Detroit Free Press*, July 1, 2008.

14. Tom Gage, "Bonderman focused on next season," *Detroit Free Press*, July 8, 2009.

15. Harold L. Klawans, *Why Michael Couldn't Hit: and Other Tales of Neurology of Sports* (New York, NY: Avon Books, 1998), 157–171.

16. WS Fields, NA Lemak, and Y Ben-Menachem, "Thoracic outlet syndrome: a review and reference to stroke in major league pitcher," *American Journal of Roentgenology* 146.4 (April 1986), 809–814.

17. H. Klawans, *Why Michael Couldn't Hit*, 163.

18. Ibid., 168.

19. Ibid., 168.

20. Ibid., 169.

21. WS Fields, NA Lemak, and Y Ben-Menachem, "Thoracic outlet syndrome: a review and reference to stroke in major league pitcher," *American Journal of Roentgenology* 146.4 (April 1986), 809–814.

22. H Klawans, *Why Michael Couldn't Hit*, 170.

23. HS Tullos, WD Erwin, GW Woods, DC Wukasch, DA Cooley, and JW King, "Unusual

lesions of the pitching arm," *Clinical Orthopedics* 88 (1972), 169–1982: Miles Coverdale Jr., *Whitey Ford: A Biography* (Jefferson, NC: McFarland, 2006), 208.

24. HS Tullos, WD Erwin, GW Woods, DC Wukasch, DA Cooley, and JW King, "Unusual lesions of the pitching arm," *Clinical Orthopedics* 88 (1972), 169–1982.

25. Ibid.

26. Coverdale, *Whitey Ford: A Biography*, 196–197.

27. HS Tullos, WD Erwin, GW Woods, DC Wukasch, DA Cooley, and JW King, "Unusual lesions of the pitching arm," *Clinical Orthopedics* 88 (1972), 169–1982.

28. Coverdale, *Whitey Ford: A Biography*, 208.

29. Pete Goodwin, "Boyd surgery success," *The Boston Globe,* August 21, 1987.

30. MJ Rohrer, PA Cardullo, AM Pappas, DA Phillips, and HB Wheeler "Axillary artery compression and thrombosis in throwing athlete," *Journal of Vascular Surgery* 11.6 (June 1990), 761–769.

31. Steve Fainaru, "Boyd accepts one-year offer from Montreal," *The Boston Globe,* December 8, 1989.

32. Larry Whiteside, "Boyd treated for blood clots," *The Boston Globe*, August 5, 1988.

33. Bob Ryan, "Boyd through for season," *The Boston Globe,* September 10, 1988.

34. Steve Fainaru, "Boyd briefed on medication," *The Boston Globe*, August 15, 1989; Steve Fainaru, "Boyd will start for Pawtucket tonight," *The Boston Globe*, August 18, 1989.

35. Dan Shaughnessy, "Risky business with Boyd and Sox," *The Boston Globe*, August 6, 1989.

36. "Names: Boyd sidelined by blood clot in shoulder," *The Boston Globe*, August 7, 1994; Nick Cafardo, "Boyd doesn't fear repercussions," *The Boston Globe*, January 18, 1995.

37. "Blood clot may sideline Wells for year," *The Washington Post*, February 27, 2008; Associated Press, "Pirates expect Wells by All-Star break," *Pittsburgh Tribune-Review*, March 7, 2006.

38. Tony DeMarco, "Wells set for surgery on blood clot," MLB.com, May 5, 2008.

39. Jack Etkin, "Padres 16, Rockies 7," *Rocky Mountain News*, August 11, 2008.

40. GJ Todd, AI Benvenisty, S Hershon, and LU Bigliani, "Aneurysms of the mid-axillary artery in major league pitchers: A report of two cases," *Journal of Vascular Surgery* 28 (1998), 702–709.

41. Ibid.

42. Lawrence K. Altman, "Baseball: No timetable set for Cone after surgery," *The New York Times*, May 11, 1996.

43. Rob Gloster, "That's what you call a comeback," *The* (Albany, NY) *Times Union*, September 3, 1996.

44. Evan Grant, "Rogers will missed rest of year," *The Dallas Morning News*, July 21, 2001;

Evan Grant, "Helling's shutout ends streak," *The Dallas Morning News*, July 31, 2001.

45. Jason Beck, "Rogers out three months after surgery," MLB.com, March 30, 2007; Patricia Anstett, "Rogers' surgeon: shoot for early July," *Detroit Free Press*, April 3, 2007; ESPN.com game stats for June 22, 2007.

46. Murray Chase, "Baseball: after aneurysm surgery, there's hope," *The New York Times*, May 24, 1996.

47. Claire Smith, "Mets Wallace has aneurysm, and faces surgery like Cone's," *The New York Times*, March 7, 1997.

48. Ibid.

49. Steve Rock, "Royals report," *Kansas City Star*, March 17, 2000.

50. Dick Kaegel, "Sports psychologist arrives at team camp: Royals notebook," *Kansas City Star*, February 25, 2000.

51. Mark Hale, "Numbness in hand sidelines Heredia," *New York Post*, March 4, 2005; David Lennon, "NOTEBOOK: Heredia too erratic on mound," *Newsday* (Melville, NY) on April 19, 2005.

52. Ben Shpigel, "Heredia suspended after test for steroids," *The New York Times*, October 19, 2005.

53. Chad Jennings, "Kennedy faces surgery for aneurysm," *Citizen's Voice* (Wilkes-Barre, PA), May 9, 2009; Associated Press, "New York Yankees right-hander Ian Kennedy still recovering from an aneurysm this year. Threw 25 pitchers off a mini-mound Tuesday and hopes to play minor league games before the season ends," *The Saratogian* (Saratoga Springs, NY), August 5, 2009; "YANKEES: Kennedy's comeback," *Newsday* (Long Island, NY), September 20, 2009.

54. John Strege, "Delucia faces surgery: ANGELS NOTES: The pitcher has an aneurysm in his right arm and may miss the rest of the season," *The Orange County Register* (CA), July 20, 1997; Maureen Delany, "DeLucia likely has aneurysm," *The Press-Enterprise* (Riverside, CA), July 20, 1997.

55. Associated Press, "DeLucia endures surgery," *Press-Telegram* (Long Beach, CA), July 22, 1997.

56. Bo Ryan, "Olerud a pro with no cons: adding veteran can only help," *The Boston Globe*, May 25, 2005; Hank Hersch, "A gentleman and a slugger," *Sports Illustrated* (SI.com), April 15, 1991.

Chapter 3

1. Tommy John with Dave Valenti, *TJ: My Twenty-six Years in Baseball* (New York, NY: Bantam Books, 1991).

2. Ibid., 143.

3. Ibid., 143.

4. Ibid., 144.

5. Ibid., 146.

6. Ibid., 149.

7. Ibid., 150.

8. Ibid., 154.

9. Ibid., 161.

10. Daniel Paulling, "Tommy John Surgery: few can cut it twice," *USA TODAY*, July 18, 2007.

11. Will Carroll and Thomas Gorman, "Inside Tommy John surgery," baseball-prospectus.com, September 22, 2004.

12. Mike Dodd, "Tommy John surgery: The pitcher's best friend," *USA TODAY*, July 28, 2003.

13. Brian Dohn, "Dreifort sidelined until next season. Injury: will have surgery on elbow for the second time in Dodger career," *Press-Telegram* (Long Beach, CA), July 4, 2001.

14. Mike Dodd, "Tommy John surgery: a career-saving procedure for many pitchers," *Baseball Digest*, May 2004.

15. Steve Kettmann, "A's clubhouse: Candiotti career a joint effort," *The San Francisco Chronicle*, May 26, 1998.

16. David Wells with Chris Kreski, *Perfect I'm Not* (New York, NY: HarperCollins, 2003), 20.

17. Ibid., 22.

18. Ibid., 167.

19. Marty Noble, "METS NOTEBOOK: Izzy has a quick recovery," *Newsday* (Melville, NY), September 28, 1996.

20. Associated Press, "Isringhausen to miss '98 season," *Vero Beach Press Journal* (FL), January 7, 1998.

21. Buster Olney, "BASBALL: Isringhausen will lose season to elbow surgery," *The New York Times*, January 6, 1998; Claire Smith, "BASEBALL: Japanese pitcher joins Mets starting staff," *The New York Times*, January 14, 1998.

22. Jeff Fletcher, "The future is now for A's Isringhausen: Ex-Met earns the closer role," *The Press Democrat* (Santa Rosa, CA), September 10, 1999.

23. Derrick Goold, "Isringhausen, Tampa Bay agree to minor-league deal," *St. Louis Post-Dispatch*, February 21, 2009.

24. Associated Press, "Demoted closer Isringhausen to undergo season ending elbow surgery," ESPN.com, September 5, 2008; Derrick Goold, "Surgery for Izzy," *St. Louis Post-Dispatch* on September 6, 2008; Bill Chastain, "Isringhausen done for season," MLB.com, June 15, 2009: Joe Smith, "Bartlett sets hits mark," *St. Petersburg Times* (FL), June 26, 2009.

25. Hal McCoy, "Pitcher Rijo considering retirement: Elbow problems have taken toll on the 33-year-old right-hander," *Dayton Daily News* (OH), April 16, 1998.

26. P Langer, P Fadale, and M Hulstyn, "Evolution of the treatment options of ulnar collateral ligament injuries," *British Journal of Sports Medicine* 40 (2006), 499–506.

27. Gary Nuhn, "Elbow has hurt Rijo for 13 years," *Dayton* (OH) *Daily News,* June 26, 1995.

28. Hal McCoy, "Rijo off to the doctor: asking

for teams' prayers," *Dayton Daily News* (OH) on July 20, 1995.

29. Ibid.

30. Jeff Horrigan, "Doctor rejects Rijo surgery, prescribes rest," *The Cincinnati Post*, July 25, 1995.

31. Hal McCoy, "Rijo's elbow gets full rebuild: ligament, tendon, nerve all figure in surgery: Reds notes," *Dayton Daily News* (OH), August 23, 1995.

32. Bill Peterson, "Rijo's rehab praised," *The Cincinnati Post*, March 18, 1996; Jeff Horrigan, "More surgery possible for Rijo," *The Cincinnati Post*, March 27, 1996; Jeff Horrigan, "Rijo's swift return suffers setback," *The Cincinnati Post*, April 5, 1996; Hal McCoy, "Rijo's setback inevitable: surgery was unavoidable," *Dayton Daily News* (OH) on April 9, 1996.

33. Jeff Horrigan, "Rijo allowed to test right elbow," *The Cincinnati Post*, May 11, 1996; Jeff Horrigan, "Frustrated Rijo considers retirement," *The Cincinnati Post*, July 2, 1996; Jeff Horrigan, "Rijo doesn't figure to return this year," *The Cincinnati Post*, August 5, 1996.

34. "Marlins sign Bonilla to multiyear deal," *The Cincinnati Post*, November 22, 1996.

35. Jeff Horrigan, "Rijo expects return in last shot," *The Cincinnati Post,* May 10, 1997; Jeff Horrigan, "Surgery halts Rijo comeback," *The Cincinnati Post*, August 15, 1997.

36. Tony Jackson, "Rijo back home: return to team unclear," *The Cincinnati Post*, May 8, 2003; Hal McCoy, "Rijo's days on the mound appear over," *Dayton Daily News* (OH), June 11, 2003.

38. Bob Lutz, "Thrown for loss, Dreifort prepares to rebuild with rebuilt elbow," *Wichita Eagle*, March 30, 1995.

39. Ken Daley, "Dreifort is advised to undergo surgery," *Daily News of Los Angeles* (CA), March 4, 1995; Ken Daley, "Dodger notes: Claire rejects demotion notion: request for farm assignment nixed," *Daily News of Los Angeles* (CA), March 15, 1995.

40. Joe Christensen, "L.A. gives Dreifort what he wanted: BASEBALL: Right-hander gets five-year deal worth $55 million, the contract he asked for all along," *Ventura County Star* (CA), December 12, 2000.

41. Brian Dohn, "Dodgers update: Dreifort outlook looks grim," *Daily News of Los Angeles* (CA), July 1, 2001.

42 Joe Christensen, "Dreifort surgery smooth: DODGERS: He still expected to miss a year after second elbow reconstruction," *The Press-Enterprise* (Riverside, CA), July 11, 2001.

43. "Dreifort's future is uncertain," *The Kansas City Star*, May 2, 2005.

44. Brian Dohn, "Dreifort sidelined until next season — injury: will have surgery on elbow for the second time in Dodger career," *Press-Telegram* (Long Beach, CA), July 4, 2001.

45. Phil Wallace, "The trials and tribulations of Darren Dreifort," LAlist.com, August 19, 2004.

46. J.D., "Brian Anderson and Tommy John surgery," draysbay.com, February 12, 2008; David Boyce, "Birthday is a little miss and hit. Sweeney welcomes daughter, not pitch that plunks him," *The Kansas City Star*, July 23, 2005.

47. Richard Durrett, "Injury puts lefty's recovery on hold. Anderson has MRI after leaving game with elbow soreness," *The Dallas Morning News,* June 7, 2006; Jan Hubbard, "Rangers Notes: Anderson re-injures elbow ligament," *Fort Worth Star-Telegram* (TX) on June 8, 2006; Bob Dutton, "Royals working to sign top pick. Team isn't discouraged about slow progress in coming to terms with Hochever," *The Kansas City Star*, July 2, 2006.

48. Maureen Mullen, "Anderson suffers career-ending injury," tampabay.rays.mlb.com/news, March 13, 2008.

49. "Vernon 'Lefty' Gomez" at latinosportslegends.com/lgomez.

50. Ben Shpigel, "A relieved Glavine says he will not need surgery," *The New York Times*, August 23, 2006; Ben Shpigel, "Glavine struggles in return, but the Mets are glad he's back," *The New York Times*, September 2, 2006.

51. David O'Brien, "Baseball Braves report: Glavine also has work on shoulder," *The Atlanta Journal-Constitution*, August 22, 2008.

52. "Baseball: Rollins, Victorino win Gold Gloves: Lidge surgery successful," *The Press of Atlantic City* (NJ), November 12, 2009.

53. Carlton Thompson, "Astros pin hopes on the future: Wagner faces surgery today," *Houston Chronicle*, June 27, 2000; Carlton Thompson, "Wagner's surgery successful," *Houston Chronicle*, June 28, 2000; Joseph Duarte, "Astros put Wagner on 15-day DL. MRI reveals closer has forearm strain," *Houston Chronicle*, June 5, 2001.

54. Associated Press, "Mets' closer Wagner could miss all of '09," *Chicago Tribune*, September 9, 2008; Ben Shpigel, "Wagner not giving up, but says Mets should move on," *The New York Times*, September 10, 2008; Brian Lewis, "It ain't over: Wagner vows to return somewhere down the line," *New York Post*, September 10, 2008.

55. P Langer, P Fadale, and M Hulstyn, "Evolution of the treatment options of ulnar collateral ligament injuries," *British Journal of Sports Medicine* 40 (2006), 499–506.

56. Ibid.

57. "Neagle has surgery: out 12–18 months," *Daily Camera* (Boulder, CO), July 31, 2003.

58. Joe Strauss, "More surgery for Carpenter," *St. Louis Post-Dispatch*, November 5, 2008; David George, "Healthy outlook for Carpenter," *The Palm Beach Post* (FL), March 1, 2009.

59. "MLB notebook: Atlanta's Soriano has elbow surgery on elbow," *El Paso Times* (TX), August 28, 2008; Marin Fennelly, "Soriano sightings rare, but he vows to be ready," *The Tampa Tribune*, March 13, 2010.

60. Joe Strauss, "Pujols has surgery. Procedure

should correct nerve problem in elbow. Situation with torn ligament is unchanged," *St. Louis Post-Dispatch*, October 14, 2008.

61. David Wilhelm, "Pujols has arthroscopic surgery on right elbow," *The Belleville* (IL) *News-Democrat*, October 22, 2009; Associated Press, "Albert has peace of mind," ESPN.com, February 21, 2010; Joe Strauss, "Pujols, Holliday arrive at Cardinals camp," *St. Louis Post-Dispatch*, February 22, 2010.

62. P Langer, P Fadale, and M Hulstyn, "Evolution of the treatment options of ulnar collateral ligament injuries," *British Journal of Sports Medicine* 40 (2006) 499–506.

63. Luke Atkinson, "Baseball Hall of Fame bid in jeopardy for Yankee pitcher and Bethany native Allie Reynolds," okgazette.com, February 10, 2010.

64. Ray Robinson, *The Greatest Yankees of Them All* (New York, NY: Putnam's, 1969), 96; Claire Smith, "Allie Reynolds, Star Pitcher for Yankees, is Dead at 79," *The New York Times* on December 28, 1994.

65. Ray Robinson, *The Greatest Yankees of Them All*, 86.

66. Milton Gross, "Reynolds' Knots 'n' Naughts surgery in 1951," *Baseball Digest*, January 1952.

67. Allen Barra, *Yogi Berra: Eternal Yankee* (New York, NY: W. W. Norton, 2009), 146; Robinson, *The Greatest Yankees of Them All*, 90–95.

68. Ed Gruver, *Koufax* (Dallas, TX: Taylor Publishing, 2000), 125–126.

69. Sandy Koufax with Ed Linn (New York, NY: Viking Press, 1966), 222.

70. Ibid., 223.

71. Ibid., 224.

72. Ibid., 225.

73. Ibid., 219.

74. Bob Hunter, "Sandy's Ailing: All's Not Well with Dodgers," *The Sporting News*, April 17, 1965.

75. Jane Leavy, *Sandy Koufax: A Lefty's Legacy* (New York, NY: HarperCollins, 2002) 159.

76. Sandy Koufax with Ed Linn, *Koufax*, 237, 238.

77. Jane Leavy, *Sandy Koufax: A Left's Legacy*, 158, 230.

78. Ed Gruver, *Koufax*, 212.

79. Bob Hunter, "One bombshell after another: Dodgers shake," *The Sporting News*, December 3, 1966.

80. KP Black and DE Taylor, "Current concepts in the treatment of common compartment syndromes in athletes," *Sports Medicine* 15.6 (June 1993), 408–418.

81. Ibid.

82. CC Tubb and D Vermillion, "Chronic exertional compartment syndrome after minor injury to lower extremity," *Military Medicine* 166.4 (April 2001), 366–368.

83. Joe Strauss, "Lohse agrees to $41 million deal," *St. Louis Post-Dispatch*, September 30, 2008.

84. Joe Strauss, "Cardinals put Lohse on hold: Notebook: Persistent arm stiffness pushes back his next start," *St. Louis Post-Dispatch*, May 28, 2009; Rick Hummel, "Lohse is on disabled list: Notebook: Pitcher is expected to be out more than 15 days," *St. Louis Post-Dispatch*, June 6, 2009.

85. Joe Strauss, "Lohse is placed on DL: Cardinals notebook: Hurler suffered groin strain Friday at San Diego," *St. Louis Post Dispatch*, August 23, 2009.

86. Joe Strauss, "Lohse has MRI on right forearm: Notebook: Pitcher says it doesn't hurt but that 'something's different here and there,'" *St. Louis Post-Dispatch*, September 15, 2009.

87. Joe Strauss, "Lohse continues his search: Notebook: Pitcher with forearm problem sees specialist today: stay on DL looks certain," *St. Louis Post-Dispatch*, May 26, 2010.

88. Matthew Leach and Micheal Bleach, "Lohse in good spirits after surgery," MLB.com, May 31, 2010.

89. Jerry Cresnick, "Lowry to have circulatory problem fixed," ESPN.com, May 19, 2009.

90. Andrew Baggarly, "Misdiagnosis of Lowry denied," *San Jose Mercury News* (CA), May 20, 2009; John Shea and Henry Schulman, "Agent, Giants at odds," *San Francisco Chronicle*, May 20, 2009.

Chapter 4

1. Nick Cafardo, "Otiz goes on DL: Sheath, not tendon, is injured in wrist," *The Boston Globe*, June 3, 2008; Amalie Benjamin, "Hoping to avoid surgery, Ortiz is cast in uncertainty," *The Boston Globe*, June 4, 2008.

2. "Ortiz in lineup despite click in wrist," *The Sun* (Lowell, MA), August 6, 2008; Jeff Horrigan, "Red Sox NOTEBOOK: All in wrist Ortiz says injury still a problem," *Boston Herald*, September 8, 2008; John Tomase, "Rays 3, Red Sox 1: BASEBALL: Frustrated Rare taste of failure for Otiz," *Boston Herald*, October 20, 2008.

3. Adam Kilgore, "Comeback or not, Ortiz in fine form," *The Boston Globe*, October 5, 2009.

4. Associated Press, "Weeks out for '09 with wrist tear," ESPN.com, May 18, 2009.

5. Tom Haudricourt, "Rickie Weeks out for season: High hopes get dashed: Leadoff hitter needs surgery on left wrist," *Milwaukee Journal Sentinel* (WI), May 19, 2009.

6. Andrew Baggarly, "Whiffs cause DeRosa to smile: New Giant is encouraged by pain-free swings," *San Jose Mercury News* (CA), March 8, 2010.

7. Joe Strauss, "DeRosa goes on the disabled list: Notebook: Wrist problem turns out to be worse than Cardinals first believed," *St. Louis Post-Dispatch*, July 8, 2009.

8. Derrick Goold, "Cards need to work on back of rotation: Baseball," *St. Louis Post-Dispatch*, October 29, 2009.

9. Carl Steward, "DeRosa says wrist surgery on tendon 'a total failure,'" *San Jose Mercury News* (CA), May 12, 2010.

10. Alex Pavlovic, "Giants update: Mark DeRosa to get another opinion on injured wrist," *The Oakland* (CA) *Tribune*, May 25, 2010.

11. Bay Area News Group, "Giants need hitter: is Fielder on the Radar," *The Oakland* (CA) *Tribune*, July 3, 2010.

12. Chico Harlan, "Johnson hurts wrist, returns for MRI exam," *The Washington* (DC) *Post*, May 15, 2008; Chic Harlan, "Johnson lands on DL-Young is called up," *The Washington* (DC) *Post*, May 16, 2008; Associated Press, "Major league baseball: Nats' Johnson could miss rest of season," *The Press of Atlantic City* (NJ), June 24, 2008.

13. George A. King III, "Wrist surgery scheduled for injury-prone Johnson," *New York Post*, May 18, 2010; George A. King III, "Sore leg keeps Swisher on bench," *New York Post*, August 26, 2010.

14. Marc Narducci, "Injury ends Burrell's season: Slugger hurt wrist in practice, will have surgery," *The Philadelphia Inquirer*, August 10, 2004; Sam Carchidi, "Burrell's rapid return features a homerun," *The Philadelphia Inquirer*, September 4, 2004; Michael Silverman, "RED SOX NOTEBOOK: Knife unlikely Doc says rest should be enough for Ortiz," *Boston Herald*, June 6, 2008.

15. AC Rettig and DV Patel, "Epidemiology of elbow, forearm, and wrist injuries in the athlete," *Clinical Sports Medicine* 14.2 (April 1995), 289–297.

16. JJ Walsh 4th and AT Bishop, "Diagnosis and management of hamate hook fractures," *Hand Clinics* 16.3 (August 2000), 397–403.

17. Tony Cooper, "Canseco's surgery a success," *The San Francisco Chronicle*, May 11, 1989.

18. Ibid.

19. Tony Cooper, "Canseco's surgery a success," *The San Francisco Chronicle*, May 11, 1989: David Bush, "Canseco requires surgery on wrist," *San Francisco Chronicle*, May 10, 1989.

20. Tony Cooper, "Canseco's surgery a success," *The San Francisco Chronicle*, May 11, 1989.

21. Tim Hips, "Conseco twins share eerie twists of fate," *The Orlando Sentinel*, July 16, 1989.

22. Ben Shpigel, "Out of Colorado, Mets' problems far from over," *The New York Times*, July 6, 2007.

23. Kelly Theiser, "Notes: Gomez reacts to Santana trade," MLB.com, January 31, 2008.

24. Barry Svrluga, "Nat's Zimmerman Breaks Bone in Wrist," *Washington Post*, November 7, 2007.

25. Mike Ritter, "Mather finished with broken wrist bone," MLB.com, September 2, 2008; Joe Strauss, "Hand surgery ends Mather's season," *St. Louis Post-Dispatch*, September 3, 2008.

26. Derrick Goold, "Wainwright's injury is one that can linger," *St. Louis Post-Dispatch*, June 22, 2008.

27. Ibid.

28. "De La Rosa's rare injury rocks rotation," *The Denver Post*, April 28, 2010; Brent Briggeman, "De La Rosa and Bucholz will rehab with Sky Sox," *The* (Colorado Springs) *Gazette*, June 19, 2010; "Stewart's six RBIs, two homers lifts Rockies," *The* (Canon City, CO) *Daily Record*, July 10, 2010.

29. "Crawford on DL, Baldelli back," blogs.tampabay.com/rays, August 10, 2008; Bill Chastain, "Crawford to have surgery on hand," MLB.com, August 12, 2008.

30. Brittany Ghiroli, "Crawford out for rest of season," MLB.com on September 18, 2008.

31. JJ Peterson and LW Bancroft, "Injuries of the fingers and thumb in an athlete," *Clinics in Sports Medicine* 25.3 (July 2006), 527–542.

32. Jason Beck, "Zumaya to have surgery," MLB.com, May 7, 2007.

33. John Lowe, "Zumaya to miss three months: Right-hand finger has ruptured tendon," *Detroit Free Press*, May 8, 2007; Jon Paul Morosi, "Zumaya glad to contribute: Miller vs. Yanks," *Detroit Free Press*, August 22, 2007.

34. Jon Paul Morosi, "Zoom gloom shoulder to blame: freak injuries follow reliever," *Detroit Free Press*, November 2, 2007.

35. Ed Gruver, *Koufax* (Dallas, Texas: Taylor Publishing, 2000), 139–145.

36. Ibid., 142.

37. Ibid., 143.

38. Ibid., 144.

39. Ibid., 144.

40. Ibid., 139–145.

Chapter 5

1. Bob Hohler, "There's concern over Schillings ankle," *The Boston Globe*, October 10, 2004.

2. Associated Press, "Ace in the hole? It looks like it," *The* (Lowell, MA) *Sun*, October 14, 2004.

3. Bob Hohler, and Raja Mishra "Morgan magic: Team doctor works wonders for Schilling," *The Boston Globe*, October 21, 2004.

4. Bob Hohler, "Two to go: with second win in hand, Red Sox head to St. Louis halfway to elusive championship: Red Sox head to St. Louis halfway home," *The Boston Globe*, October 25, 2004.

5. Bob Hohler, "Team is mum on ace: Schilling's status simply day to day," *The Boston Globe*, October 26, 2004.

6. Jeff Horrigan, "BASEBALL: All's well for Schilling after 3-hour surgery," *Boston Herald*, November 10, 2004.

7. Associated Press, "Hall enshrines Schillings bloody sock," nbcsports.msnbc.com, February 11, 2005.

8. Derrick Goold, "Freese is done for the season. Third baseman will need surgery to repair torn tissue in his ankle," *St. Louis Post-Dispatch*, August 4, 2010.

9. Joe Strauss, "Hex continues at third for Cardinals. Freese's injury puts Redbirds back at square one in six-year search for consistent production at hot corner," *St. Louis Post-Dispatch*, August 8, 2010.

10. Derrick Goold, "Freese is on better footing. Cardinals third baseman says he's progressing after surgery on both ankles," *St. Louis Post-Dispatch*, December 25, 2010.

11. H Lemont, KM Ammirati, and N Usen, "Plantar fasciitis: a degenerative process (fasciosis) without inflammation," *Journal of the American Podiatric Medical Association* 93.3 (May-June 2003), 234–237.

12. C Cole, C Seto, and J Gazewood, "Plantar fasciitis" Evidence based review of diagnosis and therapy," *American Family Physician*, 72.11 (December 1, 2005), 2237–2242.

13. George A. Sheehan, "Morton's foot," *Medical Advice for Runners* (Mountain View, CA: World Publications, 1978), 76–79.

14. "Outfielder undergoes foot surgery," *Jefferson City* (MO) *News-Tribune*, June 10, 2007.

15. C Kim, MR Cashdollar, RW Medicino, AR Catanzariti, and LFuge, "Incidence of plantar fascia ruptures following corticosteroid injections," *Foot and Ankle Specialist* 3.6 (December 2010), 335–337.

16. SK Williams and M Brage, "Heel pain: Plantar fasciitis and Achilles enthesopathy," *Clinical Sports Medicine*, 23.1 (Jan. 2004), 123–144.

17. C Cole, C Seto, and J Gazewood, "Plantar fasciitis: Evidence based review of diagnosis and therapy," *American Family Physician*, 72.11 (December 1, 2005), 2237–2242.

18. D Rabago, A Slattengren, and A Zgierska, "Prolotherapy in primary care practice," *Primary Care*, 37.1 (March 2010), 65–80.

19. L Miszezyk, B Jochymek, and J Wozniak, "Retrospective evaluation of radiotherapy in plantar fasciitis," *The British Journal of Radiology* 80. 958 (October 2007), 829–834.

20. Bart Barnes, "American Icon: Joe DiMaggio dies at 84," *Washington Post*, March 8, 1999.

21. Richard Ben Cramer, *Joe DiMaggio: The Hero's Life*, (New York, NY: Simon & Schuster, 2000), 221.

22. Jack B. Moore, *Joe DiMaggio: Baseball's Yankee Clipper* (New York, NY: Praeger, 1987), 61.

23. Richard Ben Cramer, *Joe DiMaggio: The Hero's Life*, 226.

24. Ibid., 248.

25. Ibid., 227.

26. Ibid., 249.

27. Ibid., 254.

28. Ibid., 255.

29. Jack B. Moore, *Joe DiMaggio: Baseball's Yankee Clipper*, 68.

30. Ibid., 70.

31. Ibid., 74.

32. Ibid., 73, 74.

33. Ibid., 74.

34. Ibid.

35. Richard Ben Cramer, *Joe DiMaggio: The Hero's Life*, 314.

36. "Debate surrounding McGwire, Hall of Fame intensifies," usatoday.com, December 5, 2006.

37. "McGwire has surgery on sore heel," *San Francisco Chronicle*, September 25, 1993; Steve Ketterman, "A's NOTES: McGwire undergoes surgery on left heel: recurring problem solved," *San Francisco Chronicle*, August 31, 1994; Steve Ketterman, "McGwire: Foot problems kicked. After 2 injury riddled years, slugger stays healthy," *San Francisco Chronicle*, February 14, 1995.

38. Steve Ketterman, "McGwire: Foot problems kicked. After 2 injury riddled years, slugger stays healthy," *San Francisco Chronicle* on February 14, 1995.

39. "Healthtronics Inc. receives FDA approval to market the Ossa Tron Extracorporeal shock wave device for plantar fasciitis," www.findarticles.com, October 13, 2000.

40. Derrick Goold, "Pujols foot pain flares up again," *St. Louis Post-Dispatch*, January 18, 2005.

41. H. Darr Beiser, "Pujols won't be slowed by sore heel," usatoday.com, February 20, 2005; Amy Bertrand, "FOOT FAULT: Plantar fasciitis can cramp your lifestyle, but treatments ranging from splints to shock waves can offer relief," *St. Louis Post-Dispatch*, March 21, 2005.

42. Joe Strauss, "Exodus to WBC begins for Cards," *St Louis Post-Dispatch*, March 3, 2006.

43. E-mail information from columnist Joe Strauss of *St Louis Post Dispatch*, November 26, 2007.

Chapter 6

1. Elaine M. Marieb and Jon Mallat, *Human Anatomy* 3rd Ed. (San Francisco, CA: Benjamin/Cummings Publishing, 2001), 142–143.

2. Ibid.

3. Knapp and Garrett Jr. "Stress Fractures: General Concepts," *Clinics in Sports Medicine*, 16.2, (April 1997), 339–357.

4. CM Sofka, "Imaging of Stress Fractures," *Clinics in Sports Medicine* 25.1 (January 2006), 53–62.

5. RA Snyder, MC Koester, and WR Dunn, "Epidemiology of Stress Fractures," *Clinics in Sports Medicine* 25.1 (January 2006), pages 37–52

6. GO Matheson, DB Clement, DC McKenzie, JE Taunton, DR Lloyd-Smith, and JG MacIntyre, "Stress Fractures in Athletes: A study of 320 Cases," *The American Journal of Sports Medicine* 15.1, (Jan.-Feb. 1987), 46–58.

7. Ibid.

8. GL Jones, "Upper extremity stress frac-

tures," *Clinics in Sports Medicine* 25.1 (January 2006), 159–174.

9. Buster Olney, "A stress fracture leaves O'Neill status in doubt," *The New York Times*, September 11, 2001.

10. Susan Slusser, "Reeling A's lose Mulder for season," *The San Francisco Chronicle*, August 23, 2001; Susan Slusser, "Mulder unlikely for play-offs," *The San Francisco Chronicle*, September 21, 2001.

11. Evan Grant, "Bell frustrated after being demoted. Pitcher may be out of chances to start, or play, for Rangers," *The Dallas Morning News*, August 24, 2002.

12. Unnamed article by unknown author, oklahomaredhawks.com/news, June 26, 2003; Jesse Sanchez, "Notes: Ludwig thankful," MLB.com, July 2, 2003.

13. Sean Horgan, "Ludwick on ball for quick return: Outfielder comes back from hip injury with help from regimen," *The Dallas Morning News*, February 16, 2003.

14. Maureen Fulton, "Off-season: best season for Ludwick," *The* (Cleveland, OH) *Plain Dealer*, September 15, 2004.

15. Bob Foltman, "Thomas out 8 weeks: DH hobbled by stress fracture in left foot," *Chicago Tribune*, July 17, 2004.

16. "Guillen regrets comments made about Thomas: AL beat," *Seattle Times*, April 19, 2005; "Guillen says Thomas was part of bad attitude," ESPN.com, April 18, 2004.

17. Bob Foltman, "Doctors made call to put off surgery: Schneider: Thomas not that far behind," *Chicago Tribune*, October 8, 2004.

18. "White Sox' Thomas likely done for the season," *The Washington Post*, July 31, 2005.

19. Mark Gonzales, "Thomas is out — for now. Sox slugger's return depends on health," *Chicago Tribune*, November 5, 2005.

20. Andrew Baggarly, "A's hope to put 'Big Hurts' on rivals," *The Oakland Tribune*, January 26, 2006.

21. "Thomas shelved for rest of year," *San Francisco Chronicle*, September 4, 2008.

22. John Lowe, "Consensus: The old Jack will be back," *Detroit Free Press*, July 26, 1989; Gene Guidi, "Morris on DL for first time," *Detroit Free Press* on May 26, 1989.

23. Rock Kubatko, "Good news, bad news: Orioles Loewen has a stress fracture, will be sidelined for at least 8 weeks," *The* (Baltimore) *Sun*, May 7, 2007; Mark Craig, "Orioles place Loewen on the DL: pitcher shelved, elbow soreness," *The Washington Post*, April 27, 2008.

24. Paul Sullivan, "Ramirez: MVP not in the cards," *Chicago Tribune*, September 26, 2008.

25. Joe Haakenson, "Angels notebook: Percival flexing muscles," *Daily News of Los Angeles* on April 24, 2001.

26. Juan C. Rodriguez, "Alfonseca (elbow) out

for two months," *South Florida Sun-Sentinel* (Fort Lauderdale, FA), April 23, 2005.

27. David Andriesen "Jimenez surgery set: lefty injured left elbow on Wednesday," *Seattle Post-Intelligencer* on March 10, 2007.

28. Mike Berardino and Juan Rodriguez, "Tankersley to have surgery," *Sun Sentinel* (Fort Lauderdale, FL), April 15, 2009,

29. Tom Cage, "Bats perk up in heat," *The Detroit News* July 6, 2010; Ron Beard, "Zumaya's injury is rare, yet treatable," *The Detroit News*, June 30, 2010.

30. Kat O'Brien, "Healthy Borcail rebuilding career," *Fort Worth Star-Telegram* (TX) March 4, 2004.

31. T. R. Sullivan, "McCarthy shut down for two weeks," MLB.com, August 15, 2007.

32. Joe Christensen, "More testing shows Radke has a rare stress fracture. The veteran has an injured glenoid in his shoulder, and the return for this year, or ever, is uncertain," *Star Tribune: Newspaper of the Twin Cities,* September 2, 2006.

33. John Lowe, "Tigers corner: Stress fracture latest setback for Zumaya: Reliever will be re-evaluated after resting shoulder for 6–8 weeks," *Detroit Free Press*, September 13, 2008; Associated Press, "Tigers' Zumaya has stress fracture in shoulder," sportsillustrated.com, September 12, 2008.

34. "Yanks' Hughes could be sidelined until July," *The Washington Post*, March 2, 2008.

35. Susan Slusser, "Ailing A's get a lift: Saarloos stars: Crosby on DL," *San Francisco Chronicle*, April 7, 2005.

36. Henry Shulman, "GIANTS NOTEBOOK: Injured ribs affected Morris at end of season," *San Francisco Chronicle,* October 3, 2006.

37. Gordon Edes and Amalie Benjamin, "Wakefield out with stress fracture in rib cage," *The Boston Globe,* July 20, 2006.

38. Tony Cooper "Canseco's surgery a success," *San Francisco Chronicle*, May, 11, 1989.

39. Tyler Kepner, "Baseball: Hand injury sidelines Yank's Johnson and halts rise," *The New York Times,* May 17, 2003.

40. Ken Daley, "Cordero done for season," *The Dallas Morning News,* July 1, 2001.

41. Roch Kubatko, "Good news, bad news: Orioles Loewen has a stress fracture; will be sidelined for at least 8 weeks," *The* (Baltimore) *Sun*, May 7, 2007.

42. Marc Craig, "Orioles place Loewen on the DL: pitcher shelved; elbow soreness," *The Washington Post*, April 27, 2008.

43. Marc Craig, "Good news for Loewen's left arm," *The Washington Post*, May 6, 2008.

44. Jeff Zrebiec, "O's Loewen finished as a pitcher. Elbow woes force lefty to try career as outfielder," *The* (Baltimore, MD) *Sun*, July 20, 2008; Roch Kubatko, "Crowley looks forward to working with Loewen," *The* (Baltimore, MD) *Sun*, July 23, 2008.

45. Jeff Zrebiec, "Loewen turns down O's to sign with Blue Jays," *The* (Baltimore, MD) *Sun,* October 25, 2008.

46. John Lowe, "Consensus: The old Jack will be back," *Detroit Free Press,* July 26, 1989.

47. Gene Guidi, "Morris on DL for first time," *Detroit Free Press* on May 26, 1989.

48. Kelsie Smith, "Radke joins Twins Hall of Fame: Righty pitched through pain, misses his former teammates," *St. Paul Pioneer Press,* July 12, 2009.

49. Joe Christensen, "More testing shows Radke has a rare stress fracture. The veteran has an injured glenoid in his shoulder, and the return for this year, or ever, is uncertain," *Star Tribune: Newspaper of the Twin Cities,* September 2, 2006.

50. Barry Svrtuga, "For Twins, Radke shoulders heavy load. After serious injury, righty might be pitching last game," *The Washington Post,* October 6, 2006.

51. Tom Powers, "Radke efficient in closing act," *St. Paul Pioneer Press* (MN), December 20, 2006.

52. Henry Shulman, "Aces up the sleeve: Morris, Lowry bounce back to be surprise early leaders of Giant's staff," *San Francisco Chronicle,* May 25, 2007.

53. Gordon Edes and Amalie Benjamin, "Wakefield out with stress fracture in rib cage," *The Boston Globe,* July 20, 2006.

54. Gordon Edes, "Sox left in Orioles Wake," *The Boston Globe,* September 14, 2006.

55. Kat O'Brien, "YANKEES 5, WHITE SOX 1: A not too shabby start by Hughes shows promise for next season after 4 1/2 month on sideline," *Newsday* (Long Island, NY), September 18, 2008; "Yanks Hughes could be sidelined until July," *The Washington Post,* March 2, 2008.

Chapter 7

1. Ralph Kiner and Danny Peary, *Baseball Forever: Reflections on 60 Years of Baseball* (Chicago, IL: Triumph Books USA, 2004).

2. Elliot Almond, "Johnson ok: Spring return expected," *The Seattle Times,* September 12, 1996; "Big Unit done in Big Apple? Baseball Yankees talking with several teams about a trade," *The Seattle Times,* December 26, 2006; Nick Piecoro, "Team gains welcome depth with 3 waiver acquisitions," *The* (Phoenix, AZ) *Arizona Republic,* August 5, 2007.

3. Elliot Almond, "Johnson ok: Spring return expected," *The Seattle Times,* September 12, 1996; Sarah Trotto, "Johnson at 44, hopes to create some memories," *The Arizona Daily Star* (Tucson, AZ), February 17, 2008.

4. Steve Kettmann, "Randy Johnson throws BP today," *The San Francisco Chronicle,* July 16, 1996.

5. Associated Press, "Randy Johnson back on disabled list," *The New York Times,* July 4, 2007.

6. Steve Kettmann, "Randy Johnson throws BP today," *The San Francisco Chronicle,* July 16, 1996.

7. Associated Press, "Randy Johnson back on disabled list," *The New York Times,* July 4, 2007.

8. Sarah Trotto, "Johnson at 44, hopes to create some memories," *The Arizona Daily Star* (Tucson, AZ), February 17, 2008.

9. JN Gibson and G Waddell, "Surgical interventions for lumbar disc prolapse: updated Cochrane review," *Spine* 32.16 (July 15, 2007), 1735–1747.

10. Joe Crowley, "Crede placed on DL; offence still missing: Yankees 5, White Sox 1," *The* (Aurora, IL) *Beacon News,* June 7, 2007; Joe Crowley, "Crede's career at Crossroads: Sox third baseman on DL, faces decision as to handle ailing back," *Chicago Sun-Times,* June 7, 2007; Mark Gonzales, "Losing Crede, not all hope: third baseman likely through for year: PHILLIES 7, WHITE SOX 3," *Chicago Tribune,* June 13, 2007.

11. Dave van Dyck, "Whispers" *Chicago Tribune,* November 5, 2008; Phil Rogers, "Crede a pleasant surprise for Twins: Ex-Sox third baseman making an impression," *Chicago Tribune,* March 27, 2009.

12. Associated Press, "Crede to have third back surgery," ESPN.com, September 21, 2009.

13. Toni Ginnetti, "Fractured finger sidelines Teahan," *Chicago Sun-Times,* June 2, 2010.

14. Thomas Harding, "Crede signs Minor League deal with Rockies," MLB.com, January 19, 2011.

15. Jack O'Connell, "Don Mattingly," *The Sporting News,* April 1, 1991.

16. "Mattingly out 2 weeks with two injured discs," *Detroit Free Press* on June 9, 1987.

17. Jack O'Connell, "Don Mattingly: New York Yankees," *The Sporting News,* April 1, 1991.

18. Ibid.

19. Jack O'Connell, "Mattingly: Does back pain signal end," *The Sporting News,* August 20, 1990.

20. Richard Justice, "Mattingly learning to take it easier. Slower steadier pace key to back recovery," *Washington Post,* March 11, 1991.

21. Jon Heyman, "New York Yankees," *The Sporting News,* February 3, 1997; Dick Kaegel "Kansas City Royals," *The Sporting News,* February 10, 1997.

22. David Wells with Chris Kreski, *Perfect I'm Not* (New York, NY: HarperCollins, 2003), 178.

23. Rob Oiler, "Wells, Reds overcome slow start-pitcher weathers first inning, gets support in 8–1 victory," *The Columbus Dispatch* (OH), September 15, 1995.

24. David Wells with Chris Kreski, *Perfect I'm Not,* 178.

25. Ibid., 348.

26. Ibid., 202.

27. Ibid., 371.

28. Ibid., 14.

29. Ibid.

30. Associated Press, "Canseco's problem is back again," *Chicago Tribune*, July 13, 1999.

31. Mike Klis, "From dearth to overload, Rockies pick up catcher Henandez," *The Denver Post*, January 15, 2002.

32. "Dodgers' Brown has back surgery: return uncertain," *Detroit Free Press*, June 12, 2002.

33. Associated Press, "Reds part ways with Larkin," *Chicago Tribune*, October 13, 2004.

34. Troy E Renck, "Back surgery for Helton," *The Denver Post*, September 25, 2008.

35. Associated Press, "Boston backup Kotsay undergoes back surgery," sportsillustrated.com, February 4, 2009.

36. SC Scherping Jr, "Cervical disc disease in the athlete," *Clinics in Sports Medicine* 21.1 (January 2002), 37–47; JM Rhee, T Yoon, and KD Riew, "Cervical radiculopathy," *Journal of the American Academy of Orthopedic Surgery* 15.8 (August 2007), 486–494; RJ Nasca, "Cervical radiculopathy: current diagnosis and treatment options," *Journal of Orthopedic Advances* 18.1 (Spring 2009), 13–18.

37. Carrie Muskat "Jackson fine with new hip," *USA TODAY*, September 1, 1995.

38. Joe Strauss, "Condition may explain Duncan's decline," *St. Louis Post-Dispatch*, August 3, 2008; Joe Strauss, "Surgery ends Duncan's pain: Outfielder won't be able to play until next year, but he expects to be ready to go 'full-bore' by then," *St. Louis Post-Dispatch*, August 6, 2008.

39. Joe Strauss, "Condition may explain Duncan's decline," *St. Louis Post-Dispatch*, August 3, 2008.

40. Alden Gonzales, "Duncan's return a bonus for Redbirds," MLB.com, April 2, 2009.

41. Joe Strauss, "Chris Duncan still talks a good game," *St. Louis Post-Dispatch*, April 18, 2011.

42. Ibid.

43. Patrick Saunders, "Toughing it out: Walker battling a debilitating neck injury all season, not giving in to pain because he wants one more chance at a world title," *The Denver Post*, October 4, 2005.

44. Ibid.

45. Derrick Goold, "Another shot helps Walker join line-up," *St. Louis Post-Dispatch,* September 28, 2005.

Chapter 8

1. Dr. Peter H. Gott, "Aseptic necrosis usually due to injury," *Pittsburgh Post-Gazzette*, July 31, 1991.

2. Barry Svrluga, "Nationals' Johnson suffers broken leg. Femur fractured in collision on field," *The Washington Post*, September 24, 2006

3. "A long struggle to get back up and running: 16 month after breaking leg, Nats' Johnson is ready to battle for the job at first base," *The Washington Post*, January 24, 2008.

4. David Schoen, "Ellis gone for season with

injury to shoulder," *Oakland Tribune*, April 11, 2004.

5. Frank Luksa, "Knuckler retired, but Hough busy," *The Dallas Morning News*, July 2, 1998.

6. Mark Zuckerman, "Totally disabled Belle limps away," *The Washington Times* on March 9, 2001.

7. Associated Press, "Retired All-Star Belle's hip resurfaced," sportsillustrated.com, March 15, 2007.

8. DF Amanatullah, Y Cheung, and PE Di Cesare, "Hip resurfacing arthroplasty: a review of the evidence for surgical technique, outcome, and complications," *Orthopedic Clinics of North America*, 41.2 (April 2010), 263–272.

9. HC Amstutz, MJ Le Duff, PA Campbell, TA Gruen, and LE Wisk "Clinical and radiological results of metal-on-metal hip resurfacing with a minimum ten-year follow-up," *Journal of Bone and Joint Surgery. American Volume*, 92.16 (November 2010), 2663–2271.

10. Todd Zolecki, "Hip injuries are on the rise around MLB," MLB.com, June 4, 2009.

11. Joe Strauss, "Isringhausen: Closer will undergo arthroscopic surgery on his left hip," *St. Louis Post-Dispatch* on September 20, 2006.

12. Joe Strauss, "Izzy signs 2-year extension," *St. Louis Post-Dispatch*, February 27, 2005.

13. Joe Strauss, "Izzy surgery an 'interm step,'" *St. Louis Post-Dispatch*, September 22, 2006.

14. Todd Zolecki, "Hip injuries are on the rise around MLB," MLB.com, June 4, 2009.

15. Seth Livingstone, "In baseball, hip surgery common among some stars," usatoday.com, July 1, 2009.

16. Doug Miller, "Delgado has second surgery on troubled hip," MLB.com, February 20, 2010; Jesse Sanchez, "Delgado rehabbing hip, ready for return," MLB.com, February 6, 2011.

17. Todd Zolecki, "Hip injuries are on the rise around MLB," MLB.com, June 4, 2009.

18. Ibid.

Chapter 9

1. Stan McNeal, "These side-splitters are serious business," sportingnews.com, March 15, 2007.

2. Jonathan Cluett, "Abdominal muscle strain," orthopedics.about.com.

3. Stan McNeal, "These side-splitters are serious business," sportingnews.com, March 15, 2007.

4. Stephanie Bell, "Oblique injuries strike at WBC. Or do they?" ESPN.com, March 16, 2009; Jorge Ortiz, "Oblique injuries putting strain on several major league teams," usatoday.com, July 1, 2008.

5. Matthew Leach, "Pujols out with strained oblique," MLB.com, June 3, 2006.

6. Stan McNeal, "These side-splitters are

serious business," sportingnews.com, March 15, 2007.

7. Bill Plaschke, "Suddenly, baseball is feeling side effects," *Los Angeles Times*, July 23, 2006.

8. Mark Feinsand, "Yanks' Damon leaves with sore oblique," MLB.com, July 5, 2006; Associated Press, "Indians' Blake lands on DL with strained oblique," ESPN.com on June 15, 2006.

9. Jorge Ortiz, "Oblique injuries putting strain on several major league teams," usatoday.com, July 1, 2008.

10. Ibid.

11. Anthony Castrovince, "Sabathia leaves with abdominal strain," MLB.com on April 3, 2006.

12. Associated Press, "Prior back on disabled list with strained oblique," ESPN.com, July 14, 2006.

13. Bill Plaschke, Suddenly, baseball is feeling side effects," *Los Angeles Times*, July 23, 2006.

14. Associated Press, "Hampton has oblique injury, will miss start of season," ESPN.com, March 8, 2007.

15. Jim Molony, "Astros interested in veteran Lieber," astros.com, November 6, 2007.

16. Bill Center, "Hampson rescues Padres after Young suffers injury," signonsandiego.com, July 25, 2007.

17. Lynn DeBruin "Cook not rusty from 79 day absence: Rockies starter proves he can perform again," *The Rocky Mountain News*, October 30, 2007.

18. Matthew Leach, "MRI confirms oblique tear for Carpenter," MLB.com, April 18, 2009.

19. Stephanie Bell, "Oblique injuries strike at WBC. Or do they?" ESPN.com, March 16, 2009.

20. "Blanton to start season on 15-day DL," ESPN.com, April 1, 2010.

21. Associated Press, "Angels Pineiro to miss 6–8 weeks," foxsports.com, July 28, 2010.

22. Associated Press, "Oblique strain lands Gallardo on DL," ESPN.com, July 6, 2010.

23. Richard Durnett, "Hunter out 1–2 weeks with oblique stain," ESPN.com, March 19, 2010.

24. Associated Press, "Tolbert (oblique strain) off ALDS roster," ESPN.com, October 10, 2010.

25. Jennifer Langosch "Strained oblique may spell end for Wagner," MLB.com, October 9, 2010.

26. Ibid.

27. AJ Farber and JH Wilckens, "Sports hernia: diagnosis and therapeutic approach," *Journal of the American Academy of Orthopedic Surgery* 15.8 (August 2007), 507–514.

28. V Morelli and V Smith, "Groin injuries in athletes," *American Family Physician* 64.8 (October 15, 2001), page 1405–1414.

29. LJ Fon and RA Spence, "Sportsman Hernia," *British Journal of Surgery* 87.5 (May 2000), 545–552.

30. DL Diesen and TN Pappas, "Sports Hernia," *Advances in Surgery* 41 (2007), 177–187.

31. Joe Strauss, "Duncan's season may be over," *St. Louis Post-Dispatch*, September 10, 2007.

32. "Quotable: It's worse than pl…" *Washington Post*, September 23, 2007.

33. Joe Strauss, "CARDS NOTES," *St. Louis Post-Dispatch*, September 18, 2007.

34. "Quotable: It's worse than pl…" *Washington Post*, September 23, 2007.

35. George King and Mike Puma, "Duncan leaves hospital," *New York Post*, November 21, 2007.

36. T. R. Sullivan, "Kinsler opts for season-ending surgery," MLB.com, September 5, 2008.

37. "Sizemore has sports hernia," ESPN.com, September 16, 2009.

38. Associated Press, "Lidge, Ibanez, and Eyre to have surgery," ESPN.com, November 7, 2009.

39. Associated Press, "Bautista has surgery for sports hernia," SI.com, October 21, 2010; Jordon Bastian, "Bautista undergoes surgery for sports hernia," bluejays.com, October 21, 2010.

40. Derrick Goold, "Punto is out 8–12 weeks. He will have surgery for sports hernia, which will delay plans for him to be top backup to David Freese at third base. CARDINALS," *St. Louis Post-Dispatch*, February 23, 2011.

41. Ibid.

42. Stephanie Bell, "Baseball injuries 101: Sprains, strains, and other pains," ESPN.com, February 21, 2008.

43. Freddie Fu and David A. Stone, editors, *Sports Injuries: Mechanisms, Prevention, Treatment* (Philadelphia, PA: Lippincott Williams and Wilkins, 2001), 839–888.

44. Morris B. Mellion editor, *Sports Medicine Secrets, 1st Ed.* (Philadelphia, PA: Hanley & Belfus, 1994), 212; *3rd. Ed.*, 275.

45. Kyle Nagel, "Junior's career in Cincinnati," *Dayton Daily News* (OH), August 1, 2008.

46. Tony Jackson, "Griffey vows he'll return to lineup," *The Cincinnati Post*, September 13, 2000; "Griffey expects to miss rest of Spring training: His status for Opening day in doubt," *Akron Beacon Journal* (OH), March 28, 2001.

47. Hal McCoy, "Junior's exit opens door for Deion: Griffey Jr. put on 15 day DL. Sanders headed for Cincinnati," *Dayton Daily News* (OH), April 30, 2001.

48. "MLB notes," *Akron Beacon Journal* (OH), April 8, 2002; Tony Jackson, "Griffey hurt in 4–3 loss to Angels," *The Cincinnati Post*, June 8, 2002.

49. Tony Jackson, "Griffey hurt in 4–3 loss to Angels," *The Cincinnati Post*, June 8, 2002.

50. Marc Lancaster, "Griffey's season is over: latest in string of injuries with the Reds," *The Cincinnati Post*, August 12, 2004.

51. Ibid.

52. Jim Massie, "Griffey 'miserable' after latest surgery," *The Columbus* (OH) *Dispatch*, September 10, 2004.

53. Marc Lancaster, "Griffey eager for return

to action," *The Cincinnati Post*, February 15, 2005; Gordon Edes, "It hurt being without Junior," *The Boston Globe,* April 10, 2005.

54. baseball-almanac.com/awards.

55. John Fay, "After 144 games, Griffey's year over," *The Cincinnati Enquirer,* September 21, 2007; Kyle Nagel, "Junior's career in Cincinnati," *Dayton* (OH) *Daily News*, August 1, 2008.

56. John Hickey, "Mariners still in Flux: Lineup needs big bat, but Junior just not in mix," *Seattle Post-Intelligencer,* January 23, 2009; Larry LaRue, "Griffey's career bookend," *The* (Tacoma, WA) *News Tribune*, April 6, 2009.

57. "Mariners' Griffey retires after 22 seasons," ESPN.com, June 3, 2010.

58. Lee Jenkins, "Reyes stains hamstring again," *The New York Times,* March 15, 2009; Charlie Noble, "A confident Reyes returns on fresh legs for a change," *The New York Times,* February 17, 2005.

59. Mark Hale, "Reyes sits; MRI reveals strain," *New York Post,* April 13, 2008; Bart Hubbuch, "Reyes hurt as Manuel Loses debut," *New York Post,* June 18, 2008.

60. David Lennon, "Did shoes derail Reyes? Healthy 4 years before switch to standard model. Will his early leg problems now return?" *Newsday* (Long Island New York), October 4, 2009.

61. Will Leitch, "Jose Reyes' Mad Savage Trip," newyorkmag.com, October 1, 2009.

62. A Mishra, J Woodall Jr, and A Vieira, "Treatment of tendon and muscle using platelet-rich plasma," *Clinics in Sports Medicine* 28.1 (January 2009), 113–125.

63. David Lennon, "Reyes to have surgery," *Newsday* (Long Island, NY) October 6, 2009.

64. Bart Habbuch, "Reyes set for surgery today," *New York Post* on October 15, 2009.

65. Jayson Stark, "Jose Reyes' hamstring likely to cost him," ESPN.com, August 9, 2011.

66. Bob Ryan, "Tough out for injured Garciaparra: Another tough out for injured shortstop," *The Boston Globe*, April 22, 2002.

67. Associated Press news line, ESPN.com, April 20, 2002 game.

68. L Maffey and C Emery, "What are the risks for groin strain injury in sport? A systematic review of the literature," *Sports Medicine* 37.10 (2007), 881–894.

69. "Cardinal's Grudzielank hits for cycle," *The Washington Post*, April 28, 2005.

70. Mike Kiley, "No Complications for Nomar: MRI inconclusive for Fox," *Chicago Sun-Times,* April 28, 2005.

71. "Garciaparra and Dodgers agree to deal," *The Washington Post*, December 19, 2005.

72. David Lennon, "Minor strain puts Pedro on DL," *Newsday* (Long Island, NY), August 17, 2006; ESPN.com game log, August 14, 2006.

73. Mark Hale, "Torn tendon in calf shelves Martinez," *New York Post*, September 29, 2009;

Mark Hale, "Pedro off cuff; star faces rotator cuff surgery," *New York Post*, October 1, 2009.

74. Mark Hale, "Injured El Duque complicates pitching plans," *New York Post*, October 4, 2006.

75. Joe Haakenson, "Vaughn ready to fly for Angels," *Daily News of Los Angeles*, March 2, 1999.

76. Dan Wood, "Promoting Wise a smart move: Angels notes: A starter at Edmonton, he makes an impressive major-league debut as a reliever," *The Orange County Register* (CA), August 3, 2000.

77. "Joe Haakenson, Vaughn tough on self," *Press-Telegram* (Long Beach, CA), August 13, 2000; Cheryl Rosenberg, "Mo Vaughn: His season over before it began, the injured Angel isn't looking forward to a year without baseball," *The Orange County Register* (CA), February 22, 2001.

78. Cheryl Rosenberg "No Mo-Angels first baseman is expected to be out entire season after undergoing reconstructive surgery on his left arm," *The Orange County Register* (CA), February 7, 2001.

79. Murray Chass, "Baseball: Mets land Vaughn with a twist and a tug," *The New York Times*, December 28, 2001.

80. Mark Hale, "Vaughn sticks fork in his career," *New York Post*, January 9, 2004.

81. Todd Zolecki, "MRI confirms Howard has ruptured Achilles," MLB.com, October 8, 2011.

82. Associated Press, "Ryan Howard out 5–6 months," ESPN.com, October 12, 2011.

PART II

Chapter 10

1. DH Janda, FM Hanken, and EM Wojtys, "Softball injuries: cost cause, and prevention," *American Family Physician* 33.6 (June 1986), 143–144.

2. "Braves lose game Horner for season," *The Washington Post*, August 16, 1983.

3. Tim Kurkjian, "Despite setbacks, Brave's Horner determined to play in '85," *The Dallas Morning News*, January 17, 1985.

4. Tony Fitzpatrick, "Engineer: head-first slide is quicker," newsroomstage.wustl.edu, September 25, 2008.

5. Ibid.

6. SM Kane, HO House, and KA Oveergaard, "Head-first versus feet-first sliding: a comparison of speed from base to base," *American Journal of Sports Medicine* 30.6 (Nov.-Dec. 2002), 834–836; RG Hosey, CG Mattacola, and R Shapiro, "High speed video analysis of head-first and feet-first sliding techniques in collegiate baseball players," *Clinical Journal of Sport Medicine* 13.4 (July 2003), 242–244.

7. RG Hosey, CG Mattacola, and R Shapiro, "High speed video analysis of head-first and feet-first sliding techniques in collegiate baseball play-

ers," *Clinical Journal of Sport Medicine* 13.4 (July 2003), 242–244.

8. Ibid.

9. Tony Fitzpatrick, "Engineer: head-first slide is quicker," newsroomstage.wustl.edu, September 25, 2008.

10. Phil Hersh, "Cubs learn Dunston out 4–6 weeks," *Chicago Tribune*, June 17, 1987.

11. Bob Dutton, "Royals' Gordon out 3–4 weeks because of broken thumb," *Kansas City Star*, March 8, 2010.

12. "For the Record," *Kansas City Star*, April 18, 2010.

13. Bob Dutton, "Royals' Gordon out 3–4 weeks because of broken thumb," *Kansas City Star*, March 8, 2010.

14. Tony Jackson, "Rafael Furcal breaks left thumb," ESPN.com, April 11, 2011.

15. Tony Jackson, "Rafael Furcal hurt, likely bound for DL," ESPN.com, June 3, 2011.

16. Tony Fitzpatrick, "Engineer: head-first slide is quicker," newsroomstage.wustl.edu, September 25, 2008.

17. Amy Rosewater, "Injury to Lofton was crushing blow," (Cleveland, OH) *The Plain Dealer*, October 12, 1999.

18. Paul Hoynes, "Lofton surgery expected soon," (Cleveland, OH) *The Plain Dealer* on December 13, 1999.

19. Frank Fitzpatrick, "Injury brings Dykstra's year to an early end: The Phils' leadoff hitter broke a bone in his left hand. This is his third trip to the DL this season," *The Philadelphia Inquirer*, August 17, 1992.

20. Ibid.

21. Terry Pluto, *The Curse of Rocky Colavito: A Loving Look at a Thirty Year Slump* (New York, NY: Simon & Schuster, 1994).

22. Ibid., 164.

23. Ibid., 217.

24. Ibid., 218.

25. Ibid., 219.

26. Sidney Jacobson, *Pete Reiser: The Rough-and Tumble Career of the Perfect Ballplayer* (Jefferson, NC: McFarland, 2004), 163, 188.

27. Rudy Marzano, *The Brooklyn Dodgers in the 1940s* (Jefferson, NC: McFarland, 2005), 125, 126.

28. Jacobson, *Pete Reiser*, 188.

29. Josh Leventhal, *The World Series: An Illustrated Encyclopedia of the Fall Classic* (New York, NY: Tess Press, 2006), 125–129.

30. Jacobson, *Pete Reiser*, 197.

31. Tommy Davis with Paul Gutierrez, *Tales from the Dodger Dugout* (Campaign, IL: Sports Publishing L.L.C., 2005), 139–141.

32. Davis with Gutierrez, *Tales from the Dodger Dugout*, 139.

33. Davis with Gutierrez, *Tales from the Dodger Dugout*, 141.

34. Phil Rodgers, "Ventura out 3–4 month," *Chicago Tribune*, March 22, 1997.

35. Ibid.

36. Ibid.

37. Marty Noble, "Ventura a marvel of modern medicine," MLB.com, January 11, 2008.

38. John Nadel, "Ventura brings quiet end to 16-year career," *The Daily Oklahoman* (Oklahoma City, OK), October 12, 2004.

39. Marty Noble, "Ventura a marvel of modern medicine," MLB.com, January 11, 2008.

40. Marty Noble, "Ventura a marvel of modern medicine," MLB.com, January 11, 2008; William Hageman, "Ventura's ankle a 'retread': Sox retiree finds relief through tissue transplant," *Chicago Tribune*, March 2, 2008.

41. Marty Noble, "Ventura a marvel of modern medicine," MLB.com, January 11, 2008.

42. "Padres place Bard, Young on disabled list," sportsillustrated.com, May 22, 2008.

43. Tom Krasovic, "Ever the fan, Giles wants to stay, says club couple pieces away," *The San Diego Union-Tribune*, July 25, 2008.

44. Nick Piecoro, "D-Backs lose game, Hudson," *The Arizona* (Phoenix) *Republic* on August 10, 2008.

45. Nick Piecoro, "Owings factors trade," *The Arizona* (Phoenix) *Republic*, August 13, 2008.

46. "Baseball: Silent Sammy slides badly and so do Orioles," *International Herald Tribune*, July 29, 2005.

47. Ibid.

48. Mike Sowell, *The Pitch That Killed: The Story of Carl Mays, Ray Chapman, and the Pennant Race of 1920* (Chicago, IL: Ivan R. Dee, Publisher, 1989), 22.

49. Ibid.

50. Josh Leventhal, *The World Series: An Illustrated Encyclopedia of the Fall Classic* (New York, NY: Tess Press, 2006), 92; ESPN.com's ENDOF-CENTURY 10 infamous moments.

51. Leventhal, *The World Series*, 92; ESPN.com's ENDOFCENTURY 10 infamous moments.

52. Leventhal, *The World Series*, 92.

53. Joe Morgan and David Falkner, *Joe Morgan: A Life in Baseball* (New York, NY: W. W. Norton), 67, 68.

54. Ibid.

55. Larry Dierker, *This Ain't Brain Surgery: How to Win the Pennant Without Losing Your Mind* (New York, NY: Simon & Schuster, 2000), 100.

56. Dan Shaughnessy "A-Rod in another dust-up," *The Boston Globe*, May 24, 2007.

57. Rich Marazzi, "Baseball rules corner: Rules protect middle infielder trying to launch double play," *Baseball Digest*, September 2004.

58. Ibid.

Chapter 11

1. Vahe Gregorian, "Rolen is out the rest of D'Backs series," *St. Louis Post-Dispatch*, October 5, 2002; Rick Hummel, "Minus Rolen, Cards

rolled into wall," *St. Louis Post-Dispatch*, October 16, 2002.

2. Joe Strauss, "Rolen appears headed for DL," *St. Louis Post-Dispatch*, May 12, 2005.

3. Matthew Leach, "Rolen undergoes shoulder surgery," MLB.com, May 13, 2005.

4. Joe Strauss, "Surgery on Rolen proves complicated," *St. Louis Post-Dispatch*, August 30, 2005.

5. Joe Strauss, "Surgery benefits Rolen," *St. Louis Post-Dispatch*, September 16, 2007.

6. Kristie Rieken, "Reds 3B has shoulder surgery," Associated Press Archive, August 4, 2011; Matt Snyder, "Rolen has shoulder surgery, out 4–6 weeks," cbssports.com, August 3, 2011.

7. Associated Press, "Cubs ready to place Lee on DL with broken wrist," ESPN.com, April 20, 2006.

8. "Lee returns to Cubs-Reds, Red Sox Trade pitchers," *Washington Post*, August 29, 2007.

9. Paul Sullivan, "Wrist of fate: 2 broken bones likely to bench Lee at least two months; Cubs shift options," *Chicago Tribune*, April 20, 2006.

10. Paul Sullivan, "Lee struggling to leave yard: First baseman baffled; hasn't hit homerun since June 3," *Chicago Tribune*, July 5, 2007.

11. Hank Greeenberg and Ira Berkow, *Hank Greenberg: The Story of My Life* (New York, NY: Times Books, 1989), 91.

12. Terry Pluto, *The Curse of Rocky Colavito: A Loving Look at a Thirty Year Slump* (New York, NY: Simon & Schuster, 1994).

13. Ibid., 119.

14. Antonio Gonzalez, "Posey injured in brutal collision in Giant's loss," *Associated Press State Wire*: California (CA), May 26, 2011.

15. Tyler Kepner, "Buster Posey's injury sharpens debate on collisions," *The New York Times*, June 1, 2011.

16. Joel Siegel Barbara Pinto, and Tahman Bradley, "Catcher collision ignites baseball rules debate," abcnews.com, May 28, 2011.

17. Ibid.

18. Tyler Kepner, "Buster Posey's injury sharpens debate on collisions," *The New York Times*, June 1, 2011.

19. Andrew Baggarly, "He's a catcher: Posey rehabs injury convinced his best value to team is behind the plate," *San Jose Mercury News* (CA), July 22, 2011.

20. Ibid., 118.

21. Ibid.

22. Barry Svrluga, "Nationals' Johnson suffers broken leg: Femur fractured in collision on field," *The Washington Post*, September 24, 2006.

23. Barry Svrluga, "A long struggle to get back up and running: 16 month after breaking leg, Nats' Johnson is ready to battle for the job at first base," *The Washington Post*, January 24, 2008.

24. Associated Press, "Johnson to miss season following second surgery on broken leg," ESPN. com, August 16, 2007.

25. Ben Goessling, "Johnson's season is over after surgery," *The Washington Post*, June 25, 2008.

26. Tyler Kepner, "Hand injury sidelines Yanks' Johnson and halts his rise," *The New York Times*, May 17, 2003; Chico Harlan, "Johnson hurts wrist, returns for MRI," *The Washington Post*, May 15, 2008.

27. George A. King III, "Sore leg keeps Swisher on bench," *New York Post*, August 26, 2010.

28. "David Schoen, Ellis gone for season with injury to shoulder," *Oakland Tribune*, April 11, 2004.

29. Steve Kroner, "Shoulder surgery goes well for Ellis," *San Francisco Chronicle*, September 20, 2008.

30. "Doctor's see Guillen returning to Sox," *Journal Star* (Peoria, IL), April 23, 1992.

31. Ibid.

32. Joe Goddard, "Ozzie's season over: Sox lose: Guillen tears knee in collision with Raines," *Chicago Sun-Times*, April 22, 1982.

33.. "Doctor's see Guillen returning to Sox," *Journal Star* (Peoria, IL), April 23, 1992.

34. Joe Goddard, "Guillen receives 3-year extension," *Chicago Sun-Times*, December 14, 1993.

35. Bob Teitlebaum, "Salem outfielder dies after on-field collision," *The Sporting News*, September 7, 1974; Bob Teitlebaum, "Voice on phone: 'Alfredo's dead,'" *The Sporting News*, September 7, 1974.

36. Ibid.

Chapter 12

1. Jacobson, *Pete Reiser: The Rough-and-Tumble Career of the Perfect Ballplayer* (Jefferson, NC: McFarland, 2004), 196; *Rudy* Marzano, *The Brooklyn Dodgers of the 1940s* (Jefferson, NC: McFarland, 2005), 160.

2. Jacobson, *Pete Reiser*, 201.

3. Ibid., 120.

4. Ibid., 178.

5. Ibid., 135.

6. Ibid., 166.

7. Ibid., 182.

8. Marc Lancaster, "Griffey season over: Latest in String of injuries with Reds," *The Cincinnati Post,* August 12, 2004.

9. Larry LaRue, "Griffey fractures wrist; rest of season in doubt," *The News Tribune* (Tacoma, Washington), May 27, 1995.

10. Bob Finnigan, "Prognosis for full recovery 'excellent,' Pedegana says; medical outlook: surgery goes well," *The Seattle Times* on May 28, 1995.

11. Gordon Wittenmyer, "Injury shortens Vaughn's debut," *The* (Riverside, CA) *Press-Enterprise* on April 7, 1999.

12. Joe Haakenson, "With Vaughn out, Indians rout Angels: Cleveland 9 Angels 1," *Daily Times of Los Angeles*, April 8, 1999; "Joe Haakenson, Vaughn is ready to fly for Angels," *Daily Times of Los Angeles*, April 8, 1999.

13. Joe Haakenson, "Vaughn is ready to fly for Angels," *Daily News of Los Angeles*, March 2, 1999.
14. Bob Fowler, "Injuries adding Somber Tone to Twin's Tailspin," *The Sporting News*, July 24, 1971.
15. Ibid.
16. "Information" from tonyoliva.com\bio.
17. Bob Fowler, "Fate of Swatting Star Now in Hands of Surgeons," *The Sporting News*, July 15, 1972; Bob Fowler, "Cal Expects Quilici to Lure Fans Back to the Twins," *The Sporting News*, July 22, 1972.
18. Lawrence S. Ritter and Daniel Honig, *100 Greatest Baseball Players of All Time* (New York, NY: Crown, 1981), 45.
19. Lawrence S. Ritter, *The Glory of Their Times: The Story of the Early Days of Baseball Told by the Men Who Played It* (New York, NY: William Morrow, 1981), 154.
20. Glenn Stout and Richard A. Johnson, *Red Sox Century: One Hundred Years of Red Sox Baseball* (New York, NY: Houghton Mifflin, 2000), 95.
21. Lawrence S. Ritter, *The Glory of Their Times*, 166.
22. Glenn Stout and Richard A. Johnson, *Red Sox Century*, 95.
23. Lawrence S. Ritter and Daniel Honig, *100 Greatest Baseball Players of All Time*, Introduction.

Chapter 13

1. "Rough Return for Jackson-Defeated in First Start," *The Sporting News*, May 3, 1961.
2. Gordon Verrell, "Bat Pierces Yeager's Throat," *The Sporting News*, September 25, 1976.
3. Peter S. and Joachim Horvitiz, *The Big Book of Jewish Baseball* (New York, NY: S. P. I. Books, 2001), 190.
4. Peter Morris, *A Game of Inches: The Stories Behind the Innovations That Shaped Baseball: The Game on the Field* (Chicago, IL: Ivan R. Dee Publishing, 2006), 436.
5. Tom Verducci, "The danger of maple bats is a major problem for MLB," sportsillustrated.com, June 17, 2008.
6. Troy Renck, "MLB investigating use of maple bats," *Denver Post* on June 26, 2008; Jack Curry, "Makers of maple bats face changes in rules," *The New York Times*, June 25, 2008; "Looking to get handle on maple bats," *The Washington Post*, June 25, 2008; Neil Hayes, "Battle of the bats: More players picking maple over ash," *Chicago Sun-Times*, July 6, 2008; Derrick Goold, "Notes: Busted bats abound," *St. Louis Post-Dispatch*, July 4, 2008; Barry Bloom, "MLB addressing danger of maple bats," MLB.com, June 23, 2008.
7. Peter Morris, *A Game of Inches: The Game on the Field* by Morris, 408.
8. Tom Verducci, "The danger of maple bats is a major problem for MLB," sportsillustrated.com, on June 17, 2008; "Official baseball rules" at MLB.com.

9. "Bat information" from Louisville Slugger museum website-sluggermuseum.org.
10. Tom Verducci, "The danger of maple bats is a major problem for MLB," sportsillustrated.com, on June 17, 2008; Barry Bloom, "MLB addressing danger of maple bats," MLB.com, June 23, 2008.
11. Tom Verducci, "The danger of maple bats is a major problem for MLB," sportsillustrated.com, on June 17, 2008; Ray Glier and Mel Antonen, "More players breaking their bats," usatoday.com, May 24, 2005.
12. Dejan Kovacevic, "Hitting coach escapes major injury," *Pittsburgh Post-Gazette* on April 17, 2008; Rob Biertempfel, "Maple bats becoming hazard in major leagues," *Pittsburgh Tribune-Review*, June 8, 2008.
13. Jeff Passan, "Fan's injury should force bat policy change," Yahoo Sports-sports.yahoo.com, May 30, 2008; Bill Shaikin, "Maple bats are an accident waiting to happen," *Los Angeles Times*, May 31, 2008.
14. Troy Renck, "MLB investigating use of maple bats," *Denver Post* on June 26, 2008: David Boyce, "Umpire at Royals game takes a hit from broken maple bat," *The Kansas City Star*, June 25, 2008.
15. Tom Verducci, "The danger of maple bats is a major problem for MLB," sportsillustrated.com, on June 17, 2008.
16. Paul Sullivan, "A fright to the finish: Colvin listed as stable after broken bat stabs him in finale of trip: CUBS 13, MARLINS 3," *Chicago Tribune*, September 20, 2010.
17. Paul Sullivan, "Colvin finally breathes easier," *Chicago Tribune*, October 3, 2010.
18. Jack Curry, "Makes of maple bats face changes in rules," *The New York Times*, June 25, 2008.
19. Ibid.
20. Tom Verducci, "The danger of maple bats is a major problem for MLB," sportsillustrated.com, June 17, 2008.
21. Barry Bloom, "Safety tests for maple bats mandated," MLB.com, December 9, 2008.
22. Associated Press, "MLB to step up bat quality control," sportsillustated.com, December 9, 2008.
23. Phil Rodgers, "A split decision: Company says it has solution for shattered bats; MLB is not so sure," *Chicago Tribune*, September 21, 2010.
24 Mark Yost, "Solving the broken-bat epidemic," *The Wall Street Journal*, August 17, 2011.
25. Adrian Higgins, "A race to save the ash tree," *The Washington Post*, August 30, 2007; Bobbie Dittmeier, "Ash-killing insect threatens bats future," MLB.com, April 17, 2008.
26. "Emerald Ash Borer," treeresearch.org1.html.
27. historicbaseball.com/players/r/roseboro_john.
28. John Roseboro with Bill Libby, *Glory Days*

with the Dodgers: And Other Days with Others, (New York, NY: Antheneum, 1978), 4–13.

29. Ibid., 9.

30. Tommy Davis with Paul Gutierrez, *Tales from the Dugout* (Campaign, IL: Sports Publishing L. L. C., 2005), 120.

31. "Former big leaguer Offerman arrested for melee," ESPN.com, August 15, 2007; Maureen Mullen, "Bat attack shocks Sox: Offerman known as kind, mild mannered," *Boston Herald,* August 16, 2007.

32. "Former big leaguer Offerman arrested for melee," ESPN.com, August 15, 2007.

33. Phil Rodgers, "Offerman gets new charge as manager," *Chicago Tribune,* February 1, 2009.

34. Associated Press, "Former All-star Offerman sued for minor league bat attack," sportsillustrated.com, February 12, 2009.

35. Enrique Rojas, "Offerman gets lifetime Dominican ban," ESPN.com, January 18, 2010.

Chapter 14

1. baseballlibrary.com/flashbacks/10_13_1985; Jerome Holtzman, "Coleman Sidelined by Freak Accident," *Chicago Tribune,* October 14, 1985.

2. Tony Castro, *Mickey Mantle: America's Prodigal Son* (Washington, DC: Brassey's, 2002), 113–117.

3. David Falkner, *The Last Hero: The Life of Mickey Mantle* (New York, NY: Simon & Schuster, 1995), 93–94.

4. Dan Daniel, "Big '52 Yanks Worry: Mickey's injury," *The Sporting News,* October 17, 1951.

5. David Falkner, *The Last Hero: The Life of Mickey Mantle* (New York, NY: Simon & Schuster, 1995), 93–94; "Mickey Mantle: My knee injury in 1951 series," interview at youtube.com.

6. Tony Castro, *Mickey Mantle: America's Prodigal Son,* 115.

7. Shirley Povich, "Mantle Critics Swing, Miss," *The Washington Post,* June 19, 1995.

8. Dan Daniel, "Big '52 Yanks Worry: Mickey's injury," *The Sporting News,* October 17, 1951.

9. Glenn Stout and Richard A. Johnson, *The Dodgers: 120 Years of Dodgers History* (New York, NY: Houghton Mifflin, 2004), 217.

10. Ibid., 219.

11. Roscoe McGowen, "Furillo's flareup backfires on Brooks series chances" and "Furillo says Lippy made him start for bench," *The Sporting News,* September 16, 1953.

12. Joe King, "Rocky invites the Lip to join his spar," *The Sporting News,* September 16, 1953.

13. Roscoe McGowen, "Furillo's flareup backfires on Brooks series chances" and "Furillo says Lippy made him start for bench," *The Sporting News,* September 16, 1953.

14. Joe King, "Rocky invites the Lip to join his spar," *The Sporting News,* September 16, 1953.

15. Roscoe McGowen, "Furillo's flareup backfires on Brooks series chances" and "Furillo says Lippy made him start for bench," *The Sporting News,* September 16, 1953.

16. Joe King, "Rocky invites the Lip to join his spar," *The Sporting News,* September 16, 1953.

17. Roscoe McGowen, "Furillo's flareup backfires on Brooks series chances" and "Furillo says Lippy made him start for bench," *The Sporting News,* September 16, 1953.

18. Joe King, "Rocky invites the Lip to join his spar," *The Sporting News,* September 16, 1953.

19. Roscoe McGowen, "Furillo's flareup backfires on Brooks series chances" and "Furillo says Lippy made him start for bench," *The Sporting News,* September 16, 1953.

20. Roscoe McGowen, "Furillo's flareup backfires on Brooks series chances" and "Furillo says Lippy made him start for bench," *The Sporting News,* September 16, 1953; Joe King, "Rocky invites the Lip to join his spar," *The Sporting News,* September 16, 1953; Joe Williams, "Player fights follow rules," *The Sporting News,* September 16, 1953; Tom Swope, "Furillo withdraws threat: closed incident, says Giles," *The Sporting News,* September 16, 1953; "Squabbles no substitute for victory," *The Sporting News,* September 16, 1953; Ed Burns, "Bouncing around-Now if Carl had only kept a cow," *The Sporting News,* September 16, 1953.

21. Roscoe McGowen, "Furillo's flareup backfires on Brooks series chances" and "Furillo says Lippy made him start for bench," *The Sporting News,* September 16, 1953.

22. Ibid.

23. Tom Swope, "Furillo withdraws threat: closed incident, says Giles," *The Sporting News,* September 16, 1953.

24. Joe King, "Rocky invites the Lip to join his spar," *The Sporting News,* September 16, 1953.

25. Ted Reed, *Carl Furillo: Brooklyn Dodger All-Star* (Jefferson, NC: McFarland, 2011), 96.

26. Ed Burns, "Bouncing around: Now if Carl had only kept a cow," *The Sporting News,* September 16, 1953.

27. Joe King, "Rocky invites the Lip to join his spar," *The Sporting News,* September 16, 1953.

28. Ted Reed, *Carl Furillo: Brooklyn Dodger All-Star* (Jefferson, NC: McFarland, 2011), 96.

29. Ibid.

30. Bernie Wilson, "Padres left fielder Milton Bradley tears ACL during blowup, will miss rest of season," Bernie Wilson, sports.aol.com September 24, 2007.

31. Ibid.

32. Bernie Wilson, "Padres left fielder Milton Bradley tears ACL during blowup, will miss rest of season," Bernie Wilson, sports.aol.com, September 24, 2007; Associated Press, "Bradley tears ACL during umpire spat," sportsillustrated.com, September 24, 2007; Corey Brock, "Bradley to

miss remainder of season," MLB.com, September 25, 2007.

33. Corey Brock, "Bradley to miss remainder of season," MLB.com, September 25, 2007.

34. "In brief-online," *St. Louis Post-Dispatch,* September 27, 2007.

35. Patrick Saunders, "Tulo left to wonder why: injured shortstop will try to remain positive," *Denver Post,* May 4, 2008.

36. Mark Kiszla, "$31 million, all we get was a lousy Tulo," *The Denver Post,* July 8, 2008; Patrick Saunders, "Rockies streak his wall, L.A. gives Kip Wells beating in eight-run, first inning spree Dodgers 16, Rockies 10," *The Denver Post,* July 22, 2008; Associated Press, "Tulowitzki placed on 15-day DL after cutting hand smashing bat," ESPN.com, July 5, 2008.

37. Mark Gonzales, "This Grand Slam costly to Quentin: Injured vs. Cleveland: denies punching wall," *Chicago Tribune,* September 6, 2008; Mark Gonzales, "Quentin Healing process begins: Surgery Ok: Guillen not hanging on hope," *Chicago Tribune,* September 9, 2008; Mark Gonzales, "Sox slugger Carlos Quentin to have wrist surgery," *Chicago Tribune,* September 5, 2008.

38. Ian Browne, "Pedroia wins MVP," MLB.com, November 18, 2008.

39. Tim Sullivan, "Padres go to bat against Greene: seek partial repayment over self inflicted injury," *The San Diego Union-Tribune,* October 1, 2008.

40. Derrick Goold, "Cardinals shortstop eager to bounce back," *St. Louis Post-Dispatch,* December 8, 2008; Ken Rosenthal, "Sources: Anxiety preventing Ranger's Green from reporting," foxsports.com, February 22, 2010; Associated Press, "Rangers void contract of players with social anxiety," foxsports.com, February 25, 2010.

41. John Shea, "Ortiz likely to miss rest of season," *San Francisco Chronicle,* August 22, 2007.

42. ESPN.com game log, September 3, 2004: "Brown has surgery, vows to return," *The Orland Sentinel* (FL), September 6, 2004.

43. Marty Noble, "In a tizzy over Izzy: Bad punch trashes rehab. Sidebar: Temper, temper," *Newsday* (Melville, NY), April 22, 1997; Tom Robinson, "Izzy leaves 'em dizzy with his childish behavior," *The Virginian-Pilot* (Norfolk, VA), April 24, 1997.

44. Todd Zolecki, "Madson placed on DL with broken toe," MLB.com, April 30, 2010; Associated Press, "Phils Madson needs toe surgery," foxsprts.com, May 3, 2010; Bob Brookover, "Madson has stuff to be closer. The righthander has dominated since returning from the DL," *The Philadelphia Inquirer,* September 12, 2010.

45. ESPN.com game log, April 28, 2010.

46. Sam Miller and Bill Plunkett, "Angels win the game but lose Morales," *The* (Santa Ana, CA) *Orange County Register,* May 30, 2010; Bill Plunkett, "First-base auditions begin," *The* (Santa Ana, CA) *Orange County Register,* May 31, 2010; "Morales still waiting for surgery," ESPN.com, on May 31, 2010.

Chapter 15

1. Joe Strauss, "Cards lose Molina, game catcher suffers hand injury: Gonzales homers in ninth as Arizona avoids sweep," *St. Louis Post-Dispatch,* July 8, 2005; Joe Strauss, "Molina injury will keep him out 2–3 weeks," *St. Louis Post-Dispatch,* July 20, 2005.

2. Derrick Goold, "Loss of Yadi puts Cards in bind," *St. Louis Post Dispatch,* May 31, 2007; Matthew Leach, "Molina on DL with fractured wrist," MLB.com, May 30, 2007.

3. "Unforgettable moment: hit home 39 years ago," *The Boston Globe,* August 18, 2006.

4. Maureen Mullen, "A hometown hero's fall still echoes after 40 years: Aug. 18, 1967," *The Boston Globe,* August 18, 2007.

5. David Cataneo, *Tony C: The Triumph and Tragedy of Tony Conigliaro* (Nashville, TN: Rutledge Hill Press, 1997).

6. Ibid., 137.

7. Ibid., 146.

8. Ibid., 151.

9. Ibid., 169.

10. Ibid., 206.

11. Ibid., 224.

12. Jack McCallum, "Faith, Hope and Tony C," sportsillustrated.com, July 5, 1982.

13. Lowell Reidenbaugh and editors of *The Sporting News, Baseball Hall of Fame: Cooperstown, Where Legends Live Forever* (New York, NY: Crescent Books, 1997), 54; Charlie Bevis, *Mickey Cochrane: The Life of a Baseball Hall of Fame Catcher* (Jefferson, NC: McFarland, 1998).

14. Thomas Barthel, *The Fierce Fun of Ducky Medwick* (Lanham, Maryland: Scarecrow Press, 2003).

15. Ibid., 162, 166.

16. Ibid., 166.

17. Ibid., 166, 168.

18. Ibid., 169.

19. Ibid., 171.

20. Robert W. Creamer, *Baseball and Other Matters in 1941* (Lincoln, NE: Bison Books, 2000), 75.

21. Thomas Barthel, *The Fierce Fun of Ducky Medwick,* 173, 177.

22. Bill James, The *Politics of Glory-How Baseball's Hall of Fame Really Works* (New York, NY: Macmillian, 1994), 339.

23. Barthel, *The Fierce Fun of Ducky Medwick,* 177.

24. Don Zimmer with Bill Madden, *Zim: A Baseball Life* (Kingston, NY: Total Sports Publishing, 2001), 1.

25. Ibid., 9.

26. Ibid.

27. Ibid., 13.
28. Ibid., 26.
29. Ibid., 27.
30. Ibid., 10–11.
31. Harry Shattuck, "Broadcaster joins Thon on injured list," *The Sporting News,* April 24, 1984; Ray Didinger, "The Future is as Blur for Dickie Thon," *The Sporting News,* September 24, 1984.
32. Ibid.
33. Ray Didinger, "The Future is as Blur for Dickie Thon," *The Sporting News,* September 24, 1984; Dave Anderson, "Thon looks to come back," *The San Francisco Chronicle,* March 6, 1985; "After the beaning, Thon battles back," *Washington Post,* October 14, 1986.
34. "Notes," *Chicago Tribune,* May 8, 1987: "Sports," *Chicago Tribune,* July 7, 1987.
35. Associated Press, "Baseball-poor vision finally causes Thon to retire," *The Seattle Times,* March 3, 1994; David Bush, "Recurring vision problems force A's Thon to Retire," *The San Francisco Chronicle,* March 3, 1994.
36. Mike Sowell, *The Pitch That Killed: The Story of Carl Mays, Ray Chapman, and the Pennant Race of 1920.* (Chicago, Ill: Ivan R. Dee, Publisher, 1989).
37. Ibid., 20.
38. Ibid., 22.
39. Ibid., 176.
40. Ibid., 197.
41. Ibid., 170.
42. Ibid., 173.
43. Ibid., 174.
44. Ibid., 181.
45. Ibid., 183.
46. Avani Patel and Teddy Greenstein, "Back in the box: beanball victims like Joe Girardi face uncertain road," *Chicago Tribune,* August 11, 2000.
47. Dan Schlossberg, *Baseball Gold: Mining Nuggets from our National Pastime.* (Chicago, IL: Triumph Books, 2007), 107.
48. "The Ill-fated Rookie class of 1964," rick-swaine.com/articles.
49. Peter Morris, *A Game of Inches: The Stories Behind the Innovations that Shaped Baseball: The Game on the Field* (Chicago, IL: Ivan R. Dee Publishing, 2006), 442–444.
50. Sidney Jacobson, *Pete Reiser: The Rough-and-Tumble Career of the Perfect Ballplayer* (Jefferson, NC: McFarland, 2004), 70–71.
51. Zimmer with Madden, *Zim-A Baseball Life,* page 16.
52. Associated Press, "Charlie Muse: Innovator behind modern batting helmet dies at 87," *The New York Times,* May 20, 2005.
53. Morris, *A Game of Inches-The Game on the Field,* 444.
54. Associated Press, "Batting helmet creator Muse dies," pirates.MLB.com, May 16, 2005.
55. Joe Hoppel, "Four homers in one game," *The Sporting News,* August 10, 1999.

56. Edward Prell, "Ron hospitalized with fractured cheekbone," *Chicago Tribune,* June 27, 1966; Ron Santo with Randy Minkoff, *Ron Santo: For Love of Ivy* (Chicago, IL: Bonus Books, 1993), 53–56.
57. Darcy Fast and Jonathan Kravitz, *The Missing Cub* (Longview, FL: Xulon Press, 2007) by Fast and Kravetz, 143; Dan Schlossberg, *Baseball Gold: Mining Nuggets from our National Pastime* (Chicago, IL: Triumph Books, 2007), 107.
58. "Safe at Home" by Jim Street at MLB.com on 5/6/2006.
59. Glenn Stout and Richard A. Johnson, *The Cubs: A Complete Story of Chicago Cubs Baseball* (New York, NY: Houghton Mifflin, 2007), 230; Santo with Minkoff, *Ron Santo—For Love of Ivy,* 56.
60. Rudy Marzano, *The Brooklyn Dodgers of the 1940s* (Jefferson, NC: McFarland, 2005), 44, 45; "Sports of the Times: Beanballs, Clemens, Piazza, and Medwick," *The New York Times,* July 11, 2000.
61. Marzano, *The Brooklyn Dodgers of the 1940s,* 45.
62. Larry Stone, "Fare thee well, Olerud," *The Seattle Times,* July 18, 2004.
63. Tom Singer, "Base coaches weigh in on helmet rule," MLB.com, March 2, 2008.
64. Associated Press, "Rolen put on DL: Cueto OK," ESPN.com, August 12, 2009.
65. "Wright leaves ballpark in ambulance," ESPN.com, August 15, 2009; "Wright hopes to be first wearing S100," ESPN.com, August 31, 2009.
66. Associated Press, "Gonzalez hit in the head by pitch," July 18, 2009.
67. Wright hopes to be first wearing S100," ESPN.com, August 31, 2009.
68. Tom Singer, "Reinforced helmets debuting around Majors," MLB.com, August 31, 2009.
69. Jorge L. Ortiz, "New batting helmets safer, can withstand 100 mph pitch," USAToday.com, Feb. 22, 2013.
70. Jeff Kisseloff, *Who Is Baseball's Greatest Pitcher?* (Chicago, ILL: Carus Publishing, 2003), 22–25.
71. Rick Swaine, *Beating the Breaks: Major League Ballplayers Who Overcame Disabilities* (Jefferson, NC: McFarland, 2004), 159–168.

Chapter 16

1. Bob Gibson and Lonnie Wheeler, *Stranger to the Game* (New York, NY: Penguin Books USA, 1984), 135–143.
2. dizzydean.com.
3. Vince Staten, *Ol' Diz: A Biography of Dizzy Dean* (New York, NY: HarperCollins, 1992), 181–188.
4. Jeff Kisseloff, *Who Is Baseball's Greatest Pitcher* (Chicago, IL: Carus Publishing, 2003), 89.
5. Terry Pluto, *The Curse of Rocky Colavito: A Loving Look at a Thirty Year Slump* (New York, NY: Simon & Schuster, 1994), 31.

6. Ibid., 31.

7. Ibid., 30.

8. Ibid., 31.

9. Ibid.

10. Bill Nowlin and Cecilia Tan, *'75: The Red Sox Team That Saved Baseball* (Cambridge, MA: Rounder Books, 2005), 60–62.

11. Peter Gammons, "Red Sox unraveled by injuries to key hurlers," *The Sporting News*, August 19, 1975.

12. "Dick Pole," baseballlibrary.com.

13. Nowlin and Tan, *'75: The Red Sox Team That Saved Baseball*, 60–62.

14. Gordon Edes, "Line drive puts Florie in hospital," *The Boston Globe*, September 9, 2000.

15. Larry Tye, "The waiting game for Florie: Prospects won't be clear for a while," *The Boston Globe*, September 11, 2000.

16. Bob Hohler, "Florie has 2D surgery," *The Boston Globe*, September 19, 2000.

17. Gordon Edes, "Florie's injured eye shows improvement," *The Boston Globe*, October 12, 2000.

18. Susan Slusser, "A's giving Florie chance he craved: After brutal injury, pitcher says he's ready to go," *The San Francisco Chronicle*, February 26, 2002.

19. Michael Holley, "Florie's return to baseball simply a sight to behold," *The Boston Globe*, June 29, 2001; Associated Press, "Florie pitches for first time since getting hit in face," ESPN.com, June 28, 2001.

20. "Red Sox give up on Florie," *The Seattle Times*, July 31, 2001.

21. Susan Slusser, "A's giving Florie chance he craved: After brutal injury, pitcher says he's ready to go," *The San Francisco Chronicle*, February 26, 2002.

22. Gordon Edes, "Sox get scare as line drive hits Clement: Pitcher will be reevaluated today," *The Boston Globe*, July 27, 2005.

23. Ken Rosenthal, "Selig should be proactive," *The Sporting News*, October 2, 2000; Gordon Edes, "Sox get scare as line drive hits Clement," *The Boston Globe*, July 27, 2005.

24. Corey Brock, "Young set for mound return," MLB.com, July 29, 2008; Joe Strauss, "Pujols: It did bother' Cardinals slugger overwhelmed after line drive hits Padres pitcher Chris Young in the face in Wednesday night's game," *St. Louis Post-Dispatch*, May 23, 2008.

25. Barry Bloom, "Shots to the head a scary risk to players," MLB.com, August 28, 2009.

26. Joe Strauss, "Hawksworth 'thankful after injury': Notebook: Pitcher probably done for the season but could have been hurt worse," *St. Louis Post-Dispatch*, September 27, 2010; Associated Press, "Cards' Blake Hawksworth out of hospital," ESPN.com, September 26, 2010.

27. Associated Press, "Rockies' Juan Nicasio has neck surgery," ESPN.com, August 6, 2011.

28. Ibid.

29. "Rockies' Nicasio feels luck to be alive," Associated Press Archive, August 17, 2011.

30. Gary Klein, DiGiovanna and Dylan Hernandez, "Baseball explores ways to keep players' heads in the game, literally," *Los Angeles Times*, Feb. 26, 2013.

31. "Montreal Expos vs. Colorado Rockies," ESPN.com game recap, August 20, 2004.

32. "Expos Johnson likely done for season," *The Washington Post*, August 22, 2004; "For the record," *The Kansas City Star*, September 15, 2004.

33. Barry Svrluga, "Johnson agrees to one-year deal," *The Washington Post*, January 15, 2005.

34. Associated Press, "Encarnacion hit in face by foul, out for season," sportsillustrated.com, September 1, 2007.

35. Derrick Goold, "Career in Jeopardy? Surgery, uncertainty await Encarnacion," *St. Louis Post-Dispatch*, September 2, 2007.

36. Joe Strauss, "Cards meet with White Sox assistant GM Rick Hahn," *St. Louis Post-Dispatch*, October 13, 2007.

37. Derrick Goold, "Mariners will interview Oquendo," *St. Louis Post-Dispatch*, Nov. 11, 2008.

38. David O'Brien, "Salazar's head injury not as bad as feared: Braves minor league manager hit in face by liner while in dugout," *The Atlanta Journal-Constitution*, March 10, 2011.

39. David O'Brien, "McCann still shaken as Salazar has surgery: Minor league manager might lose left eye after being hit by line drive," *The Atlanta Journal-Constitution*, March 11, 2011.

40. Mark, Bowman, "Progress for Salazar; more surgery planned," MLB.com, March 11, 2011.

41. David O'Brien, "Despite surgeons' efforts, Salazar loses left eye," *The Atlanta Journal-Constitution*, March 17, 2011.

42. Associated Press, "Luis Salazar returns to Braves camp," ESPN.com, March 23, 2011.

43. Associated Press, "Burst blood vessel in neck killed coach," *The New York Times*, July 26, 2007; "Coach who died hit in neck," *Detroit Free Press*, July 26, 2007; Associated Press, "Coroner: Ball hit Coolbaugh on neck, ruptured artery," at ESPN.com, July 25, 2007.

44. Bob Dutton, "Former Royals minor-leaguer Coolbaugh dies when hit by line drive," *Kansas City Star*, July 24, 2007.

45. "Coolbaugh, 35, dies after struck by ball," ESPN.com, July 24, 2007.

46. Teddy Kider, "Line drive strikes and kills former major leaguer," *The New York Times*, July 24, 2007.

47. Tom Singer, "Base coaches weigh in on helmet rule," MLB.com, March 2, 2008.

48. Information on bat exit speeds, http://www.efastball.com/hitting/average-bat-speed-exit-speed-by-age-group, April 23, 2012.

Chapter 17

1. "Muhammad Ali and his battle," *The Guardian* (UK), March 20, 2009; Harold Kawans, *Why Michael Couldn't Hit: and Other Tales of the Neurology of Sport* (New York, NY: Avon Books, 1996), 117–147.

2. Morris B. Mellion, Margo Putukian, and Christopher C. Madden, *Sports Medicine Secrets, 3rd Ed.*, (Philadelphia, PA: Hanley and Belfus, 2003), 287.

3. C Toth, S McNeil, and T Feasby, "Central nervous system injuries in sport and recommendations, a systematic review," *Sports Medicine* 35.8 (2005), 685–715.

4. "Concussion are a fact of life in today's sports world," sports-concussion.com.

5. Morris B. Mellion, *Sports Medicine Secrets, 1st Ed.* (Philadelphia, PS: Hanley and Belfus, 1994), 218.

6. Wills and Leathem, "A review: Sports related brain injury research: methodological difficulties associated with ambiguous terminology," *Brian Injury* 15.7 (July 2001), 645–648.

7. Mellion, Putukian, and Madden, *Sports Medicine Secrets, 3rd Ed.*, 287.

8. "Head concussions — causes, prevention, management, and recommendations," www.medcoathletics.com/education/head_concussions/print_out.htm.

9. Ibid.
10. Ibid.
11. Ibid.

12. MP McClincy, MR Lovell, J Pardini, and MK Spore, "Recovery from sports concussion in high school and Collegiate athletes," *Brain Injury* 21.1 (January 2006), 33–39.

13. N Biasca and WL Maxwell, "Minor traumatic brain injury: a review in order to prevent neurologic sequelae," *Progressive Brain Research* 161 (2007), 263–291.

14. Ibid.
15. Ibid.

16. Don Zimmer with Bill Madden, *Zim: A Baseball Life* (Kingston, NY: Total Sports Publishing, 2001), 13.

17. Marcia C. Smith, "Baseball recognizing concussions effects," *The Orange County Register* (Santa Ana, CA), June 19, 2007.

18. Mellion, Putukian, and Madden, *Sports Medicine Secrets, 3rd Ed.*, 287.

19. LM Ryan and DL Warden, "Post concussion syndrome," *International Review of Psychiatry* 15.4 (November 2003), 310–316.

20. Matthew Leach, "Edmonds exits early against White Sox," MLB.com, June 21, 2006.

21. Matthew Leach, "Notes: Edmonds out indefinitely," MLB.com, August 17, 2006; Matthew Leach, "Notes: Edmonds could sit a while," MLB.com August 29, 2006.

22. Joe Strauss and Derrick Goold, "Edmonds,

Cards agree on two-year extension," *St. Louis Post-Dispatch*, November 11, 2006.

23. "Cardinals' Jim Edmonds announces retirement," MLB.com, February 18, 2011.

24. Barry M. Bloom, "MLB must look at head injuries," MLB.com, October 4, 2006; Jerry Crasnick, "Much still unknown about concussions," ESPN.com, August 31, 2010.

25. Rick Braun, "BREWERS NOTES: Koskie sits out again. Third baseman suffering from effects of a concussion," *Milwaukee Journal Sentinel*, July 9, 2006.

26. Dennis Semrau, "Head injury still bothering Koskie," *The Capital Times* (Madison, WI), July 25, 2006.

27. Tom Haudricourt, "Nightmare living: Koskie struggles to return from head injury," *Milwaukee Journal Sentinel*, February 22, 2007.

28. Jerry Crasnick, "Concussion related issues having an impact on the diamond," ESPN.com, March 23, 2007.

29. Ibid.

30. Jerry Crasnick, "Much still unknown about concussions," ESPN.com, August 31, 2010.

31. Associated Press, "Koskie opts to retire after setback," ESPN.com, March 21, 2009.

32. Andrew Baggarly, "Concussions KO durable Matheny," *Oakland (CA) Tribune*, June 3, 2006.

33. Janie McCauley, "Dangerous job: Matheny's season over after too many blows to his head," *Deseret News* (Salt Lake City, Utah), August 20, 2006.

34. Associated Press, "Concussion symptoms force Matheny to retire," ESPN.com, February 1, 2007.

35. John Shipley, "Morneau copes with concussion: Blow to the head the second of his big-league career," *St. Paul Pioneer Press* (MN), July 9, 2010; Jerry Crasnick, "Much still unknown about concussions," ESPN.com, August 31, 2010.

36. John Shipley, "Cleanup sitter: Morneau's return up in the air after his cutback in his rehab," *St. Paul Pioneer Press* (MN), August 14, 2010.

37. Alden Gonzales, "Bay, Morneau fighting concussions together," MLB.com, March 11, 2011; La Velle E. Neal III, "Morneau says so far, so good this spring," *StarTribune* (Minneapolis, MN), March 29, 2011.

38. Joe LaPointe, "Concussion symptoms developed late for Bay," *The New York Times*, July 28, 2010; Alden Gonzales, "Bay, Morneau fighting concussions together," MLB.com, March 11, 2011.

39. David Waldstein, "Bay's concussion may signal need for change in Mets' protocol," *The New York Times*, August 15, 2010.

40. Dan Martin, "Mets' Bay feels better heading into next season," *New York Post*, December 15, 2010; Jerry Crasnick, "Much still unknown about concussions," ESPN.com, August 31, 2010.

41. Alden Gonzales, "Bay, Morneau fight-

ing concussions together," MLB.com, March 11, 2011.

42. Anthony DiComo, "Bay sidelined with left rib discomfort," MLB.com, March 29, 2011.

Conclusion

1. Paul McCardell and Jeff Zrebiec, "The games, the times, The Ripken legacy: Chronology," *The* (Baltimore) *Sun,* October 7, 2001.

2. Paul McCardell and Jeff Zrebiec, "The games, the times, the Ripken legacy: Chronology," *The* (Baltimore) *Sun,* October 7, 2001; Cal Ripken Jr. and Mike Bryan, *The Only Way I Know* (New York, NY: Penguin Books USA, 1997).

3. Paul McCardell and Jeff Zrebiec, "The games, the times, the Ripken legacy: Chronology," *The* (Baltimore) *Sun,* October 7, 2001.

4. Ibid.

5. Cal Ripken Jr. and Mike Bryan, *The Only Way I Know,* 263.

6. Ibid., 266.

7. Ibid., 268.

8. Joe Strauss, "His last years were a pain, injuries: A remarkable run ended after back began to cause him problems in 1997: The Ripken Legacy: Health," *The* (Baltimore) *Sun,* October 10, 2001.

9. Ibid.

10. Ken Rosenthal, "For Ripken, year of pain, year of grit," *The* (Baltimore) *Sun,* September 23, 1999.

11. Joe Strauss, "Ripken eligible, not able, to return," *The* (Baltimore) *Sun,* August 18, 1999.

12. Joe Strauss, "O's expecting Ripken back after successful operation," *The* (Baltimore) *Sun,* September 24, 1999.

13. Joe Strauss, "Ripken reinvigorated, but resigned to surgery," *The* (Baltimore) *Sun* on May 16, 1999.

14. Joe Strauss, "O's expecting Ripken back after successful operation," *The* (Baltimore) *Sun,* September 24, 1999.

15. Peter Schmuck, "Ripken gets a shot of 'good news': Injection has him ready," *The* (Baltimore) *Sun,* May 17, 2000.

16. Joe Strauss and Roch Kubatko, "Pain again drives Ripken from field," *The* (Baltimore) *Sun,* June 29, 2000.

17. Roch Kubatko, "Ripken returns at return of month-Infielder to come off DL as roster expands Friday," *The* (Baltimore) *Sun,* August 26, 2000.

18. Joe Strauss, "Hargrove: O's to play Ripken less," *The* (Baltimore) *Sun* April 25, 2001; Joe Strauss, "His last years were a pain, injuries: A remarkable run ended after back began to cause him problems in 1997; The Ripken Legacy: Health," *The* (Baltimore) *Sun,* October 10, 2001.

19. Nolan Ryan with T. R. Sullivan and Mickey Herskowitz, *Nolan Ryan: The Road to Cooperstown* (Lenexa, KS: Addax Publishing Group, 1999), 32.

20. Nolan Ryan and Harvey Frommer, *Throwing Heat* (New York, NY: Avon Books, 1990), 42.

21. Ibid., 48.

22. Ibid., 134.

23. "Astros' Ryan on shelf again-sore elbow," *The San Francisco Chronicle,* July 31, 1986; Nolan Ryan, T. R. Sullivan, and Mickey Herskowitz, *Nolan Ryan: The Road to Cooperstown* by Ryan, 44.

24. Gerry Fraley, "Knee injury sidelines Ryan," *The Dallas Morning News,* April 16, 1993.

25. Ibid.

26. Gerry Fraley, "Injury ends Ryan's career: Start at Seattle results in major elbow damage," *The Dallas Morning News,* September 23, 1993; Nolan Ryan, T. R. Sullivan, and Mickey Herskowitz, *Nolan Ryan: The Road to Cooperstown,* 55.

27. Jonathan Eig, *Luckiest Man: The Life and Death of Lou Gehrig* (New York, NY: Simon & Schuster, 2005), 209.

28. Ibid., 184.

29. Ibid.

30. Ibid., 185.

31. Ray Robinson, *The Iron Horse: Lou Gehrig in His Time* (New York, NY: W. W. Norton, 1990), 207.

32. Jonathan Eig, *Luckiest Man: The Life and Death of Lou Gehrig,* 186, 187.

33. Ibid.

34. Ibid.

35. Ibid.

36. Ibid., 199.

37. Ibid., 125.

38. Ibid., 152.

Appendix

1. Tommy John and Valenti *TJ: My 26 Years in Baseball* (New York, NY: Bantam Books, 1991)

2. Jimmy Greenfield and Phil Ridgers, "Once something special, 'Tommy John' surgery has become almost commonplace among major league pitchers, such as Cub's Kerry Wood: Elbow room," *Chicago Tribune,* February 24, 2000.

3. Jimmy Greenfield and Phil Ridgers, "Once something special, 'Tommy John' surgery has become almost commonplace among major league pitchers, such as Cub's Kerry Wood: Elbow room," *Chicago Tribune,* February 24, 2000.

4. Jimmy Greenfield and Phil Ridgers, "Once something special, 'Tommy John' surgery has become almost commonplace among major league pitchers, such as Cub's Kerry Wood: Elbow room," *Chicago Tribune,* February 24, 2000.

5. Mike Dodd, "Tommy John: surgery a career saving procedure for many pitchers," *Baseball Digest,* November, 2004; Marc Carig, "Mariano Rivera, Tommy John and an old question answered," *The Star-Ledger* (NJ.com), August 15, 2009.

6. John Romano, "Reyes a singular closer," tampabay.com, May 7, 2007.

7. Brain Dohn, "Dreifort sidelined until next season-injury: will have surgery on elbow for second time in his Dodger career," *Press-Telegram* (Long Beach, CA), July 4, 2001.

8. Hal McCoy, "Rijo's elbow gets full rebuild-ligament, tendon, nerve all figure in surgery Reds notes," *Dayton Daily News* (OH), August 23, 1995.

9. Jimmy Greenfield and Phil Ridgers, "Once something special, 'Tommy John' surgery has become almost commonplace among major league pitchers, such as Cub's Kerry Wood: Elbow room," *Chicago Tribune*, February 24, 2000.

10. Mike Dodd, "Tommy John: surgery a career saving procedure for many pitchers," *Baseball Digest*, November, 2004; Rich Hammond, "Gagne gets some good news: closer doesn't need second Tommy John surgery," *Daily News of Los Angeles* (CA), June 25, 2005.

11. David Haugh, "Surgery not always cure: Tommy John surgery has saved careers, but it hasn't worked for everyone," *Chicago Tribune*, May 4, 2005; Bill Chastain, "Isringhausen done for season," MLB.com, June 15, 2009.

12. Daniel Paulling, "Pitcher gets familiar with Tommy John," *USA TODAY*, July 18, 2007.

13. Mike Dodd, "Tommy John: surgery a career saving procedure for many pitchers," *Baseball Digest*, November, 2004.

14. David Haugh, "Surgery not always cure: Tommy John surgery has saved careers, but it hasn't worked for everyone," *Chicago Tribune*, May 4, 2005.

15. Jimmy Greenfield and Phil Ridgers, "Once something special, 'Tommy John' surgery has become almost commonplace among major league pitchers, such as Cub's Kerry Wood: Elbow room," *Chicago Tribune*, February 24, 2000.

16. Chris Jenkins, "Tommy John, lesser of two evils," *San Diego Union-Tribune*, June 7, 2000.

17. Jimmy Greenfield and Phil Rodgers, "Once something special, 'Tommy John' surgery has become common place among major league pitchers, such as Cubs' Kerry Wood: elbow room," *Chicago Tribune*, February 24, 2000.

18. Chris Jenkins, "Tommy John, lesser of two evils," *San Diego Union-Tribune*, June 7, 2000.

19. Josh Palley, "John Smoltz, pitcher for Atlanta Braves," WebMD.com, July 26, 2004.

20. Chris Jenkins, "Tommy John, lesser of two evils," *San Diego Union-Tribune*, June 7, 2000.

21. "Benson to have reconstructive elbow surgery," *Erie Times-News* (PA), May 19, 2001.

22. Associated Press, "Yankee OF Nady to have Tommy John surgery," SportingNews.com, July 1, 2009.

23. Mike Dodd, "Tommy John: surgery a career saving procedure for many pitchers," *Baseball Digest*, November 2004.

24. Kathleen O'Brien, "Healthy Brocail rebuilding career," *Fort-Worth Star Telegram* (TX), March 4, 2004.

25. Jayson Stark, "Tommy John surgery: cutting edge to common place," ESPN.com, August 13, 2003.

26. T. R. Sullivan, "NOTES: Zimmerman undergoes second elbow surgery," *Fort Worth Star-Telegram* (TX), July 17, 2004.

27. Joe Strauss, "Ankiel is slated to start rehab duty at Class A," *Saint Louis Post-Dispatch*, July 27, 2004.

28. David Haugh, "Surgery not always cure: Tommy John surgery has saved careers, but it hasn't worked for everyone," *Chicago Tribune*, May 4, 2005.

29. David Haugh, "Surgery not always cure: Tommy John surgery has saved careers, but it hasn't worked for everyone," *Chicago Tribune*, May 4, 2005.

30. Mike Berardino, "Burnett faces tough road back–Smoltz, Tejera among surgery success stories," *Sun-Sentinel* (South FL), April 30, 2003.

31. "Brown has surgery, vows to return," *The Orlando Sentinel*, September 6, 2004.

32. David Haugh, "Byrd just baffling," *Chicago Tribune*, October 12, 2005.

33. "Neagle has surgery, out 12–18 months," *Daily Camera* (Boulder, CO), July 31, 2003.

34. Martin Fennelly, "Soriano sighting rare, but he vows to be ready," *The Tampa Tribune* (FL), March 13, 2010.

35. Ken Gurnick, "Izturis eager to force decision at short," MLB.com on February 16, 2006.

36. Maureen Mullen, "Anderson suffers career-ending injury," raysbaseball.com, May 13, 2008.

37. Susan Slusser, "A's report: Dotel's surgery goes well; he could pitch opening day," *San Francisco Chronicle* on June 9, 2005.

38. David Bush, "A's report: Durazo's season is over, faces 'Tommy John' surgery," *San Francisco Chronicle*, July 20, 2005.

39. "Wolf undergoes Tommy John procedure," *Pittsburgh Tribune-Review* (PA), July 1, 2005.

40. Associated Press, "Hampton out until '07 after Tommy John surgery," ESPN.com, September 20, 2005.

41. Joe Christensen "Team notes: Liriano plays it cool on eve of 2008 debut," *Star-Tribune* (Minneapolis, MN), April 13, 2008.

42. Mike Ritter, "Kinney works way back to Cardinals," MLB.com, September 2, 2008.

43. Pete Grathoff, "Thirty-fifth anniversary of Tommy John surgery," *The Kansas City Star* on October 19, 2009.

44. John Shipley, "After 28 starts Pavano is optimistic," *St. Paul Pioneer Press* (MN), September 12, 2009.

45. Pete Grathoff, "Thirty-fifth anniversary of Tommy John surgery," *The Kansas City Star*, October 19, 2009.

46. Associated Press, "Wagner needs elbow surgery, will miss all of 2009 season," SI.com, September 8, 2008.

47. Mike Dodd, "Tommy John: surgery a career saving procedure for many pitchers," *Baseball Digest*, November 2004.

48. David O'Brien, "Baseball: Hudson concedes need to have elbow surgery," *Atlanta Journal-Constitution*, August 3, 2008.

49. Jordan Bastian, "Marcum flirts with no-no before Jays fall," MLB.com, April 5, 2010.

50. Associated Press, "Volquez faces 12 months of rehab," ESPN.com, August 3, 2009.

51. Anthony Castrovince, "Reyes undergoes two elbow surgeries," MLB.com, June 12, 2010.

52. Bob Dutton, "Royals Aviles scheduled for major elbow surgery, looking 9–12 months of rehab," *The Kansas City Star*, July 2, 2009.

53. Adam Kligore, "Zimmerman looks sharp as Nationals lose to Mets," *The Washington Post*, October 2, 2010.

54. Kelly Thesier, "Nathan undergoes Tommy John surgery," MLB.com, March 26, 2010.

55. "Rockies briefs," *The Denver Post*, September 2, 2010.

56. Adam Kilgore, "Strasburg focused on return: Nationals: After Tommy John surgery, Phenom not likely to pitch in majors again until 2012," *The* (Baltimore, MD) *Sun*, August 28, 2010.

57. Todd Zolecki, "Moyer to have elbow surgery, eyes 2012 return," MLB.com, November 30, 2010.

58. Matthew Leach, "Wainwright to undergo Tommy John surgery," MLB.com, February 24, 2011.

59. Associated Press, "Joba has torn elbow ligament," SI.com, June 9, 2011.

60. "Rockies' Jorge De La Rosa out for year," ESPN.com, May 25, 2011.

61. "John Lackey to have elbow surgery," ESPN.com, October 25, 2011.

62. Bob Dutton, "Royal's Soria diagnosed with ligament damage in elbow," *The Kansas City Star*, March 19, 2012.

63. Stephanie Bell, "Spring Notes: Three relievers hit the shelf," ESPN.com, March 26, 2012.

64. Associated Press, "A's lose Joey Devine for season," ESPN.com, April 10, 2012.

65. Carl Steward, "Giants' Brian Wilson will have Tommy John surgery," *San Jose* (CA) *Mercury News*, April 18, 2012.

Bibliography

Andrews, James R., Bertram Zarins, and Kevin E. Wilk. *Injuries in Baseball*. Philadelphia: Lippincott-Raven, 1998.

Barra, Allen. *Yogi Berra: Eternal Yankee*. New York: W. W. Norton, 2009.

Barthel, Thomas. *The Fierce Fun of Ducky Medwick*. Lanham, MD: Scarecrow Press, 2003.

Bevis, Charlie. *Mickey Cochrane: The Life of a Baseball Hall of Fame Catcher*. Jefferson, NC: McFarland, 1998.

Canseco, Jose. *Juiced: Wild Times, Rampant 'Roids, Smash Hits, and How Baseball Got Big*. New York: HarperCollins, 2005. 1998. ?

Castro, Tony. *Mickey Mantle: America's Prodigal Son*. Washington, DC: Brassey's, 2002.

Cataneo, David. *Tony C: The Triumph and Tragedy of Tony Conigliaro*. Nashville: Rutledge Hill Press, 1997.

Clemens, Roger, and Peter Gammons. *Rocket Man: The Roger Clemens Story*. Lexington, MA: Stephen Greene Press, 1987.

Coverdale, Miles. *Whitey Ford: A Biography*. Jefferson, NC: McFarland, 2006.

Cramer, Richard Ben. *Joe DiMaggio: The Hero's Life*. New York: Simon & Schuster, 2000.

Creamer, Robert W. *Baseball and Other Matters in 1941*. Lincoln, NE: Bison Books, 2000.

Davis, Tommy, and Paul Gutierrez. *Tales from the Dodger Dugout*. Campaign, IL: Sports Publishing, 2005.

Deford, Frank. *The Old Ball Game: How John McGraw, Christy Mathewson, and the New York Giants Created Modern Baseball*. New York: Atlantic Monthly Press, 2005.

Dierker, Larry. *This Ain't Brain Surgery: How to Win a Pennant Without Losing Your Mind*. New York: Simon & Schuster, 2003.

Drysdale, Don, and Bob Verdi. *Once a Bum, Always a Dodger*. New York: St. Martin's Press, 1990.

Eig, Jonathan. *Luckiest Man: The Life and Death of Lou Gehrig*. New York: Simon & Schuster, 2005.

Falkner, David. *The Last Hero: The Life of Mickey Mantle*. New York: Simon & Schuster, 1995.

Fast, Darcy, and Jonathan Kravetz. *The Missing Cub*. Longwood, FL: Xulon Press, 2007.

Fu, Freddie H., and David A. Stone. *Sports Injuries: Mechanisms, Prevention, Treatment*. Philadelphia: Lippincott Williams & Wilkins, 2001.

Gibson, Bob, and Lonnie Wheeler. *Stranger to the Game*. New York: Penguin Books USA, 1984.

Greenberg, Hank and Ira Berkow. *Hank Greenberg: The Story of My Life*. New York: Times Books, 1989.

Gruver, Ed. *Koufax*. Dallas, Texas: Taylor Publishing, 2000.

Horvitz, Peter S., and Joachim Horvitz. *The Big Book of Jewish Baseball*. New York: S.P.I. Books, 2001.

Jacobson, Sidney. *Pete Reiser: The Rough-and-Tumble Career of the Perfect Ballplayer*. Jefferson, NC: McFarland, 2004.

James, Bill. *The Politics of Glory: How Baseball's Hall of Fame Really Works*. New York: Macmillan, 1994.

John, Tommy, and Dan Valenti. *TJ: My 26 Years in Baseball*. New York: Bantam Books, 1991.

Kiner, Ralph, and Danny Peary. *Baseball Forever: Reflections on 60 Years of Baseball*. Chicago: Triumph Books, 2004.

Kisseloff, Jeff. *Who Is Baseball's Greatest Pitcher?* Chicago: Carus Publishing, 2003.

Klawans, Harold L. *Why Michael Couldn't Hit: And Other Tales of the Neurology of Sports*. New York: Avon Books, 1998.

Koufax, Sandy, and Ed Linn. *Koufax*. New York: Viking Press, 1966.

Leavy, Jane. *Sandy Koufax: A Lefty's Legacy*. New York: HarperCollins, 2002.

Leventhal, Josh. *The World Series: An Illustrated Encyclopedia of the Fall Classic*. New York: Tess Press, 2006.

Marieb, Elaine M., and Jon Mallat. *Human Anatomy*, 3rd ed. San Francisco: Benjamin/Cummings Publishing, 2001.

Marzano, Rudy. *The Brooklyn Dodgers of the 1940s*. Jefferson, NC: McFarland, 2005.

Mellion, Morris B. *Sports Medicine Secrets. 1st Ed*. Philadelphia: Hanley & Belfus, 1994.

_____, Margot Putukian and Christopher C. Madden. *Sports Medicine Secrets*, 3rd ed. Philadelphia: Hanley & Belfus, 2003.

Moore, Jack B. *Joe DiMaggio: Baseball's Yankee Clipper*. New York: Praeger, 1987.

Morgan, Joe, and David Falkner. *Joe Morgan: A Life in Baseball*. New York: W. W. Norton, 1993.

Morris, Peter. *A Game of Inches: The Stories Behind the Innovations That Shaped Baseball: The Game Behind the Scenes*. Chicago: Ivan R. Dee, 2006.

Nowlin, Bill, and Cecilia Tan. *'75: The Red Sox Team That Saved Baseball*. Cambridge, MA: Rounder Books, 2005.

Pecina, Marko M., and Ivan Bojanic. *Overuse Injuries of the Musculoskeletal System*, 2nd ed. Boca Raton, FL: CRC Press, 2004.

Pluto, Terry. *The Curse of Rocky Colavito: A Loving Look at a Thirty Year Slump*. New York: Simon & Schuster, 1994.

Reed, Ted. *Carl Furillo: Brooklyn Dodger All-Star*. Jefferson, NC: McFarland, 2011.

Reidenbaugh, Lowell, and Sporting News. *Baseball's Hall of Fame: Cooperstown, Where Legends Live Forever*. New York: Crescent Books, 1997.

Ripken, Cal, Jr., and Mike Bryan. *The Only Way I Know*. New York:Penguin Books USA, 1997.

Ritter, Lawrence S. *The Glory of Their Times: The Story of the Early Days of Baseball Told by the Men Who Played It*. New York: William Morrow, 1992.

_____, and Donald Honig. *The 100 Greatest Baseball Players of All Time*. New York: Crown, 1981.

Robinson, Ray. *Matty: An American Hero, Christy Mathewson of the New York Giants*. New York: Oxford University Press, 1993.

_____. *The Greatest Yankees of Them All*. New York: Putnam's, 1969.

_____. *Iron Horse: Lou Gehrig in His Time*. New York: W. W. Norton, 1990.

Roseboro, John, and Bill Libby. *Glory Days with the Dodgers, and Other Days with Others*. New York: Atheneum, 1978.

Ryan, Nolan, and Harvey Frommer. *Throwing Heat*. New York: Avon Books, 1990.

Ryan, Nolan, T.R. Sullivan, and Mickey Herskowitz. *Nolan Ryan: The Road to Cooperstown*. Lenexa, KS: Addax Publishing, 1999.

Santo, Ron, and Randy Minkoff. *Ron Santo: For Love of Ivy*. Chicago: Bonus Books, 1993.

Schlossberg, Dan. *Baseball Gold: Mining Nugget's from our National Pastime*. Chicago: Triumph Books, 2007.

Scott, W. Norman. *Arthroscopy of the Knee: Diagnosis and Treatment*. Philadelphia: W. B. Saunders, 1990.

Sheehan, George A. *Dr. George Sheehan's Medical Advice for Runners*. Mountain View, CA: World Publications, 1978.

Smiles, Jack. *Big Ed Wash: The Life and Times of a Spitballing Hall of Famer*. Jefferson, NC: McFarland, 2008.

Sowell, Mike. *The Pitch That Killed: The Story of Carl Mays, Ray Chapman, and the Pennant Race of 1920*. Chicago: Ivan R. Dee, 1989.

Staten, Vince. *Ol' Diz: A Biography of Dizzy Dean*. New York: HarperCollins, 1992.

Stout, Glenn, and Richard A. Johnson. *The Cubs: The Complete Story of Chicago Cubs Baseball*. New York: Houghton Mifflin, 2007.

_____. *The Dodgers: 120 Years of Dodger Baseball*. New York: Houghton Mifflin, 2004.

_____. *Red Sox Century: One Hundred Years of Red Sox Baseball*. New York: Houghton Mifflin, 2000.

Swaine, Rick. *Beating the Breaks: Major League Ballplayers Who Overcame Disabilities*. Jefferson, NC: McFarland, 2004.

Wells, David and Chris Kreski. *Perfect I'm Not*. New York: HarperCollins, 2003.

Zimmer, Don, and Bill Madden. *Zim: A Baseball Life*. Kingston, NY: Total Sports Publishing, 2001.

Websites

In numerous articles, statistics obtained from www.baseball-reference.com

Index

Numbers in *bold italics* indicate pages with photographs.